PRESCRIBING SKILLS WORKBOOK

Daniel Norton
MBBS BSc (Hons)
F2 Foundation Doctor, Addenbrooke's Hospital,
Cambridge University Hospitals NHS Trust, Cambridge, UK

Nicholas Norton
MBBS BSc (Hons) MSc DTM&H MRCP (UK)
CT2 Core Medical Trainee, Southampton General Hospital,
University Hospital Southampton NHS Foundation Trust, Southampton, UK

Jane Caisley
BPharm MRPharmS
Formulary Pharmacist, Maidstone and Tunbridge Wells NHS Trust, Maidstone, UK

Rosie Furner
BSc (Hons) MSc IP MRPharmS
Community Services Pharmacist, East Sussex Healthcare NHS Trust, Bexhill, UK

Elizabeth Hamilton
MBChB BSc (Hons) MRCP (UK) MRCP (Acute) PGDipMedEd
Consultant in Acute and General Medicine,
Norfolk and Norwich University Hospitals NHS Foundation Trust, Norwich, UK

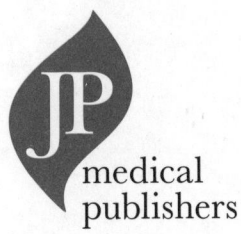

JP
medical
publishers

D1339033

© 2014 JP Medical Ltd.

Published by JP Medical Ltd, 83 Victoria Street, London, SW1H 0HW, UK

Tel: +44 (0)20 3170 8910   Fax: +44 (0)20 3008 6180

Email: info@jpmedpub.com   Web: www.jpmedpub.com

ISBN: 978-19-0781-6-86-4

British Library Cataloguing in Publication Data

A catalogue record for this book is available from the British Library

Library of Congress Cataloging in Publication Data

A catalog record for this book is available from the Library of Congress

JP Medical Ltd is a subsidiary of Jaypee Brothers Medical Publishers (P) Ltd, New Delhi, India.

Publisher: Richard Furn

Development Editors: Thomas Fletcher, Alison Whitehouse

Editorial Assistant: Sophie Woolven

Design: Designers Collective Ltd

Typeset, printed and bound in India.

Foreword

Prescribing any drug a patient might need – including controlled ones – is an entitlement that more or less defines a doctor. With that right comes a responsibility to prescribe well. Both right and responsibility are endowed at the moment of licensure, with very little preparation. From an educational perspective, that needs to change.

Alongside the high of being able to practise, recently qualified doctors experience strong negative emotions. Prescribing is often their worst stressor. No amount of book-learning can substitute for first-hand experience of ill-defined patient problems and the difficult conditions in which they sometimes have to be handled. But, by providing opportunities to complete drug charts in the context of realistic clinical scenarios, the authors have paved the way to prescribing for real and provided a valuable adjunct to clinical experience.

Patients will have reason to be thankful that the authors have also supplied authoritative advice on safe and effective practice to help young doctors keep their nerve when first prescribing in busy on-call situations.

I wouldn't be surprised if students who use this book to habituate themselves conscientiously to the conditions in which they will prescribe continue to refer back to it long after their first experiences of prescribing for real.

Tim Dornan
Professor of Medical Education
Maastricht University
March 2014

Preface

Prescribing is a routine task for doctors, yet medical students and junior doctors receive little preparation or teaching on the practicalities. The potential for error and harm to patients is large, and this is recognised by the introduction of a national Prescribing Safety Assessment (PSA) in the UK. All final year medical students approaching exams and later clinical work will recognise the anxiety associated with being underprepared for prescribing for patients.

This book addresses the need for more thorough preparation before heading out on to the wards. It contains 45 exercises designed to build readers' confidence in completing a drug chart, by presenting them with a scenario and a drug chart, and asking them to write up the appropriate prescription themselves. In each exercise we use our experiences to highlight common scenarios, pitfalls and useful tips, while introductory sections provide background on the basics of prescribing. The book is a collaborative effort between doctors and pharmacists, which we hope adds valuable realism.

Above all, we hope this book reinforces the old maxim: first, do no harm.

Daniel Norton
Nicholas Norton
Jane Caisley
Rosie Furner
Elizabeth Hamilton
March 2014

Dates and abbreviations

We don't know in which year you will be reading this book. For this reason, in the scenarios we have used YYYY to denote the year in admissions dates and for birth years (alongside a note of each patient's current age). Standard abbreviations for routes and frequencies are given below. All other abbreviations are defined in the text.

Route:

BE	both eyes
INH	inhaled
IV	intravenous
IM	intramuscular
JEJ	by jejunostomy tube
LE	left eye
NEB	nebuliser
NG	by nasogastric tube
PEG	by PEG tube
PO	oral
PR	rectal
PV	vaginal
RE	right eye
SC	subcutaneous
S/L	sublingual
TOP	topical

Frequency:

o.d.	once daily (omni die)
b.d.	twice daily (bis die)
o.m./mane	in the morning
o.n./nocte	at night
p.r.n.	as required (pro re nata)
q.d.s.	four times daily (quater die sumendum)
stat	immediately (statim)
Ṫ	one dose
T̈	two doses
t.d.s.	three times daily (ter die sumendum)

Other terms:

NBM nil-by-mouth

NKDA no known drug allergies

R/V for review

Contents

Foreword   iii
Preface   iii
Dates and abbreviations   iv
How to use this book   vi
Introduction to prescribing   1
   Filling in drug charts   1
   Practical tips   2
   Fluids   2
   Antibiotics   5
   Analgesics   6
   Antiemetics   7
   Thromboprophylaxis   7
   Oxygen   8
   The role of the hospital pharmacy team   9
   Prescribing in pregnancy, lactation and renal failure   9

Exercises
1   Basic skills   10
2   Maintenance fluids   18
3   Awkward medications   26
4   Preoperative assessment   34
5   Postoperative complications   42
6   Elective operations   50
7   Vomiting   58
8   Renal failure   66
9   Chest pain   74
10 Warfarin interactions   82
11 Dysphagia   90
12 Anaphylaxis   98
13 Shortness of breath   106
14 Fluid prescribing in hypotension   114
15 Paediatric fluid prescribing   122
16 Fluid prescribing in epigastric pain   130
17 Prescribing blood   138
18 Electrolyte replacement   146
19 Heparin infusions   154
20 Paracetamol overdose   162
21 Hyperkalaemia   170
22 Hypovolaemic shock   178
23 Preoperative assessment in diabetes   186
24 Prescribing in pregnancy   194
25 Breastfeeding   202
26 Poor oral intake   210
27 Atrial fibrillation   218
28 Acute coronary syndrome   226
29 Alcoholic liver disease   234
30 Antibiotics   242
31 Regular medications   250
32 Nil-by-mouth patient   258
33 Warfarin therapy   266
34 Prescribing gentamicin   274
35 Headache   282
36 Paediatric prescribing   290
37 Palliative care   298
38 Sore throat   306
39 Thromboprophylaxis   314
40 Pain management   322
41 Oliguria   330
42 Confusion in the elderly   338
43 Analgesia   346
44 Insomnia   354
45 Unresponsive patient   362

How to use this book

Prescribing Skills Workbook presents 45 case-based exercises that allow you to practise your prescribing. Each exercise presents a clinical scenario which you should read carefully. Jot down notes if necessary in the space provided. Once you have read the scenario and reviewed any medication already in the patient's chart, complete the exercise as follows:

- **Step 1:** starting on the page facing the scenario, fill in the prescription, adding drugs as needed and stopping a drug when appropriate.

- **Step 2:** once you have completed the whole chart, turn to the answer page for a brief explanation of the exercise.

- **Step 3:** compare your work with the checklist in the DRUGCHARTS table (see example below) and with the correctly completed drug chart on the facing and following pages. For the sake of clarity, blue handwriting under the name Alex Lewis is always used to denote a correctly completed prescription, or correct amendments to an existing prescription.

The DRUGCHARTS table (**Table 1**) reminds you of the key considerations for prescribing in each scenario. There is then more detailed discussion in the subsequent Rationale section.

Table 1 DRUGCHARTS: a reminder of key considerations in prescribing

D	**Details**	Does the chart include the correct patient details? (name, address, birth date, hospital number, etc.) Are block capitals used? Are abbreviations either universally recognised ones or avoided altogether?	☐
R	**Regular medications**	Write up any regular medications. Do any regular medications need to be stopped? Check the date on repeat prescriptions: are they still in use?	☐
U	**Unpleasant reactions**	Document allergies and sensitivities and take this into account when prescribing	☐
G	**Gravid?**	Is the patient pregnant? Do the prescribed medications have adverse effects in pregnancy?	☐
C	**Contra-indications**	What are the contraindications for the drug you are about to prescribe? What are the contraindications of the drugs already prescribed? Are these drugs still appropriate?	☐
H	**Hydration**	What is this patient's fluid requirement? Nil-by-mouth or oral intake? Consider urea and electrolytes, and rule out heart failure and urinary retention	☐
A	**Analgesia**	Is the patient in pain now? Is it likely that analgesia will be needed in the future (prescribe p.r.n.)? Prescribe analgesia according to the WHO pain ladder (see Figure 3 on page 6)	☐
R	**Renal function**	Is the drug renally excreted? Is it nephrotoxic? Does the dose need adjusting because of renal impairment?	☐
T	**Thrombo-prophylaxis**	Does this patient need thromboprophylaxis?	☐
S	**Signature box**	It is essential to record your details on the chart	☐

Introduction to prescribing

Filling in drug charts

A drug chart is a communication between you, other doctors, the nursing staff and the pharmacist. It brings together all current prescriptions for a patient, including those from his or her general practitioner (GP). Different staff members need to access and act on the information at different times, sometimes under considerable time pressure. So it is vital that you make your communication unambiguous, write in block capitals and in black ink, and avoid abbreviations (or only use universally recognised abbreviations). For clarity, however, in exercises 1–45 we use blue ink to show correctly completed prescriptions.

Always review the whole chart, even if you are being asked to address only one specific aspect.

Starting a drug

Don't prescribe a drug until you have checked it is safe, even if someone asks you to do it. If there is an *Additional Instructions* box, document why a drug was started and whether it needs to be reviewed (see **Figure 1**); recording this information provides vital clarity for clinicians subsequently treating the patient, both in hospital and in the community.

Ensure the rest of the prescription is unambiguous too. For example, if you write a prescription for regular paracetamol q.d.s. on the chart at 10am, it is advisable to enter a cross against the earlier 8am dose so it can't be given by mistake (in practice, however, today's 8am box would often be left empty). If you withhold a drug, e.g. perioperatively, cross off the appropriate doses.

Changing the dose or frequency of a drug

When up-titrating the frequency of administration of a drug, write the dose opposite the additional time(s) when it should be given (see **Figure 1**). When changing a dose, you must re-prescribe the drug: do not 'edit' the original dose.

Stopping a drug

The following must be recorded on the chart when you stop a drug:

- the word 'STOP'
- the date and your signature
- the reason why
- unambiguous lines scoring out the original drug but not obscuring its name. In this book we have used thick blue lines (see **Figure 1**)

Reviewing a drug

If you need to show that a drug must be reviewed before being continued, draw a box and write 'R/V' (for review) or 'REVIEW' in the space for the required time and date (see **Figure 1**).

Recording allergies and sensitivities

Document all allergies and sensitivities in the *Allergies* box. If there are none, write 'NKDA' for No Known Drug Allergies. Remember that although a rash caused by penicillin 20 years ago is clearly less significant than an anaphylactic reaction that required hospitalisation 3 years ago, both should be recorded.

NAME OF DRUG FUROSEMIDE	TIME	DATE → DOSE ↓	1/2	2/2	3/2	4/2	5/2
						REVIEW	
ADDITIONAL INSTRUCTIONS STARTED: FLUID OVERLOAD. R/V ON 4/2	08:00	40MG	RN	RN	TJ	————	————
DATE 1/2/YYYY ROUTE PO	12:00	40MG	X	RN	TJ	————	————
PRESCRIBER'S SIGNATURE BFord	18:00	EJones				STOP EUVOLAEMIC ALewis 4/2/YYYY	
PRESCRIBER'S NAME AND BLEEP BEN FORD 1569	22:00						

Figure 1: Initiating, uptitrating frequency, reviewing and stopping a drug. Ben Ford initiated furosemide once daily on 1 February, with a requirement for review after a further 3 days. The frequency was increased on 2 February by Emma Jones. At review on 4 February, Alex Lewis stopped furosemide because the patient had achieved euvolaemia. (Throughout this book, correct completed prescriptions are always shown under the name Alex Lewis and written in blue to differentiate from the existing prescriptions.)

Confirm the nature of the allergies and document both the drug and the reaction.

As well as taking an allergy and sensitivity history, check previous drug charts, prescriptions, discharge letters and GP notes for a history of allergy.

Considerations when prescribing

Use reminders such as the DRUGCHARTS mnemonic on page vi to remember the most important considerations when prescribing.

Rewriting a drug chart

This is a common on-call request and junior doctors are often asked to rewrite charts for patients they have never met. On the new drug chart it is helpful to write 'REWRITTEN' and the date somewhere prominent, such as across the top of the front page of the chart. Cross through all pages in the old chart to prevent mistakes while maintaining legibility. If the chart you are rewriting contains antibiotics, carry across the review dates and use the original start dates. If no review dates have been entered, insert these on the appropriate dates (see **Figure 1**). This prompts a review on the relevant date, regardless of which staff are looking after the patient at the time.

Practical tips

Drug formularies and local and national guidelines

Ensure you know how to make best use of the relevant drug formulary (in the UK the *British National Formulary* – the *BNF*). You may find yourself under pressure to navigate the formulary with proficiency in very limited time, so you need to be familiar with it. Select the dose carefully; in the *BNF*, doses are listed by indication, route and patient group. Read the whole of the dose section, ensure you are not missing anything and take into account the clinical condition of the patient.

Familiarise yourself with guidance on prescribing for special patient groups. For example, prescribing for the elderly must take into account pharmacokinetic changes with age, notably reduced renal clearance and hepatic metabolism: susceptibility to adverse reactions and nephrotoxicity is raised, and polypharmacy increases potential for interactions.

Remember to use formularies in combination with both national and local guidelines; the latter apply especially to antibiotics.

Paediatric formularies

Paediatric prescribing requires great care because normal physiology changes enormously during childhood. Check *all* drugs for paediatric dosage before prescribing. In the UK, always refer to the latest *BNF for Children*.

Dosage is often calculated according to the child's age and weight. This sometimes results in very specific

doses being required. Childrens' medicines are often liquid formulations: you will need to know the concentration to calculate a dose that provides a volume suitable to be measured by the parent. Some drugs may have to be made up from a mixture of tablets to achieve the required dose. Others may be available only in standard amounts and it may not be physically possible to prepare, for example, a fifth of a tablet. When entering the dose in the chart, the decision to round up or down is a clinical one and advice should be sought from a more senior clinician if you are unsure.

Writing up a GP prescription

Many patients are admitted to hospital via their GP and arrive with a letter containing their drug history. This is often a computer-generated print-out and is usually split into acute and repeat prescriptions:

- **Acute medications:** check the date and whether the patient is still taking the drug

- **Repeat prescription:** check what date the drug was last issued and check the dose

Doses on a GP prescription are usually written for patients rather than medical staff, e.g. 'take two tablets twice daily' along with a line stating '15mg tablets'. Look out for this and convert to the appropriate dosage, e.g. '30mg b.d.'

Generic vs brand names

Use the generic (non-proprietary) drug name wherever possible. This allows the pharmacy to dispense whatever brand is in stock, saving time and money.

However, remember that some drugs should be prescribed by brand (proprietary) name, either because there is a difference in the clinical effect of two or more brands, even though they contain the same drug, or to remove ambiguity. This applies, for example, to insulins, inhalers and some controlled release preparations such as calcium channel blockers.

Fluids

Intravenous fluid prescribing is a routine task for junior doctors but there is no universal prescription regimen. Few aspects of physiology are unaffected by fluid and electrolyte status, hence each fluid prescription has to be individually tailored.

Fluid compartments

Fluid prescribing requires an understanding of fluid compartments and the movement of fluid between them. Fluid is distributed between compartments according to its protein and electrolyte content, with the capillary wall and cell membranes acting as selective barriers to movement between compartments (**Figure 2**). Thus the content of an infused fluid (**Table 1**) determines which compartment it can expand.

Fluid balance can be disrupted in disease, causing fluid shifts. For example, 'third spacing' occurs when

	PROTEIN	Na$^+$ (mmol/L)	Cl$^-$ (mmol/L)	K$^+$ (mmol/L)	Ca^{2+} (mmol/L)	LACTATE (mmol/L)
PLASMA	0	135–145	95–105	3.5–5.0	2.2–2.6	0.6–2.4
5% DEXTROSE	0	0	0	0	0	0
0.9% N SALINE	0	154	154	0	0	0
HARTMANN'S SOLUTION	0	131	111	5	2	29
Gelofusin (colloid) contains 40g gelatin, 154 mmol/L Na$^+$, 120 mmol/L Cl$^-$						

Table 1: Content of fluids for intravenous infusion. Saline should be written as '0.9% sodium chloride' when prescribing but is often written as 'Saline'.

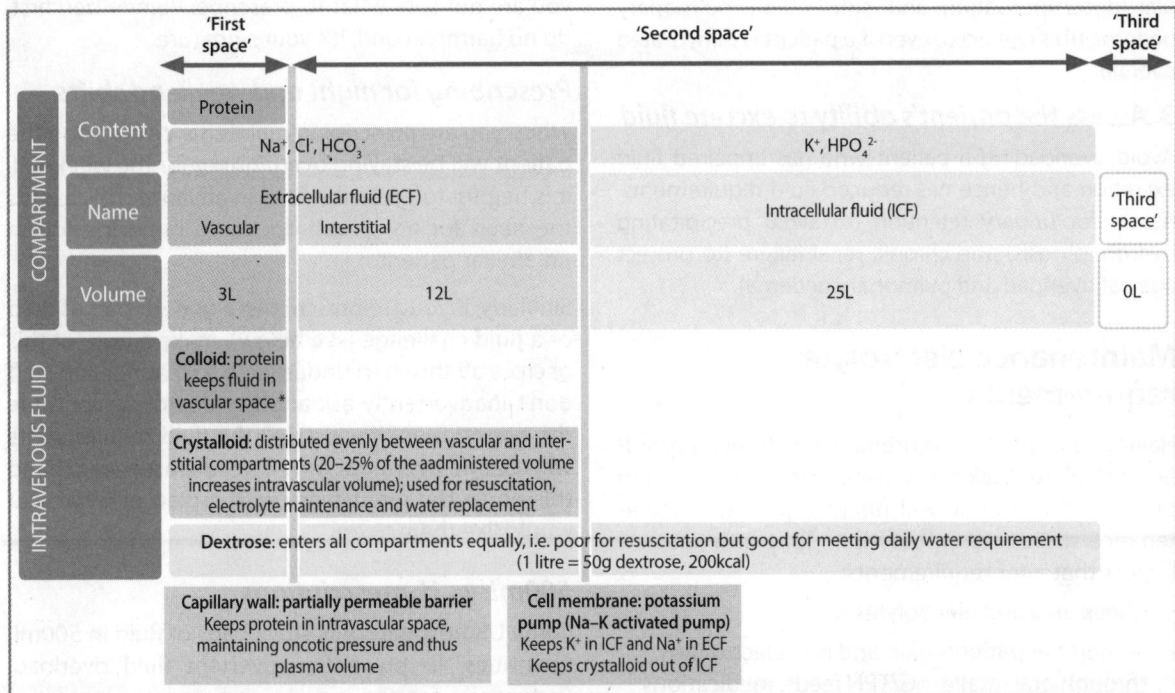

Figure 2: Fluid compartments and the distribution of infused fluids. *Colloid has electrolyte content but its protein content (gelatin) holds it in the vascular compartment. Current evidence has created a movement away from the use of colloid solutions in preference for crystalloid solutions. In the UK, the only colloid that is still in routine use is human albumin solution (HAS).

fluid collects in a significant quantity in a space where it is not usually present, for example the peritoneal or pleural cavities. The depleted 'first' and 'second spaces' (corresponding to vascular, interstitial and intracellular compartments) may require fluid replacement. Causes of 'third spacing' include sepsis, burns, pancreatitis, peritonitis, pleural effusion and prolonged surgery.

Maintenance volume requirements

Assess the patient's fluid status and requirements in a systematic approach, using clinical signs and serum biochemistry.

1. Calculate volume requirements

- *Check maintenance fluid requirements by body weight* (**Table 2**)
- *Clinically assess volume status.* Check the patient is not dehydrated or overloaded: examine vital signs, mucous membranes, skin turgor, urine output and peripheral oedema. Record the fluid balance (intake, urine output and net fluid

balance) on a nursing chart

- *Check if fluid intake is possible by a non-intravenous route*, e.g. nasogastric (NG) tube, PEG tube or oral. If oral intake is possible, encourage it. Alternative routes decrease the intravenous volume you need to prescribe
- *Check for causes of increased fluid loss*, which increase intravenous fluid requirement, e.g. diarrhoea, vomiting, stomas and high-output drains

MAINTENANCE VOLUME

If the patient is euvolaemic, calculate maintenance volume requirements. The often quoted 1500–2400mL of water over 24 hours is too broad to be useful: the required 25–35mL/kg/24 hours is 2700mL for a 90kg patient (30mL x 90kg) and just 1500mL for a 50kg patient. Understanding this concept is key to avoiding overloading frail elderly patients.

Water	25–35mL/kg (1500–2500mL)
Sodium	50–100mmol
Potassium	40–80mmol

Table 2: Adult fluid and electrolyte requirements over 24 hours.

2. Assess the 'pump'

Check if the patient has heart failure. Giving too much fluid too quickly overloads the heart and overwhelms the Frank–Starling relationship, precipitating ventricular decompensation and subsequent pulmonary oedema (this can occur even if a patient is dehydrated overall).

3. Assess the patient's ability to excrete fluid

Avoid overloading a patient who has impaired fluid excretion and hence has reduced fluid requirements. Assess for urinary retention (to avoid precipitating hydronephrosis) and chronic renal failure (to protect against overload and pulmonary oedema).

Maintenance electrolyte requirements

Having calculated maintenance volume, consider electrolyte intake. If there is none other than in prescribed fluid, you will need to prescribe maintenance sodium and potassium. Take into account factors that alter requirements:

- Check urea and electrolytes
- Remember patients gain and lose electrolytes through oral intake, NG/TPN feeds, medications and pathological states
- Remember some drugs alter serum biochemistry by virtue of their action, e.g. ACE inhibitors cause hyperkalaemia, or by their 'ingredients', e.g. a drug presented as a sodium salt contains high levels of sodium

Fluid prescribing tips

Patients on diuretics

Before prescribing fluids, remember to check if a patient is taking diuretics. In general you should not prescribe diuretics and fluids concomitantly as they have opposing effects. Reassess the patient's volume status and discuss this with a senior doctor if in doubt.

Prescribing fluids for unfamiliar patients

This is a common task for junior doctors. When you are unfamiliar with the patient, the chance of error is increased. The safest way to prescribe is to assess the patient fully, but time constraints may make this challenging. Ask the nursing staff about the patient. What was the reason for the patient's admission? Why are fluids being given and what is the current regimen? Compare this to your expectation for this patient's age and weight: is it unusual? There is a big difference between a 19-year-old who is fasting preoperatively and an 89-year-old with renal failure and atrial fibrillation.

If you do prescribe, ensure there will be enough fluid to cover the patient until the patient's usual team returns to the ward, and write 'REVIEW' underneath, so the prescription does not continue infinitely. However, do not succumb to pressure to prescribe if you are not sure what to prescribe. Remember: first, do no harm; second, it's your signature.

Prescribing for night and weekend shifts

When you are prescribing maintenance fluid and the patient will be staying overnight or for the weekend, it is helpful to prescribe fluid in advance. This avoids the need for an on-call doctor to prescribe for an unfamiliar patient.

Similarly, if you are prescribing a one-off bag of fluid or a fluid challenge (see below), make a note of this or cross off the chart underneath so that nursing staff don't inadvertently ask another doctor to continue the prescription. If you think the fluid requirements will change overnight or will need reassessing, hand this on to the night team with a plan of what you would like them to do.

500mL vs 1L prescriptions

Some UK hospitals only stock bags of fluid in 500mL quantities, to prevent inadvertent fluid overload. Particularly for the elderly and underweight, it is often safer to prescribe in 500mL quantities than 1L.

Choosing between Hartmann's and normal saline

In practice, for most stable patients there is little clinical consequence to choosing one of these rather than the other, and they are equally valuable in resuscitation scenarios. However, because the sodium and chloride content of normal saline is higher than the more 'physiological' Hartmann's (**Table 1**), there is a greater risk of hypernatraemia or hyperchloraemic acidosis if normal saline is used in excess. When considering specific electrolyte adjustment, you will need to bear this in mind.

The fluid challenge

The fluid challenge is a bolus of fluid delivered as quickly as possible, for example 250mL over 5 minutes, to see if a transient rise in blood pressure is elicited (i.e. if the patient is a fluid responder) and to guide further fluid resuscitation. Make sure the nursing staff know it is to be administered in this way and not just through the quickest pump setting (often half an hour), which can negate the effect entirely.

Antibiotics

In most hospitals there are local antibiotic guidelines, drawn up by the microbiology department. Generally, they suggest:

- First-line empirical therapies for common infections seen at that hospital
- Alternatives for patients who are allergic to penicillins

Local guidance takes into account the local flora and the patterns of antibiotic resistance in the area, with the result that it may differ from national guidance.

Choosing the correct antibiotic

Choosing the correct antibiotic is critical to effective treatment and requires answers to the following questions:

- What is the likely causative organism?
- Which antibiotic(s) will cover this?
- By what route should the antibiotic(s) be given?
- Are there side effects or contraindications?

Causative organism

Bear in mind that the site of the infection provides key information about the causative organism. It suggests major characteristics of the species; for example, an uncomplicated chest infection is unlikely to be caused by a strict anaerobe, because the lungs are full of air.

Consider also which organisms are constituents of the normal flora at the infection site. For example *Staphylococcus aureus* and *Streptococcus pyogenes* are both present in the normal skin flora and are responsible for the majority of skin and soft tissue infections.

Check the patient's history for clues to the likely pathogen. A history of immunosuppression, for example, dramatically changes the range of potential organisms. Another example is that intravenous drug users are predisposed to tricuspid endocarditis, *Staphylococcus aureus* pneumonias and infection by relatively rare organisms such as *Clostridium botulinum*.

Antibiotic cover for the organism

The next step is to choose an antibiotic or combination of antibiotics that is effective against the organism(s). Antibiotic effect is dependent not only on the susceptibility of the target organism but also on the concentration achieved at the site of infection, for example:

- penicillins do not readily cross the blood–brain barrier; drugs that do cross, such as the third generation cephalosporin ceftriaxone, are used instead
- urinary tract infection requires antibiotics that are excreted unchanged in the urine where they can have their effect

Route

It is a common misconception that antibiotics administered intravenously are in some way 'stronger' than oral antibiotics. It is bioavailability that differs, being between 50 and 100% for the oral route, depending on the antibiotic. Antibiotics administered intravenously have a bioavailability of 100% and are not affected by food or other drugs in the gastrointestinal tract, which allows more predictable tissue concentrations to be achieved. Because of this, intravenous antibiotics are favoured in severe infection. The intravenous route is also used for antibiotics that have particularly poor oral absorption (e.g. aminoglycosides and carbapenems).

For antibiotics that can be administered by either route, remember that the dose may differ depending on the route. For example, co-amoxiclav 1.2g IV and 625mg PO, and metronidazole 500mg IV and 400mg PO.

All patients should be switched to oral therapy as soon as possible to reduce risk, nursing time and costs associated with intravenous administration: remember that intravenous therapy may require the patient to be in hospital.

Side effects and contraindications

Side effects are common, in addition to the impact that antibiotics have on each patient's normal flora. Examples include nephrotoxicity (gentamicin – see below), peripheral neuropathy (isoniazid), cholestatic jaundice (clarithromycin) and bone marrow failure (co-trimoxazole).

Excessive broad-spectrum antibiotic usage allows resistant organisms such as *Clostridium difficile* to proliferate. Prescribe the antibiotic with the narrowest spectrum that will cover the infection being treated. Whenever possible, prescribing should be guided by culture and sensitivity results and the local antibiotic guidelines.

Monitoring antibiotics

Some intravenous antibiotics require monitoring and dose adjustment to minimise the likelihood of toxicity while maintaining an effective dose. The examples you will encounter most commonly are the aminoglycoside gentamicin and the glycopeptide vancomycin. Both groups have the potential for renal and oto-toxicity, and gentamicin should be used

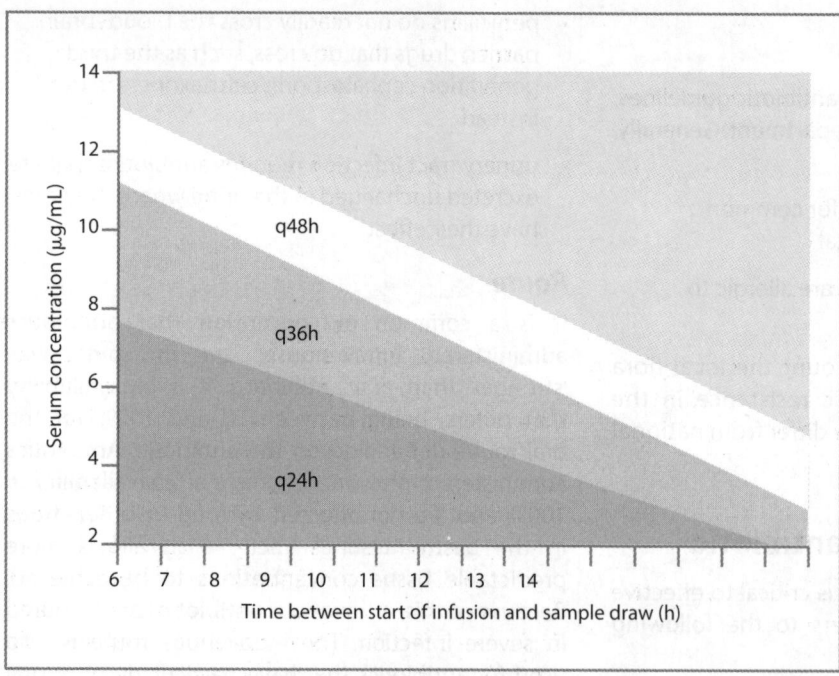

Figure 3: The Hartford nomogram for monitoring 'once-daily' gentamicin. Gentamicin is administered intravenously at a dose of 5–7mg/kg per time period. The serum gentamicin level is checked 6–14 hours after the first infusion was started: its position on the nomogram indicates the frequency at which the dose should be repeated – every 24, 36 or 48 hours. The level is checked again on day 5 if gentamicin is to be continued beyond that point.

with caution in renal impairment (if a decline in renal function occurs, change the treatment).

Gentamicin is administered intravenously and may be given in once daily or three times daily dosing. The once daily regimen is more common as it is equally effective and simpler to manage: monitoring for this regimen is shown in **Figure 3**. Eight-hourly dosing is reserved for infective endocarditis.

Intravenous vancomycin is given twice daily. Monitoring of levels is often a source of confusion: a sample for determining the trough level should be obtained *immediately prior* to giving the third dose. The third dose should not be delayed to await the result. The target level is 10–15mg/L. The effect of vancomycin is dependent on the *length of time* the bacteria are exposed to a level above their minimum inhibitory concentration: if the level is too high, reduce the dose rather than increasing the dosing interval.

MRSA infection

Staphylococcus aureus resistant to flucloxacillin is synonymous with meticillin-resistant *S. aureus* (meticillin itself is no longer used in clinical practice). In the UK, MRSA swabs are taken for all patients on admission to hospital. If the result is positive, a hospital prescribing policy is usually enacted for the patient, including topical washes to clear the bacteria.

Analgesics

The most widely recognised model for effective analgesia is the World Health Organization pain ladder (**Figure 4**), which encourages a stepwise approach to regular pain relief. Patients move up or down a step according to their pain relief requirements.

Non-opioids are continued regardless of the patient's position on the ladder. For most patients the non-opioid is paracetamol. Non-steroidal anti-inflammatory drugs (NSAIDs) such as aspirin and ibuprofen have side effects of a nature that makes them better suited for short courses and for younger patients (see below).

If a non-opioid is insufficient, then a weak opioid is added. If this does not achieve control, there is no value in combining weak opioids, for example pain relief is unlikely to be improved by adding tramadol to regular codeine. Instead, the next step is to substitute a strong opioid such as morphine (there is no benefit in using a strong and a weak opioid together). The most commonly used strong opioid

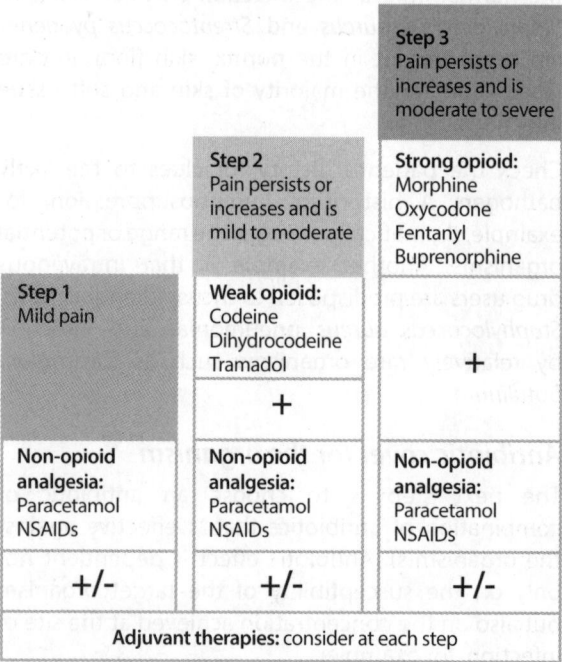

Figure 4: The World Health Organization pain ladder for adults. NSAID, non-steroidal anti-inflammatory drug.

is morphine, given in an oral liquid formulation of 10mg in 5mL.

When prescribing simple analgesia such as paracetamol a useful tip is to write more than one route in the chart, e.g. PO/PR/IV. This gives the nurse more than one option without requiring a new prescription if one route becomes unavailable.

For the patient, this avoids waiting for pain relief. Remember that bioavailability is greater via the intravenous route, so check for any dose adjustment first.

Generally, the oral route is preferable as it is easiest and cheapest. Switch route if the patient can't take oral medication.

As-required analgesia

This extra pain relief is given for 'breakthrough' pain, i.e. pain that is not controlled by the patient's regular medication, or to cover a particularly painful activity such as physiotherapy or dressing changes. It is selected from one step above the patient's current medication, for example a small dose of a strong opioid for a patient who is on regular paracetamol and codeine.

Adjuvant therapies

Not all pain responds to 'traditional' analgesia. Adjuvant therapies include a wide range of techniques from cold compresses to radiologically guided nerve blocks. The most common use of pharmacological adjuvants is in the setting of neuropathic pain, for example a tricyclic antidepressant with or without the addition of an anticonvulsant.

NSAIDs

NSAIDs have a number of side effects that limit their use (**Table 3**). They are best avoided in older patients, who often have pre-existing renal or cardiovascular disease. Specific NSAIDs are used with caution or are contraindicated in cardiac, gastric, renal and hepatic impairment in all age groups. Despite this there are a number of indications for which NSAIDs are extremely useful, for example as first-line analgesic and anti-inflammatory agents for inflammatory arthritis, pericarditis, gout, renal colic and migraine. Long-term NSAIDs are always prescribed with a proton pump inhibitor to reduce the risk of gastric ulceration.

System	Raised risks
Gastrointestinal	Gastric and duodenal ulceration; enteropathy
Renal	Interstitial nephritis
Cardiovascular	Myocardial infarction, stroke

Table 3: Principal side effects of non-steroidal anti-inflammatory drugs.

Antiemetics

Nausea and vomiting are common, particularly postoperatively and in patients receiving chemotherapy. Different antiemetics have different mechanisms of action (**Table 4**): if a patient receiving one antiemetic is still showing symptoms, it makes sense to add a second that acts by a different mechanism. Adding two drugs from the same group is more likely to increase the risk of side effects than improve the patient's symptoms.

Most antiemetics are available in a variety of formulations and can be given via different routes: this is especially important if the patient is vomiting. For most purposes, the first-line antiemetic is cyclizine because it is cheap and well tolerated. In some settings dopamine antagonists are first-line treatments; for example in vomiting caused by gastric stasis or paralytic ileus, they can be extremely useful because they increase gut motility.

Thromboprophylaxis

Deep vein thrombosis and pulmonary embolus cause significant morbidity and mortality among hospitalised patients. In the UK it is mandatory for the risk of venous thromboembolism to be assessed and documented for every patient admitted to hospital. Medical patients who can move freely around the ward do not need thromboprophylaxis. All other patients require assessment of risk factors for both thromboembolism and haemorrhage: most will need thromboprophylaxis unless they have a significant risk of bleeding. Patients who are anticoagulated, e.g. with warfarin, do not need thromboprophylaxis.

H_1 receptor antagonists	Dopamine antagonists	$5HT_3$ antagonists
Cyclizine	Domperidone	Ondansetron
Promethazine	Metoclopramide	
	Prochlorperazine	
	Haloperidol	
	Levomepromazine	

Table 4: Antiemetic mechanisms of action.

Mechanical thromboprophylaxis

This employs devices to improve venous return from the legs, usually compression stockings but sometimes an intermittent pneumatic compression device. Some hospitals require mechanical prophylaxis to be prescribed on the drug chart, although this is not universal.

Low molecular weight heparins

Low molecular weight heparins (e.g. enoxaparin, dalteparin) are the mainstay of pharmacological thromboprophylaxis and are given subcutaneously in the early evening. In this book enoxaparin is used throughout, although dalteparin or tinzaparin would be equally acceptable. The prophylactic dose of enoxaparin for a patient with normal renal function is 40mg. A patient with a glomerular filtration rate less than $30mL/min/1.73m^2$ should have half this dose.

Oral anticoagulants

Warfarin remains the mainstay: be familiar with prescribing and monitoring requirements. Alternatives that require less monitoring are increasingly being used. Currently licensed in the UK are rivaroxaban (factor Xa inhibitor), apixaban (factor Xa inhibitor) and dabigatran (direct thrombin inhibitor).

Oxygen

Oxygen is a drug and requires prescription except in an emergency (when it can be given without prescription and documented afterwards). Most drug charts contain an oxygen section (**Figure 5**). Record the target saturation (SaO_2) and specify the mode of delivery (**Table 5**). Review the prescription daily and aim to wean the patient off oxygen when SaO_2 reaches the target level.

Practical tips for oxygen prescribing

- Patients with chronic obstructive pulmonary disease (COPD) are often in type 2 respiratory failure, and a proportion will rely on hypoxic drive (rather than hypercapnia) to stimulate respiratory effort. High-dose oxygen aiming for SaO_2 94–98% risks obliterating this drive and causing respiratory arrest, therefore the 88–92% target is commonly chosen. However, hypoxia kills before hypercapnia. In a critically ill patient with suspected COPD, start with high-flow oxygen and then down-titrate the dose according to arterial blood gas results until saturations of 88–92% are achieved.

- Young people and non-smokers should saturate at 94–98%. If they do not, exclude pathology.

- Oxygen is a treatment for hypoxaemia, not breathlessness: if SaO_2 is normal without oxygen, discontinue it.

Oxygen Therapy								
1. Target SaO_2 % – Rate and method of O_2 delivery must be adjusted and documented by nursing staff	DATE →							
	TIME ↓							
88-92% ☐ OR 94-98% ☐ OR MIN.....% MAX.....%	**06:00**							
Is Venturi delivery essential? Yes ☐ No ☐	**12:00**							
Additional Instructions:	**18:00**							
PRESCRIBER'S SIGNATURE AND BLEEP	**22:00**							
2. Target SaO_2 % – Rate and method of O_2 delivery must be adjusted and documented by nursing staff	DATE →							
	TIME ↓							
88-92% ☐ OR 94-98% ☐	**06:00**							

Figure 5: Oxygen prescription.

Venturi device	Non-Venturi device
BLUE – 24% (2–4L/min)	Nasal cannulae 1L/min
WHITE – 28% (4–6L/min)	Nasal cannulae 2L/min
YELLOW – 35% (8–10L/min)	Nasal cannulae 4L/min
RED – 40% (10–12L/min)	Simple face mask 5–6L/min
GREEN – 60% (12–15L/min)	Simple face mask 7–10L/min
Reservoir mask at 15L/min	

Table 5: Oxygen administration devices, flow rates and equivalent steps. A Venturi device is colour-coded according to the maximum percentage of oxygen it can deliver.

The role of the hospital pharmacy team

The team supports the safe use of medicines. A pharmacist is available on most wards in acute hospitals and ideally visits daily, usually at the same time each day. Find out who this is, and the time, so you can raise prescribing issues without delay.

For each admission a pharmacist clinically screens the chart and a pharmacy technician undertakes medicines reconciliation with the patient's medical and medication history. Discrepancies are checked with the GP and prescribing doctor. The pharmacist identifies parameters which require monitoring, e.g. renal function, and prior to dispensing checks all discharge prescriptions.

Pharmacists have access to patient notes and laboratory test results and use these to support their work. Prescriptions are checked for:

- accurate dosing
- accurate transcribing of information
- appropriate administration
- potential drug interactions
- drug level monitoring
- appropriate drug choice
- course lengths
- adherence to local and national prescribing guidance

Pharmacists often use green pen to write information on prescription charts, so that it is easy to spot.

One role of the ward pharmacist is to support your prescribing, helping you with medication-related problems, such as simple questions on dose, administering injections and complicated prescribing (e.g. in pregnancy). When you need advice contact the pharmacist as soon as possible, preferably before writing the prescription; this avoids treatment delays while the pharmacist chases you for information or a new prescription. The pharmacist may seem like a gatekeeper but will welcome the opportunity to work with you.

Most hospitals also have a medicines information department to deal with more complex queries.

Prescribing in pregnancy, lactation and renal failure

The pharmacist is a valuable source of help in these complex areas. Details are beyond the scope of this book but useful references include:

Ashley C, Currie A (ed). The renal drug handbook, 3rd edn. Radcliffe Publishing, 2009.

Briggs G, Freeman R, Yaffe S. Drugs in pregnancy and lactation, 9th edn. Lippincott, Williams & Wilkins, 2011.

Hale T. Medications and mothers' milk, 15th edn. Hale Publishing, 2012.

Schaefer C, Peters P, Miller R (ed). Drugs during pregnancy and lactation. Elsevier, 2007.

Robert Smith (hospital number: 456723, DOB 16/09/YYYY [63 years old], address: 32 Vicoli Street, Longbury LB2 3DP), has been admitted to the medical assessment ward for an elective procedure. He feels well, and has brought a bag containing his regular medication, which he has not taken today. He has no allergies and takes no over-the-counter medication. Thromboprophylaxis prescription is not required. He weighs 76kg and his consultant is Dr Erin Johnson.

Your task is to prescribe the regular medication.
It is 07:00 on Wednesday 07th March. Presume the medication labels are in date.

Trimethoprim 100mg tablets

Take ONE tablet EACH DAY

Take at regular intervals. Complete the prescribed course unless otherwise directed

Mrs Elizabeth Smith
Qty 28

05 Mar YYYY

Ramipril 2.5mg capsules

Take ONE capsule EACH DAY

Mr Robert Smith
Qty 28

05 Mar YYYY

Methotrexate 2.5mg tablets

Take EIGHT tablets EACH WEEK on Saturdays

Mr Robert Smith
Qty 32

05 Mar YYYY

Prednisolone 5mg tablets

Take ONE tablet EACH DAY

Take with or just after food or a meal

Mr Robert Smith
Qty 28

05 Mar YYYY

Notes

LONGBURY HOSPITAL TRUST	HOSPITAL NUMBER SURNAME FIRST NAME ADDRESS D.O.B		

DATE OF ADMISSION		ADMISSION WEIGHT (KG)		WARD	
ALLERGIES			CONSULTANT		
			CHART NO		...OF...

ONCE ONLY PRESCRIPTIONS

DATE	TIME	NAME OF DRUG	DOSE	ROUTE	PRESCRIBER'S SIGNATURE	GIVEN BY	TIME GIVEN

REGULAR MEDICATIONS

NAME OF DRUG		TIME	DATE → DOSE ↓				
ADDITIONAL INSTRUCTIONS		08:00					
DATE	ROUTE	12:00					
PRESCRIBER'S SIGNATURE		18:00					
PRESCRIBER'S NAME AND BLEEP		22:00					

NAME OF DRUG		TIME	DATE → DOSE ↓				
ADDITIONAL INSTRUCTIONS		08:00					
DATE	ROUTE	12:00					
PRESCRIBER'S SIGNATURE		18:00					
PRESCRIBER'S NAME AND BLEEP		22:00					

NAME OF DRUG		TIME	DATE → DOSE ↓				
ADDITIONAL INSTRUCTIONS		08:00					
DATE	ROUTE	12:00					
PRESCRIBER'S SIGNATURE		18:00					
PRESCRIBER'S NAME AND BLEEP		22:00					

PATIENT NAME   HOSPITAL NO.

NAME OF DRUG		TIME	DATE → DOSE ↓					
ADDITIONAL INSTRUCTIONS		08:00						
DATE	ROUTE	12:00						
PRESCRIBER'S SIGNATURE								
		18:00						
PRESCRIBER'S NAME AND BLEEP		22:00						

NAME OF DRUG		TIME	DATE → DOSE ↓					
ADDITIONAL INSTRUCTIONS		08:00						
DATE	ROUTE	12:00						
PRESCRIBER'S SIGNATURE								
		18:00						
PRESCRIBER'S NAME AND BLEEP		22:00						

NAME OF DRUG		TIME	DATE → DOSE ↓					
ADDITIONAL INSTRUCTIONS		08:00						
DATE	ROUTE	12:00						
PRESCRIBER'S SIGNATURE								
		18:00						
PRESCRIBER'S NAME AND BLEEP		22:00						

AS REQUIRED PRESCRIPTIONS

NAME OF DRUG		DATE					
INDICATION/ INSTRUCTION	DOSE	TIME					
FREQUENCY	ROUTE	DOSE					
PRESCRIBER'S SIGNATURE		ROUTE					
PRESCRIBER'S NAME AND BLEEP		GIVEN BY					
START DATE	STOP DATE						

PATIENT NAME   HOSPITAL NO.

NAME OF DRUG		DATE						
INDICATION/INSTRUCTION	DOSE	TIME						
FREQUENCY	ROUTE	DOSE						
PRESCRIBER'S SIGNATURE		ROUTE						
PRESCRIBER'S NAME AND BLEEP		GIVEN BY						
START DATE	STOP DATE							

INTRAVENOUS FLUIDS

DATE	FLUID	ADDITIVE & DOSE	VOLUME	RATE/DURATION	PRESCRIBER'S SIGNATURE	GIVEN BY	START TIME	END TIME

Record of signatures. ALL prescribers MUST complete.

DATE	NAME	DESIGNATION	SIGNATURE	BLEEP NUMBER

Answer 1

This scenario highlights the potential for harm to patients, even when carrying out a simple task. Converting boxes of drugs and general practitioner medication lists that patients bring with them into hospital prescriptions is a routine task, but often done in a hurry. Taking time to methodically check each drug is an essential part of safe prescribing. Always check the details on every drug that a patient brings to hospital.

Step 3: Compare your answer to the checklist below and the chart opposite ☑

D Details	Checked patient details. Used capital letters throughout. Used correct abbreviations. Noticed that not all prescriptions are for the patient	☐
R Regular medications	Prescribed: – methotrexate 20mg once weekly, calculated correct doses from patient packet – prednisolone 5mg daily – ramipril 2.5mg daily	☐
U Unpleasant reactions	Wrote NKDA or equivalent	☐
G Gravid?	N/A	☐

C Contra-indications	Noticed that the trimethoprim prescription is not for this patient and did not prescribe it	☐
H Hydration	Not required	☐
A Analgesia	Not required	☐
R Renal function	Not required	☐
T Thrombo-prophylaxis	Not required	☐
S Signature box	Signed signature box	☐

Rationale

This patient mistakenly brought in his wife's trimethoprim. Prescribing trimethoprim with methotrexate can have serious consequences: both inhibit folic acid metabolism and their use together increases the risk of haematological toxicity.

Methotrexate is a cytotoxic drug used in a range of inflammatory diseases, e.g. rheumatoid arthritis. In some hospitals, its prescription is restricted to senior doctors. Check you are authorised to prescribe it before doing so. Make it clear that methotrexate is given once weekly: to avoid erroneous daily administration, cross off the days it should not be given.

This scenario also highlights the need to ensure the correct dose is prescribed. Notice that the label instructs 8 tablets on Saturdays, i.e. 8 × 2.5mg = 20mg. On the chart this should be prescribed as a single dose of 20mg.

It is unusual for once-weekly methotrexate to be prescribed without weekly folic acid. Furthermore, this patient did not present a methotrexate or steroid card. This raises the suspicion that he may not have brought all of his medications. The best way to seek clarification of a patient's regular medication is to speak to the patient's general practitioner.

KEY POINTS

- Check the details for every drug a patient brings to hospital
- Methotrexate and trimethoprim produce a clinically significant interaction
- Cross off days that you definitely do not want a drug to be administered on

LONGBURY HOSPITAL TRUST			HOSPITAL NUMBER	456723		
			SURNAME	SMITH		
			FIRST NAME	ROBERT		
			ADDRESS	32 VICOLI STREET, LONGBURY LB2 3DP		
			D.O.B	16/09/YYYY (63 YEARS AGO)		
DATE OF ADMISSION	07/03/YYYY	ADMISSION WEIGHT (KG)	76kg	WARD	MEDICAL ASSESSMENT	
ALLERGIES			CONSULTANT		ERIN JOHNSON	
NO KNOWN ALLERGIES (NKDA)			CHART NO		1…OF…1	

ONCE ONLY PRESCRIPTIONS

DATE	TIME	NAME OF DRUG	DOSE	ROUTE	PRESCRIBER'S SIGNATURE	GIVEN BY	TIME GIVEN

REGULAR MEDICATIONS

NAME OF DRUG RAMIPRIL	TIME	DATE → DOSE ↓	07/03				
ADDITIONAL INSTRUCTIONS	08:00	2.5mg					
DATE 07/03 ROUTE PO	12:00						
PRESCRIBER'S SIGNATURE ALewis	18:00						
PRESCRIBER'S NAME AND BLEEP ALEX LEWIS 4567	22:00						

NAME OF DRUG PREDNISOLONE	TIME	DATE → DOSE ↓	07/03				
ADDITIONAL INSTRUCTIONS	08:00	5mg					
DATE 07/03 ROUTE PO	12:00						
PRESCRIBER'S SIGNATURE ALewis	18:00						
PRESCRIBER'S NAME AND BLEEP ALEX LEWIS 4567	22:00						

NAME OF DRUG METHOTREXATE	TIME	DATE → DOSE ↓	07/03	08/03	09/03	10/03 SATURDAY	11/03
ADDITIONAL INSTRUCTIONS 20mg ONCE WEEKLY, SATURDAYS	08:00	20mg (8 X 2.5mg)	X	X	X		X
DATE 07/03 ROUTE PO	12:00						
PRESCRIBER'S SIGNATURE ALewis	18:00						
PRESCRIBER'S NAME AND BLEEP ALEX LEWIS 4567	22:00						

PATIENT NAME *ROBERT SMITH*   HOSPITAL NO.   456723

NAME OF DRUG		TIME	DATE → DOSE ↓					
ADDITIONAL INSTRUCTIONS		08:00						
DATE	ROUTE	12:00						
PRESCRIBER'S SIGNATURE		18:00						
PRESCRIBER'S NAME AND BLEEP		22:00						

NAME OF DRUG		TIME	DATE → DOSE ↓					
ADDITIONAL INSTRUCTIONS		08:00						
DATE	ROUTE	12:00						
PRESCRIBER'S SIGNATURE		18:00						
PRESCRIBER'S NAME AND BLEEP		22:00						

NAME OF DRUG		TIME	DATE → DOSE ↓					
ADDITIONAL INSTRUCTIONS		08:00						
DATE	ROUTE	12:00						
PRESCRIBER'S SIGNATURE		18:00						
PRESCRIBER'S NAME AND BLEEP		22:00						

AS REQUIRED PRESCRIPTIONS

NAME OF DRUG		DATE					
INDICATION/ INSTRUCTION	DOSE	TIME					
FREQUENCY	ROUTE	DOSE					
PRESCRIBER'S SIGNATURE		ROUTE					
PRESCRIBER'S NAME AND BLEEP		GIVEN BY					
START DATE	STOP DATE						

PATIENT NAME *ROBERT SMITH*   HOSPITAL NO.   *456723*

NAME OF DRUG		DATE					
INDICATION/ INSTRUCTION	DOSE	TIME					
FREQUENCY	ROUTE	DOSE					
PRESCRIBER'S SIGNATURE		ROUTE					
PRESCRIBER'S NAME AND BLEEP		GIVEN BY					
START DATE	STOP DATE						

INTRAVENOUS FLUIDS

DATE	FLUID	ADDITIVE & DOSE	VOLUME	RATE/ DURATION	PRESCRIBER'S SIGNATURE	GIVEN BY	START TIME	END TIME

Record of signatures. ALL prescribers MUST complete.

DATE	NAME	DESIGNATION	SIGNATURE	BLEEP NUMBER
07/03	ALEX LEWIS	F1	ALewis	4567

Grace Parker (hospital number: 435090, DOB 12/04/YYYY [92 years old], address: 60 Terrance Place, Longbury LB19 6JO) has dementia and is receiving treatment for aspiration pneumonia. She is frail and weighs 45kg. Her urine output has been good but she is refusing to drink or eat. She is euvolaemic.

Blood test results:
Sodium 131mmol/L
Potassium 3.9mmol/L
Urea 4.5mmol/L
Creatinine 45µmol/L
eGFR 52mL/min/1.73m^2

As the evening F1 doctor on call for the medical wards, your task is to prescribe maintenance fluid.
It is 18:00 on 10th July.

Notes

Step 1: Complete your answers in the drug chart opposite and overleaf

LONGBURY HOSPITAL TRUST		HOSPITAL NUMBER	435090
		SURNAME	PARKER
		FIRST NAME	GRACE
		ADDRESS	60 TERRANCE PLACE, LONGBURY LB19 6J0
		D.O.B	12/04/YYYY (92 YEARS AGO)

DATE OF ADMISSION	10/07/YYYY	ADMISSION WEIGHT (KG)	45kg	WARD	MEDICAL ASSESSMENT
ALLERGIES NKDA				CONSULTANT	ERIN JOHNSON
				CHART NO	1...OF...1

ONCE ONLY PRESCRIPTIONS

DATE	TIME	NAME OF DRUG	DOSE	ROUTE	PRESCRIBER'S SIGNATURE	GIVEN BY	TIME GIVEN

REGULAR MEDICATIONS

NAME OF DRUG / details	TIME	DATE → / DOSE ↓	10/07				14/07
NAME OF DRUG TAZOCIN	06:00	4.5g	HS				
ADDITIONAL INSTRUCTIONS FOR LRTI	08:00						
DATE 10/07 ROUTE IV	12:00						
PRESCRIBER'S SIGNATURE KCho	14:00	4.5g	SS				
	18:00						REVIEW
PRESCRIBER'S NAME AND BLEEP KENNETH CHO 5765	22:00	4.5g					

NAME OF DRUG / details	TIME	DATE → / DOSE ↓	10/07				
NAME OF DRUG RAMIPRIL							
ADDITIONAL INSTRUCTIONS	08:00	2.5mg	HS				
DATE 10/07 ROUTE PO	12:00						
PRESCRIBER'S SIGNATURE KCho							
	18:00						
PRESCRIBER'S NAME AND BLEEP KENNETH CHO 5765	22:00						

NAME OF DRUG / details	TIME	DATE → / DOSE ↓	10/07				
NAME OF DRUG DONEPEZIL							
ADDITIONAL INSTRUCTIONS	08:00						
DATE 10/07 ROUTE PO	12:00						
PRESCRIBER'S SIGNATURE KCho							
	18:00						
PRESCRIBER'S NAME AND BLEEP KENNETH CHO 5765	22:00	10mg					

PATIENT NAME GRACE PARKER   HOSPITAL NO.   435090

NAME OF DRUG		TIME	DATE → DOSE ↓					
ADDITIONAL INSTRUCTIONS		08:00						
DATE	ROUTE	12:00						
PRESCRIBER'S SIGNATURE								
		18:00						
PRESCRIBER'S NAME AND BLEEP								
		22:00						

NAME OF DRUG		TIME	DATE → DOSE ↓					
ADDITIONAL INSTRUCTIONS		08:00						
DATE	ROUTE	12:00						
PRESCRIBER'S SIGNATURE								
		18:00						
PRESCRIBER'S NAME AND BLEEP								
		22:00						

NAME OF DRUG		TIME	DATE → DOSE ↓					
ADDITIONAL INSTRUCTIONS		08:00						
DATE	ROUTE	12:00						
PRESCRIBER'S SIGNATURE								
		18:00						
PRESCRIBER'S NAME AND BLEEP								
		22:00						

AS REQUIRED PRESCRIPTIONS

NAME OF DRUG		DATE					
INDICATION/ INSTRUCTION	DOSE	TIME					
FREQUENCY	ROUTE	DOSE					
PRESCRIBER'S SIGNATURE		ROUTE					
PRESCRIBER'S NAME AND BLEEP							
START DATE	STOP DATE	GIVEN BY					

PATIENT NAME GRACE PARKER   HOSPITAL NO.   435090

NAME OF DRUG		DATE					
INDICATION/ INSTRUCTION	DOSE	TIME					
FREQUENCY	ROUTE	DOSE					
PRESCRIBER'S SIGNATURE		ROUTE					
PRESCRIBER'S NAME AND BLEEP		GIVEN BY					
START DATE	STOP DATE						

INTRAVENOUS FLUIDS

DATE	FLUID	ADDITIVE & DOSE	VOLUME	RATE/ DURATION	PRESCRIBER'S SIGNATURE	GIVEN BY	START TIME	END TIME

Record of signatures. ALL prescribers MUST complete.

DATE	NAME	DESIGNATION	SIGNATURE	BLEEP NUMBER
10/07	KENNETH CHO	F2	KCho	5765

Step 2: Now check your work overleaf

Answer 2

The key to correctly prescribing this patient's fluids is to recognise that her frailty and low body weight mean she will have a reduced fluid requirement and be more susceptible to fluid overload. There is no standard fluid regime and accurate prescription requires a complete overview of the patient, taking into account their serum electrolytes and the medications they are taking.

Step 3: Compare your answer to the checklist below and the chart opposite ☑

D	Details	Checked patient details Used capital letters throughout Used correct abbreviations	☐
R	Regular medications	Continued the regular medications	☐
U	Unpleasant reactions	No change	☐
G	Gravid?	No	☐

C	Contra-indications	Noted no serious drug interactions	☐
H	Hydration	Prescribed 1.5–2L to be given over 24 hours with at least 40mmol of potassium	☐
A	Analgesia	Not required	☐
R	Renal function	Noted moderate renal impairment, but no changes to any medications necessary	☐
T	Thrombo-prophylaxis	Recognised the need for thromboprophylaxis and prescribed enoxaparin 40mg	☐
S	Signature box	Signed signature box	☐

Rationale

This patient's maintenance fluid requirement is 25–35mL/kg/24h and her weight is 45kg, so her daily volume requirement is 1125–1575mL. In this case 1.5L of fluid has been prescribed over a 24-hour period as three 500mL bags of fluid, which will automatically be given in turn. However, a fluid prescription of 2L in 24 hours would be safe. Bags of fluid usually come in either 500mL or 1L volumes. 500mL bags are commonly stocked on wards for the elderly, to prevent too much fluid being given.

The second consideration is what type of fluid to give. There is no rule but the aim is to maintain electrolyte values in the normal range. Sodium requirements are approximately 70mmol daily and potassium 40–80mmol. A 500mL bag of 0.9% normal saline contains 77mmol sodium, so no more is required in this scenario. The patient's 24-hour potassium requirement has been prescribed as 20mmol additives to two of the fluid bags. This ensures that potassium will enter the patient's circulation at an acceptably slow rate. Given this patient's normal electrolytes and moderate renal impairment it would be acceptable to prescribe 1L of normal saline or Hartmann's with 500mL dextrose over 24 hours. Ramipril will cause potassium retention. However, the ramipril has been continued because patient is euvolaemic and her potassium is within the normal range.

A complicating issue is the use of the antibiotic piperacillin-tazobactam (Tazocin), an antibiotic known for its high sodium content. A normal 4.5g t.d.s. regime would equate to an extra sodium delivery of approximately 33mmol per day. Here, the addition of 33mmol to the 77mmol in the saline prescription is acceptable. Tazocin-derived sodium is more often a problem when hypernatraemia is accompanied by reduced kidney function. This patient was not prescribed thromboprophylaxis. It is important to assess whether the patient will require thromboprophylaxis and prescribe it if necessary. In this case 40mg enoxaparin has been prescribed because this elderly patient is likely to be immobile while hospitalised with a chest infection and is therefore at risk of venous thromboembolism.

KEY POINTS

- Approach each patient individually when prescribing fluids: assess their physiology, medications and current requirements
- Remember that elderly patients often have reduced maintenance requirements

LONGBURY HOSPITAL TRUST		HOSPITAL NUMBER	435090
		SURNAME	PARKER
		FIRST NAME	GRACE
		ADDRESS	60 TERRANCE PLACE, LONGBURY LB19 6JO

			D.O.B	12/04/YYYY (92 YEARS AGO)	
DATE OF ADMISSION	10/07/YYYY	ADMISSION WEIGHT (KG)	45kg	WARD	MEDICAL ASSESSMENT
ALLERGIES			CONSULTANT		ERIN JOHNSON
NKDA			CHART NO		1...OF...1

ONCE ONLY PRESCRIPTIONS

DATE	TIME	NAME OF DRUG	DOSE	ROUTE	PRESCRIBER'S SIGNATURE	GIVEN BY	TIME GIVEN

REGULAR MEDICATIONS

NAME OF DRUG	TIME	DATE → / DOSE ↓	10/07				14/07
TAZOCIN	06:00	4.5g	HS				
ADDITIONAL INSTRUCTIONS FOR LRTI	08:00						
DATE 10/07 ROUTE IV	12:00						
PRESCRIBER'S SIGNATURE KCho	14:00	4.5g	SS				
	18:00						REVIEW
PRESCRIBER'S NAME AND BLEEP KENNETH CHO 5765	22:00	4.5g					

NAME OF DRUG	TIME	DATE → / DOSE ↓	10/07				
RAMIPRIL							
ADDITIONAL INSTRUCTIONS	08:00	2.5mg	HS				
DATE 10/07 ROUTE PO	12:00						
PRESCRIBER'S SIGNATURE KCho	18:00						
PRESCRIBER'S NAME AND BLEEP KENNETH CHO 5765	22:00						

NAME OF DRUG	TIME	DATE → / DOSE ↓	10/07				
DONEPEZIL							
ADDITIONAL INSTRUCTIONS	08:00						
DATE 10/07 ROUTE PO	12:00						
PRESCRIBER'S SIGNATURE KCho	18:00						
PRESCRIBER'S NAME AND BLEEP KENNETH CHO 5765	22:00	10mg					

PATIENT NAME GRACE PARKER   HOSPITAL NO. 435090

NAME OF DRUG ENOXAPARIN		TIME	DATE → DOSE ↓						
ADDITIONAL INSTRUCTIONS		08:00							
DATE 10/07	ROUTE S/C	12:00							
PRESCRIBER'S SIGNATURE ALewis		18:00	40mg						
PRESCRIBER'S NAME AND BLEEP ALEX LEWIS 4567		22:00							

NAME OF DRUG		TIME	DATE → DOSE ↓						
ADDITIONAL INSTRUCTIONS		08:00							
DATE	ROUTE	12:00							
PRESCRIBER'S SIGNATURE		18:00							
PRESCRIBER'S NAME AND BLEEP		22:00							

NAME OF DRUG		TIME	DATE → DOSE ↓						
ADDITIONAL INSTRUCTIONS		08:00							
DATE	ROUTE	12:00							
PRESCRIBER'S SIGNATURE		18:00							
PRESCRIBER'S NAME AND BLEEP		22:00							

AS REQUIRED PRESCRIPTIONS

NAME OF DRUG		DATE					
INDICATION/ INSTRUCTION	DOSE	TIME					
FREQUENCY	ROUTE	DOSE					
PRESCRIBER'S SIGNATURE		ROUTE					
PRESCRIBER'S NAME AND BLEEP		GIVEN BY					
START DATE	STOP DATE						

PATIENT NAME GRACE PARKER   HOSPITAL NO.   435090

NAME OF DRUG		DATE					
INDICATION/ INSTRUCTION	DOSE	TIME					
FREQUENCY	ROUTE	DOSE					
PRESCRIBER'S SIGNATURE		ROUTE					
PRESCRIBER'S NAME AND BLEEP		GIVEN BY					
START DATE	STOP DATE						

INTRAVENOUS FLUIDS

DATE	FLUID	ADDITIVE & DOSE	VOLUME	RATE/ DURATION	PRESCRIBER'S SIGNATURE	GIVEN BY	START TIME	END TIME
10/07	N.SALINE	20mmol KCl	500ml	8hr	ALewis			
10/07	5% DEXTROSE	20mmol KCl	500ml	8hr	ALewis			
10/07	5% DEXTROSE	——————	500ml	8hr	ALewis			

Record of signatures. ALL prescribers MUST complete.

DATE	NAME	DESIGNATION	SIGNATURE	BLEEP NUMBER
10/07	KENNETH CHO	F2	KCho	5765
10/07	ALEX LEWIS	F1	ALewis	4567

James Dulson (hospital number: 752011, DOB 12/10/YYYY [49 years old], address: 1 Upper Court, Longbury LB9 1NR) has been admitted with an injured ankle. He is currently experiencing mild pain. His past medical history includes psoriasis and glaucoma, which he treats with the list of creams, eye drops and co-codamol he has brought in. He says he once had a rash after taking co-amoxiclav for a urinary tract infection. His admission weight is 82kg. He is on the surgical ward and his consultant is Mr Joshua Gibb.

Regular medications:
Co-codamol 8/500 one tablet four times a day
Diprobase cream for left arm, once daily
Calcipotriol ointment for left elbow, twice daily
Viscotears eye drops, for both eyes as required
Timoptol 0.25% drops for the left eye twice daily

Your task is to prescribe regular medications and start analgesia.
It is 09:45 on 14th November.

Notes

Step 1: Complete your answers in the drug chart opposite and overleaf

LONGBURY HOSPITAL TRUST	HOSPITAL NUMBER SURNAME FIRST NAME ADDRESS D.O.B		
DATE OF ADMISSION		ADMISSION WEIGHT (KG)	WARD	
ALLERGIES		CONSULTANT		
		CHART NO	...OF...

ONCE ONLY PRESCRIPTIONS

DATE	TIME	NAME OF DRUG	DOSE	ROUTE	PRESCRIBER'S SIGNATURE	GIVEN BY	TIME GIVEN

REGULAR MEDICATIONS

NAME OF DRUG		**TIME**	DATE → DOSE ↓				
ADDITIONAL INSTRUCTIONS		**08:00**					
DATE	ROUTE	**12:00**					
PRESCRIBER'S SIGNATURE		**18:00**					
PRESCRIBER'S NAME AND BLEEP		**22:00**					

NAME OF DRUG		**TIME**	DATE → DOSE ↓				
ADDITIONAL INSTRUCTIONS		**08:00**					
DATE	ROUTE	**12:00**					
PRESCRIBER'S SIGNATURE		**18:00**					
PRESCRIBER'S NAME AND BLEEP		**22:00**					

NAME OF DRUG		**TIME**	DATE → DOSE ↓				
ADDITIONAL INSTRUCTIONS		**08:00**					
DATE	ROUTE	**12:00**					
PRESCRIBER'S SIGNATURE		**18 :00**					
PRESCRIBER'S NAME AND BLEEP		**22:00**					

PATIENT NAME   HOSPITAL NO.

NAME OF DRUG		TIME	DATE → DOSE ↓					
ADDITIONAL INSTRUCTIONS		08:00						
DATE	ROUTE	12:00						
PRESCRIBER'S SIGNATURE								
		18:00						
PRESCRIBER'S NAME AND BLEEP								
		22:00						

NAME OF DRUG		TIME	DATE → DOSE ↓					
ADDITIONAL INSTRUCTIONS		08:00						
DATE	ROUTE	12:00						
PRESCRIBER'S SIGNATURE								
		18:00						
PRESCRIBER'S NAME AND BLEEP								
		22:00						

NAME OF DRUG		TIME	DATE → DOSE ↓					
ADDITIONAL INSTRUCTIONS		08:00						
DATE	ROUTE	12:00						
PRESCRIBER'S SIGNATURE								
		18:00						
PRESCRIBER'S NAME AND BLEEP								
		22:00						

AS REQUIRED PRESCRIPTIONS

NAME OF DRUG		DATE					
INDICATION/ INSTRUCTION	DOSE	TIME					
FREQUENCY	ROUTE	DOSE					
PRESCRIBER'S SIGNATURE		ROUTE					
PRESCRIBER'S NAME AND BLEEP		GIVEN BY					
START DATE	STOP DATE						

PATIENT NAME   HOSPITAL NO.

NAME OF DRUG		DATE						
INDICATION/ INSTRUCTION	DOSE	TIME						
FREQUENCY	ROUTE	DOSE						
PRESCRIBER'S SIGNATURE		ROUTE						
PRESCRIBER'S NAME AND BLEEP		GIVEN BY						
START DATE	STOP DATE							

INTRAVENOUS FLUIDS

DATE	FLUID	ADDITIVE & DOSE	VOLUME	RATE/ DURATION	PRESCRIBER'S SIGNATURE	GIVEN BY	START TIME	END TIME

Record of signatures. ALL prescribers MUST complete.

DATE	NAME	DESIGNATION	SIGNATURE	BLEEP NUMBER

Answer 3

Admitting doctors are often charged with writing up a patient's regular medications. Some of these will be unfamiliar and it can be unclear exactly how to convert the patient's regimen into a safe prescription on a hospital chart.

This exercise is about demonstrating the skills for dealing with brand names and physically prescribing drugs via the less used routes. Here 'awkward' medications must be prescribed clearly on the drug chart, with the aim of making the prescription as clear and as safe as possible.

Step 3: Compare your answer to the checklist below and the chart opposite ☑

D	Details	Checked patient details Used capital letters throughout Used correct abbreviations	☐
R	Regular medications	Prescribed: – diprobase cream for left arm o.d. – calcipotriol ointment for left elbow b.d. – viscotears eye drops, for both eyes p.r.n. – timolol maleate 0.25% drops for the left eye b.d. – codeine 30mg q.d.s. – paracetamol 1g q.d.s.	☐
U	Unpleasant reactions	Noticed penicillin allergy	☐
G	Gravid?	Not required	☐

C	Contra-indications	Recognised co-codamol 8/500 and paracetamol 1g q.d.s	☐
H	Hydration	Not required	☐
A	Analgesia	See regular medications	☐
R	Renal function	Not required	☐
T	Thrombo-prophylaxis	Not required	☐
S	Signature box	Signed signature box	☐

Rationale

This man is taking co-codamol 8/500 q.d.s. (8mg codeine, 500mg paracetamol). Prescribing an additional 1g of paracetamol q.d.s. would create an overdose. It is clearest to refrain from prescribing co-codamol and instead prescribe paracetamol and codeine separately. Alternatively, it would be safe to prescribe co-codamol 30/500 instead (one or two tablets q.d.s.).

When writing up creams, it is useful to use $\dot{T}$ (T with a dot above it) to symbolise a dose. $\dot{T}$ means one application, tablet or drop, depending on the medication. In the route section, TOP indicates a topical formulation. Some drug charts will have additional boxes for directions, in which it is appropriate to specify where the cream is to be applied.

When prescribing eye drops ensure that there are clear instructions as to whether the drops are bilateral or for one eye only. Do this in the route section, e.g. LEFT EYE, or BOTH EYES, or in the additional instruction box. The strength of the drug is often specified as a percentage, and one drop is denoted by the $\dot{T}$ symbol. Systemic absorption can occur with eye drops, and drops containing the beta-blocker timolol are contraindicated in asthma.

KEY POINTS

- Before prescribing paracetamol, check the patient is not already receiving it in another form
- The abbreviation TOP is used to indicate topical application and specify clearly where the drug is to be applied

LONGBURY HOSPITALS TRUST		HOSPITAL NUMBER	752011

		HOSPITAL NUMBER	752011
		SURNAME	DULSON
		FIRST NAME	JAMES
		ADDRESS	1 UPPER COURT, LONGBURY LB9 1NR
		D.O.B	12/10/YYYY (49 YEARS AGO)

DATE OF ADMISSION	14/11/YYYY	ADMISSION WEIGHT (KG)	82kg	WARD	SURGICAL
ALLERGIES				CONSULTANT	JOSHUA GIBB
PENICILLIN - RASH				CHART NO	1...OF...1

ONCE ONLY PRESCRIPTIONS

DATE	TIME	NAME OF DRUG	DOSE	ROUTE	PRESCRIBER'S SIGNATURE	GIVEN BY	TIME GIVEN

REGULAR MEDICATIONS

NAME OF DRUG PARACETAMOL	TIME	DATE → DOSE ↓	14/11				
ADDITIONAL INSTRUCTIONS	08:00	1g	X				
DATE 14/11 ROUTE PO	12:00	1g					
PRESCRIBER'S SIGNATURE ALewis	18:00	1g					
PRESCRIBER'S NAME AND BLEEP ALEX LEWIS 4567	22:00	1g					

NAME OF DRUG CODEINE	TIME	DATE → DOSE ↓	14/11				
ADDITIONAL INSTRUCTIONS	08:00	30mg	X				
DATE 14/11 ROUTE PO	12:00	30mg					
PRESCRIBER'S SIGNATURE ALewis	18:00	30mg					
PRESCRIBER'S NAME AND BLEEP ALEX LEWIS 4567	22:00	30mg					

NAME OF DRUG DIPROBASE	TIME	DATE → DOSE ↓	14/11				
ADDITIONAL INSTRUCTIONS LEFT ARM	08:00	T	X				
DATE 14/11 ROUTE TOP	12:00						
PRESCRIBER'S SIGNATURE ALewis	18:00						
PRESCRIBER'S NAME AND BLEEP ALEX LEWIS 4567	22:00						

PATIENT NAME *JAMES DULSON* HOSPITAL NO. *752011*

NAME OF DRUG *CALCIPOTRIOL OINTMENT*		TIME	DATE → DOSE ↓	*14/11*				
ADDITIONAL INSTRUCTIONS *LEFT ELBOW*		08:00	Ṫ	X				
DATE *14/11*	ROUTE *TOP*	12:00						
PRESCRIBER'S SIGNATURE *ALewis*		18:00						
PRESCRIBER'S NAME AND BLEEP *ALEX LEWIS 4567*		22:00	Ṫ					

NAME OF DRUG *TIMOLOL MALEATE 0.25%*		TIME	DATE → DOSE ↓	*14/11*				
ADDITIONAL INSTRUCTIONS *LEFT EYE*		08:00	Ṫ	X				
DATE *14/11*	ROUTE *EYE*	12:00						
PRESCRIBER'S SIGNATURE *ALewis*		18:00						
PRESCRIBER'S NAME AND BLEEP *ALEX LEWIS 4567*		22:00	Ṫ					

NAME OF DRUG		TIME	DATE → DOSE ↓					
ADDITIONAL INSTRUCTIONS		08:00						
DATE	ROUTE	12:00						
PRESCRIBER'S SIGNATURE		18:00						
PRESCRIBER'S NAME AND BLEEP		22:00						

AS REQUIRED PRESCRIPTIONS

NAME OF DRUG *VISCOTEARS*		DATE					
INDICATION/ INSTRUCTION *DRY EYES*	DOSE *Ṫ*	TIME					
FREQUENCY *QDS*	ROUTE *BOTH EYES*	DOSE					
PRESCRIBER'S SIGNATURE *ALewis*		ROUTE					
PRESCRIBER'S NAME AND BLEEP *ALEX LEWIS 4567*		GIVEN BY					
START DATE *14/11*	STOP DATE						

PATIENT NAME *JAMES DULSON*   HOSPITAL NO.   *752011*

NAME OF DRUG		DATE						
INDICATION/ INSTRUCTION	DOSE	TIME						
FREQUENCY	ROUTE	DOSE						
PRESCRIBER'S SIGNATURE		ROUTE						
PRESCRIBER'S NAME AND BLEEP		GIVEN BY						
START DATE	STOP DATE							

INTRAVENOUS FLUIDS

DATE	FLUID	ADDITIVE & DOSE	VOLUME	RATE/ DURATION	PRESCRIBER'S SIGNATURE	GIVEN BY	START TIME	END TIME

Record of signatures. ALL prescribers MUST complete.

DATE	NAME	DESIGNATION	SIGNATURE	BLEEP NUMBER
14/11	ALEX LEWIS	F1	ALewis	4567

Jessica Wilson (hospital number: 329170, DOB 13/02/YYYY [72 years old], address: 44 Jersey Street, Longbury LB4 5YY), is coming in for an elective knee replacement in 2 weeks' time. She had a non-ST elevation myocardial infarction 10 months ago but has recovered well and has no symptoms. Today she is attending the orthopaedic preoperative assessment clinic.

Her admission weight is 75kg. She is on the surgical ward and her consultant is Mr Joshua Gibb.

Examination is normal. Mrs Wilson supplies a list of her tablets, mentioning that she is allergic to Elastoplast. She will be admitted the night before her operation.

Mrs Wilson's tablets:

Breakfast:

Plavix 75mg in the morning

Co-amilofruse 5/40, one in the morning

Mini aspirin, one a day

Bedtime:

Diprobase, for dry feet before bed

Simvastatin 20mg, two at night

As the F1 doctor running the clinic, your task is to prescribe the medications prior to admission planned for 12th May.

It is 30th April.

Notes

Step 1: Complete your answers in the drug chart opposite and overleaf

LONGBURY HOSPITAL TRUST	HOSPITAL NUMBER SURNAME FIRST NAME ADDRESS D.O.B		

DATE OF ADMISSION		ADMISSION WEIGHT (KG)		WARD	
ALLERGIES			CONSULTANT		
			CHART NO		…OF…

ONCE ONLY PRESCRIPTIONS

DATE	TIME	NAME OF DRUG	DOSE	ROUTE	PRESCRIBER'S SIGNATURE	GIVEN BY	TIME GIVEN

REGULAR MEDICATIONS

NAME OF DRUG		TIME	DATE → DOSE ↓				
ADDITIONAL INSTRUCTIONS		08:00					
DATE	ROUTE	12:00					
PRESCRIBER'S SIGNATURE		18:00					
PRESCRIBER'S NAME AND BLEEP		22:00					

NAME OF DRUG		TIME	DATE → DOSE ↓				
ADDITIONAL INSTRUCTIONS		08:00					
DATE	ROUTE	12:00					
PRESCRIBER'S SIGNATURE		18:00					
PRESCRIBER'S NAME AND BLEEP		22:00					

NAME OF DRUG		TIME	DATE → DOSE ↓				
ADDITIONAL INSTRUCTIONS		08:00					
DATE	ROUTE	12:00					
PRESCRIBER'S SIGNATURE		18:00					
PRESCRIBER'S NAME AND BLEEP		22:00					

PATIENT NAME   HOSPITAL NO.

NAME OF DRUG		TIME	DATE → DOSE ↓					
ADDITIONAL INSTRUCTIONS		08:00						
DATE	ROUTE	12:00						
PRESCRIBER'S SIGNATURE								
		18:00						
PRESCRIBER'S NAME AND BLEEP								
		22:00						

NAME OF DRUG		TIME	DATE → DOSE ↓					
ADDITIONAL INSTRUCTIONS		08:00						
DATE	ROUTE	12:00						
PRESCRIBER'S SIGNATURE								
		18:00						
PRESCRIBER'S NAME AND BLEEP								
		22:00						

NAME OF DRUG		TIME	DATE → DOSE ↓					
ADDITIONAL INSTRUCTIONS		08:00						
DATE	ROUTE	12:00						
PRESCRIBER'S SIGNATURE								
		18:00						
PRESCRIBER'S NAME AND BLEEP								
		22:00						

NAME OF DRUG		TIME	DATE → DOSE ↓					
ADDITIONAL INSTRUCTIONS		08:00						
DATE	ROUTE	12:00						
PRESCRIBER'S SIGNATURE								
		18:00						
PRESCRIBER'S NAME AND BLEEP								
		22:00						

PATIENT NAME   HOSPITAL NO.

AS REQUIRED PRESCRIPTIONS

NAME OF DRUG		DATE					
INDICATION/ INSTRUCTION	DOSE	TIME					
FREQUENCY	ROUTE	DOSE					
PRESCRIBER'S SIGNATURE		ROUTE					
PRESCRIBER'S NAME AND BLEEP		GIVEN BY					
START DATE	STOP DATE						

NAME OF DRUG		DATE					
INDICATION/ INSTRUCTION	DOSE	TIME					
FREQUENCY	ROUTE	DOSE					
PRESCRIBER'S SIGNATURE		ROUTE					
PRESCRIBER'S NAME AND BLEEP		GIVEN BY					
START DATE	STOP DATE						

INTRAVENOUS FLUIDS

DATE	FLUID	ADDITIVE & DOSE	VOLUME	RATE/ DURATION	PRESCRIBER'S SIGNATURE	GIVEN BY	START TIME	END TIME

Record of signatures. ALL prescribers MUST complete.

DATE	NAME	DESIGNATION	SIGNATURE	BLEEP NUMBER

Step 2: Now check your work overleaf

Answer 4

It is not uncommon to encounter medications with unfamiliar names. This exercise highlights the importance of finding out about a drug you do not recognise before you prescribe it. Certain medications, particularly those that affect blood clotting, should be withheld before surgery.

Step 3: Compare your answer to the checklist below and the chart opposite ☑

D Details	Checked patient details Used capital letters throughout Used correct abbreviations	☐
R Regular medications	Prescribed co-amilofruse, diprobase and simvastatin 40mg	☐
U Unpleasant reactions	Documented Elastoplast reaction	☐
G Gravid?	No	☐

C Contra-indications	Omitted clopidogrel (Plavix) and aspirin	☐
H Hydration	Not required	☐
A Analgesia	Prescribed regular paracetamol and codeine and Oramorph PRN	☐
R Renal function	Not required	☐
T Thrombo-prophylaxis	Prescribed enoxaparin 40mg SC	☐
S Signature box	Signed signature box	☐

Rationale

Check drugs that you do not recognise before prescribing them: often patients will refer to their medications by the brand name on the box or by what colour the tablet is. Here, the patient had been taking a branded version of clopidogrel (Plavix) and a combined potassium sparing diuretic (amiloride) and loop diuretic (furosemide). Combined tablets are sometimes used where compliance is a problem. Avoid using brand names when prescribing; some exceptions to this rule are insulin, topical products (e.g. Dovobet) and contraceptive pills, and some modified release products, e.g. theophylline and nifedipine.

Patients should take the majority of their tablets preoperatively. However, clopidogrel and aspirin have not been prescribed: these antiplatelet agents are commonly avoided preoperatively to prevent perioperative blood loss and patients are often asked to stop them 1 week before an operation. There are exceptions to this rule, such as recent coronary or cerebral stenting (check if unsure). The decision to restart should be taken after the operation. Writing the drugs into the drug chart with a note explaining they are withheld perioperatively helps prevent them being forgotten afterwards.

Notice that the patient is actually taking 40mg of simvastatin, as she is taking two 20mg tablets.

Pre-emptive analgesic prescribing can be done preoperatively, as has been done here. Don't forget laxatives if prescribing opiates regularly.

KEY POINTS

- Check unfamiliar drugs in the formulary or with the pharmacist
- Stop antiplatelets such as clopidogrel preoperatively unless there is a known reason to do otherwise
- Prescribe postoperative analgesia pre-emptively where possible

LONGBURY HOSPITALS TRUST

HOSPITAL NUMBER	329170
SURNAME	WILSON
FIRST NAME	JESSICA
ADDRESS	44 JERSEY STREET, LONGBURY LB4 5YY
D.O.B	13/02/YYYY (72 YEARS AGO)

DATE OF ADMISSION	12/05/YYYY	ADMISSION WEIGHT (KG)	75kg	WARD	SURGICAL

ALLERGIES		CONSULTANT	JOSHUA GIBB
ELASTOPLAST		CHART NO	1...OF...1

ONCE ONLY PRESCRIPTIONS

DATE	TIME	NAME OF DRUG	DOSE	ROUTE	PRESCRIBER'S SIGNATURE	GIVEN BY	TIME GIVEN

REGULAR MEDICATIONS

NAME OF DRUG CO-AMILOFRUSE 5/40	TIME	DATE → DOSE ↓	12/05				
ADDITIONAL INSTRUCTIONS	08:00	ONE					
DATE 30/04 ROUTE PO	12:00						
PRESCRIBER'S SIGNATURE ALewis	18:00						
PRESCRIBER'S NAME AND BLEEP ALEX LEWIS 4567	22:00						

NAME OF DRUG DIPROBASE CREAM	TIME	DATE → DOSE ↓	12/05				
ADDITIONAL INSTRUCTIONS BOTH FEET	08:00						
DATE 30/04 ROUTE TOP	12:00						
PRESCRIBER'S SIGNATURE ALewis	18:00						
PRESCRIBER'S NAME AND BLEEP ALEX LEWIS 4567	22:00	T					

NAME OF DRUG SIMVASTATIN	TIME	DATE → DOSE ↓	12/05				
ADDITIONAL INSTRUCTIONS	08:00						
DATE 30/04 ROUTE PO	12:00						
PRESCRIBER'S SIGNATURE ALewis	18:00						
PRESCRIBER'S NAME AND BLEEP ALEX LEWIS 4567	22:00	40mg					

PATIENT NAME *JESSICA WILSON* HOSPITAL NO. *329170*

NAME OF DRUG PARACETAMOL	TIME	DATE → DOSE ↓	12/05				
ADDITIONAL INSTRUCTIONS	08:00	1g					
DATE 30/04 ROUTE PO/IV/PR	12:00	1g					
PRESCRIBER'S SIGNATURE ALewis	18:00	1g					
PRESCRIBER'S NAME AND BLEEP ALEX LEWIS 4567	22:00	1g					

NAME OF DRUG CODEINE PHOSPHATE	TIME	DATE → DOSE ↓	12/05				
ADDITIONAL INSTRUCTIONS	08:00	30–60mg					
DATE 30/04 ROUTE PO	12:00	30–60mg					
PRESCRIBER'S SIGNATURE ALewis	18:00	30–60mg					
PRESCRIBER'S NAME AND BLEEP ALEX LEWIS 4567	22:00	30–60mg					

NAME OF DRUG ENOXAPARIN	TIME	DATE → DOSE ↓	12/05				
ADDITIONAL INSTRUCTIONS	08:00						
DATE 30/04 ROUTE S/C	12:00						
PRESCRIBER'S SIGNATURE ALewis	18:00	40mg					
PRESCRIBER'S NAME AND BLEEP ALEX LEWIS 4567	22:00						

NAME OF DRUG SENNA	TIME	DATE → DOSE ↓	12/05				
ADDITIONAL INSTRUCTIONS	08:00						
DATE 30/04 ROUTE PO	12:00						
PRESCRIBER'S SIGNATURE ALewis	18:00						
PRESCRIBER'S NAME AND BLEEP ALEX LEWIS 4567	22:00	15mg					

PATIENT NAME *JESSICA WILSON*   HOSPITAL NO.   *329170*

AS REQUIRED PRESCRIPTIONS

NAME OF DRUG ORAMORPH		DATE					
INDICATION/ INSTRUCTION PAIN	DOSE 5-10mg	TIME					
FREQUENCY 4HRLY	ROUTE PO	DOSE					
PRESCRIBER'S SIGNATURE ALewis		ROUTE					
PRESCRIBER'S NAME AND BLEEP ALEX LEWIS 4567		GIVEN BY					
START DATE 12/05	STOP DATE						
NAME OF DRUG CYCLIZINE		DATE					
INDICATION/ INSTRUCTION NAUSEA	DOSE 50mg	TIME					
FREQUENCY TDS	ROUTE IM/IV/PO	DOSE					
PRESCRIBER'S SIGNATURE ALewis		ROUTE					
PRESCRIBER'S NAME AND BLEEP ALEX LEWIS 4567		GIVEN BY					
START DATE 12/05	STOP DATE						

INTRAVENOUS FLUIDS

DATE	FLUID	ADDITIVE & DOSE	VOLUME	RATE/ DURATION	PRESCRIBER'S SIGNATURE	GIVEN BY	START TIME	END TIME

Record of signatures. ALL prescribers MUST complete.

DATE	NAME	DESIGNATION	SIGNATURE	BLEEP NUMBER
30/04	ALEX LEWIS	F1	ALewis	4567

Rosalind Drury (hospital number: 215213, DOB 12/05/YYYY [85 years old], address: 28 Oakwood Drive, Longbury LB12 8YQ) is on the surgical ward after a left hip hemiarthroplasty 2 days ago. Her nurses feel that she has become more confused over the course of the day. She was previously independent and was admitted after falling and fracturing the neck of her left femur. She was hypotensive after the operation and received a small fluid challenge. She is known to have atrial fibrillation.

On examination Mrs Drury is found to be drowsy, with coarse bilateral chest crepitations and pitting oedema to the thigh.

Observations:
SaO$_2$ 92% on air
Temperature 36.6°C
Blood pressure 118/78mmHg
Pulse 92bpm, irregular
Respiratory rate 24 breaths/minute

Chest X-ray: diffuse bilateral shadowing in keeping with pulmonary oedema

Electrocardiogram: left ventricular hypertrophy, atrial fibrillation, no acute changes

Blood tests: normal

Arterial blood gases: type 1 respiratory failure

Your task is to prescribe appropriate immediate treatment.
Assume that the patient will be prescribed appropriate oxygen therapy.
It is 12:15 on 16th October.

Notes

Step 1: Complete your answers in the drug chart opposite and overleaf

LONGBURY HOSPITAL TRUST

HOSPITAL NUMBER	215213
SURNAME	DRURY
FIRST NAME	ROSALIND
ADDRESS	28 OAKWOOD DRIVE, LONGBURY LB12 8YQ
D.O.B	12/05/YYYY (85 YEARS AGO)

DATE OF ADMISSION	14/10/YYYY	ADMISSION WEIGHT (KG)	60kg	WARD	SURGICAL

ALLERGIES	CONSULTANT	JOSHUA GIBB
NO KNOWN ALLERGIES (NKDA)	CHART NO	1...OF...1

ONCE ONLY PRESCRIPTIONS

DATE	TIME	NAME OF DRUG	DOSE	ROUTE	PRESCRIBER'S SIGNATURE	GIVEN BY	TIME GIVEN

REGULAR MEDICATIONS

NAME OF DRUG	TIME	DATE → DOSE ↓	14/10	15/10	16/10		
DIGOXIN							
ADDITIONAL INSTRUCTIONS	08:00	125 micrograms	HS	HS	WP		
DATE 14/10 ROUTE PO	12:00						
PRESCRIBER'S SIGNATURE MHughes	18:00						
PRESCRIBER'S NAME AND BLEEP MICHELLE HUGHES 2357	22:00						

NAME OF DRUG	TIME	DATE → DOSE ↓	14/10	15/10	16/10		
ENOXAPARIN							
ADDITIONAL INSTRUCTIONS	08:00						
DATE 14/10 ROUTE S/C	12:00						
PRESCRIBER'S SIGNATURE MHughes	18:00	40mg	———	HS			
PRESCRIBER'S NAME AND BLEEP MICHELLE HUGHES 2357	22:00		PRE-OP				

NAME OF DRUG	TIME	DATE → DOSE ↓					
ADDITIONAL INSTRUCTIONS	08:00						
DATE ROUTE	12:00						
PRESCRIBER'S SIGNATURE	18:00						
PRESCRIBER'S NAME AND BLEEP	22:00						

PATIENT NAME ROSALIND DRURY   HOSPITAL NO.   215213

NAME OF DRUG	TIME	DATE → DOSE ↓				
ADDITIONAL INSTRUCTIONS	08:00					
DATE	ROUTE	12:00					
PRESCRIBER'S SIGNATURE						
	18:00					
PRESCRIBER'S NAME AND BLEEP	22:00					

NAME OF DRUG	TIME	DATE → DOSE ↓				
ADDITIONAL INSTRUCTIONS	08:00					
DATE	ROUTE	12:00					
PRESCRIBER'S SIGNATURE						
	18:00					
PRESCRIBER'S NAME AND BLEEP	22:00					

NAME OF DRUG	TIME	DATE → DOSE ↓				
ADDITIONAL INSTRUCTIONS	08:00					
DATE	ROUTE	12:00					
PRESCRIBER'S SIGNATURE						
	18:00					
PRESCRIBER'S NAME AND BLEEP	22:00					

AS REQUIRED PRESCRIPTIONS

NAME OF DRUG ORAMORPH		DATE	15/10	16/10	16/10		
INDICATION/ INSTRUCTION PAIN	DOSE 10mg	TIME	2300	0600	1200		
FREQUENCY 2-4 HRLY	ROUTE PO	DOSE	10mg	10mg	10mg		
PRESCRIBER'S SIGNATURE MHughes		ROUTE	PO	PO	PO		
PRESCRIBER'S NAME AND BLEEP MICHELLE HUGHES 2357		GIVEN BY	CB	CB	WP		
START DATE 14/10	STOP DATE						

PATIENT NAME ROSALIND DRURY   HOSPITAL NO.   215213

NAME OF DRUG			DATE						
INDICATION/ INSTRUCTION	DOSE		TIME						
FREQUENCY	ROUTE		DOSE						
PRESCRIBER'S SIGNATURE			ROUTE						
PRESCRIBER'S NAME AND BLEEP			GIVEN BY						
START DATE	STOP DATE								

INTRAVENOUS FLUIDS

DATE	FLUID	ADDITIVE & DOSE	VOLUME	RATE/ DURATION	PRESCRIBER'S SIGNATURE	GIVEN BY	START TIME	END TIME
15/10	N. SALINE	————————	250ml	STAT	MHughes	CB	0730	0800
15/10	N. SALINE	20 mmol KCl	1l	8 hrs	MHughes	HS	0800	1600
15/10	HARTMANN'S	————————	1l	8 hrs	NShah	HS	1630	0030
16/10	N. SALINE	————————	1l	8 hrs	NShah	CB	0200	1000
16/10	HARTMANN'S	————————	1l	8 hrs	NShah	WP	1200	

Record of signatures. ALL prescribers MUST complete.

DATE	NAME	DESIGNATION	SIGNATURE	BLEEP NUMBER
14/10	MICHELLE HUGHES	F1	MHughes	2357
15/10	NAZIA SHAH	F1	NShah	9761

Answer 5

This patient has been 'pushed into' pulmonary oedema by excessive fluid prescribing. It looks as though she was prescribed a fluid challenge followed by 1L of fluid in 8 hours for postoperative hypotension, and this has then been continued by the next prescriber, causing fluid overload. This exercise demonstrates the harm unclear prescriptions can cause and the importance of reviewing a chart for drugs worsening a patient's condition.

Step 3: Compare your answer to the checklist below and the chart opposite ☑

D	Details	Checked patient details Used capital letters throughout Used correct abbreviations	☐
R	Regular medications	Did not change digoxin, prescribed regular paracetamol, codeine and senna	☐
U	Unpleasant reactions	Wrote NKDA or equivalent	☐
G	Gravid?	N/A	☐

C	Contra-indications	No absolute contraindications	☐
H	Hydration	Stopped all fluid Prescribed stat dose of furosemide	☐
A	Analgesia	Stopped or reduced Oramorph and continued the paracetamol and codeine	☐
R	Renal function	Not required, but it will be important to check this postanaesthetic	☐
T	Thrombo-prophylaxis	Noticed the patient is on enoxaparin already	☐
S	Signature box	Signed signature box	☐

Rationale

For this patient, furosemide 40mg is an appropriate acute prescription to reduce the fluid overload. She should also be sat up and be given high-flow oxygen therapy. Remember oxygen is a drug and needs to be prescribed.

This scenario demonstrates the potential for iatrogenic harm to a patient through unclear prescribing. Dr Hughes could have avoided precipitating pulmonary oedema by either writing REVIEW under the 8-hourly bag or prescribing much slower fluids to follow. Dr Shah, who may have been unfamiliar with the patient, should have reviewed the patient before simply repeating Dr Hughes's regimen.

The patient had also been given significant quantities of Oramorph, which is a respiratory depressant and has contributed to the drowsiness. She has not been prescribed analgesia according to the WHO pain ladder, which explains her high demand for morphine. A more suitable regimen is regular paracetamol and codeine, using as-required Oramorph for breakthrough pain only after review has established that drowsiness is no longer a problem.

KEY POINTS

- Make fluid prescriptions clear. Are they to be continued? Should the patient be reviewed before the next bag? Is this a fluid challenge?
- Review the whole chart to check for drugs that may be contributing to a patient's condition

LONGBURY HOSPITAL TRUST			HOSPITAL NUMBER	215213
			SURNAME	DRURY
			FIRST NAME	ROSALIND
			ADDRESS	28 OAKWOOD DRIVE, LONGBURY LB12 8YQ
			D.O.B	12/05/YYYY (85 YEARS AGO)

DATE OF ADMISSION	13/10/YYYY	ADMISSION WEIGHT (KG)	60kg	WARD	SURGICAL
ALLERGIES			CONSULTANT		JOSHUA GIBB
NO KNOWN ALLERGIES (NKDA)			CHART NO		1...OF...1

ONCE ONLY PRESCRIPTIONS

DATE	TIME	NAME OF DRUG	DOSE	ROUTE	PRESCRIBER'S SIGNATURE	GIVEN BY	TIME GIVEN
16/10	STAT	FUROSEMIDE	40mg	IV	ALewis		

REGULAR MEDICATIONS

NAME OF DRUG DIGOXIN	TIME	DATE → DOSE ↓	14/10	15/10	16/10		
ADDITIONAL INSTRUCTIONS	08:00	125 micrograms	HS	HS	WP		
DATE 13/10 ROUTE PO	12:00						
PRESCRIBER'S SIGNATURE MHughes	18:00						
PRESCRIBER'S NAME AND BLEEP MICHELLE HUGHES 2357	22:00						

NAME OF DRUG ENOXAPARIN	TIME	DATE → DOSE ↓	14/10	15/10	16/10		
ADDITIONAL INSTRUCTIONS	08:00						
DATE 13/10 ROUTE S/C	12:00						
PRESCRIBER'S SIGNATURE MHughes	18:00	40mg	——	HS			
PRESCRIBER'S NAME AND BLEEP MICHELLE HUGHES 2357	22:00		PRE-OP				

NAME OF DRUG PARACETAMOL	TIME	DATE → DOSE ↓			16/10		
ADDITIONAL INSTRUCTIONS	08:00	1g					
DATE 16/10 ROUTE PO/ IV/PR	12:00	1g					
PRESCRIBER'S SIGNATURE ALewis	18:00	1g					
PRESCRIBER'S NAME AND BLEEP ALEX LEWIS 4567	22:00	1g					

PATIENT NAME ROSALIND DRURY   HOSPITAL NO.   215213

NAME OF DRUG CODEINE PHOSPHATE	TIME	DATE → DOSE ↓			16/10		
ADDITIONAL INSTRUCTIONS	08:00	30-60mg					
DATE 16/10 ROUTE PO	12:00	30-60mg					
PRESCRIBER'S SIGNATURE ALewis	18:00	30-60mg					
PRESCRIBER'S NAME AND BLEEP ALEX LEWIS 4567	22:00	30-60mg					

NAME OF DRUG SENNA	TIME	DATE → DOSE ↓			16/10		
ADDITIONAL INSTRUCTIONS	08:00						
DATE 16/10 ROUTE PO	12:00						
PRESCRIBER'S SIGNATURE ALewis	18:00						
PRESCRIBER'S NAME AND BLEEP ALEX LEWIS 4567	22:00	Ṫ					

NAME OF DRUG	TIME	DATE → DOSE ↓					
ADDITIONAL INSTRUCTIONS	08:00						
DATE ROUTE	12:00						
PRESCRIBER'S SIGNATURE	18:00						
PRESCRIBER'S NAME AND BLEEP	22:00						

AS REQUIRED PRESCRIPTIONS

NAME OF DRUG ORAMORPH		DATE	15/10	16/10	16/10	REVIEW – DROWSY ALewis 16/10
INDICATION/ INSTRUCTION PAIN	DOSE 10mg	TIME	2300	0600	1200	
FREQUENCY 2-4 HRLY	ROUTE PO	DOSE	10mg	10mg	10mg	
PRESCRIBER'S SIGNATURE MHughes		ROUTE	PO	PO	PO	
PRESCRIBER'S NAME AND BLEEP MICHELLE HUGHES 2357		GIVEN BY	CB	CB	WP	
START DATE 14/10	STOP DATE					

PATIENT NAME ROSALIND DRURY   HOSPITAL NO.   215213

NAME OF DRUG			DATE						
INDICATION/ INSTRUCTION	DOSE		TIME						
FREQUENCY	ROUTE		DOSE						
PRESCRIBER'S SIGNATURE			ROUTE						
PRESCRIBER'S NAME AND BLEEP			GIVEN BY						
START DATE	STOP DATE								

INTRAVENOUS FLUIDS

DATE	FLUID	ADDITIVE & DOSE	VOLUME	RATE/ DURATION	PRESCRIBER'S SIGNATURE	GIVEN BY	START TIME	END TIME
15/10	N. SALINE	————	250ML	STAT	MHughes	CB	0730	0800
15/10	N. SALINE	20 mmol KCL	1L	8 HRS	MHughes	HS	0800	1600
15/10	HARTMANN'S	————	1L	8 HRS	NShah	HS	1630	0030
16/10	N. SALINE	————	1L	8 HRS	NShah	CB	0200	1000
16/10	HARTMANN'S	————	1L	8 HRS	NShah	WP	1200	
		STOP – ALewis, 12:20 16/10. BLEEP 4567						

Record of signatures. ALL prescribers MUST complete.

DATE	NAME	DESIGNATION	SIGNATURE	BLEEP NUMBER
14/10	MICHELLE HUGHES	F1	MHughes	2357
15/10	NAZIA SHAH	F1	NShah	9761
16/10	ALEX LEWIS	F1	ALewis	4567

Exercise 6 | Elective operations

Emily Hawkings (hospital number: 786665, DOB 02/03/YYYY [70 years old], address: 120 Lyonsdown Road, Longbury LB20 0UV) is being admitted to the surgical ward for an elective total hip replacement. She is well with no significant medical history. She is allergic to penicillin, which brings her out in a rash, and says she sometimes takes over-the-counter ibuprofen tablets for the pain in her hip. She takes '20mg of silverstantin at night for cholesterol' and a mini-aspirin, which she stopped 7 days ago for this operation. The nurses weighed her: she is 67kg. Mrs Hawkings' consultant is Mr Joshua Gibb.

Your task is to prescribe appropriate perioperative treatment.
It is 09:00 on 13th May.

Notes

Step 1: Complete your answers in the drug chart opposite and overleaf

LONGBURY HOSPITAL TRUST					HOSPITAL NUMBER SURNAME FIRST NAME ADDRESS			
					D.O.B			
DATE OF ADMISSION			ADMISSION WEIGHT (KG)				WARD	
ALLERGIES					CONSULTANT			
					CHART NO			…OF…

ONCE ONLY PRESCRIPTIONS

DATE	TIME	NAME OF DRUG	DOSE	ROUTE	PRESCRIBER'S SIGNATURE	GIVEN BY	TIME GIVEN

REGULAR MEDICATIONS

NAME OF DRUG		TIME	DATE → DOSE ↓					
ADDITIONAL INSTRUCTIONS		08:00						
DATE	ROUTE	12:00						
PRESCRIBER'S SIGNATURE								
		18:00						
PRESCRIBER'S NAME AND BLEEP								
		22:00						

NAME OF DRUG		TIME	DATE → DOSE ↓					
ADDITIONAL INSTRUCTIONS		08:00						
DATE	ROUTE	12:00						
PRESCRIBER'S SIGNATURE								
		18:00						
PRESCRIBER'S NAME AND BLEEP								
		22:00						

NAME OF DRUG		TIME	DATE → DOSE ↓					
ADDITIONAL INSTRUCTIONS		08:00						
DATE	ROUTE	12:00						
PRESCRIBER'S SIGNATURE								
		18:00						
PRESCRIBER'S NAME AND BLEEP								
		22:00						

PATIENT NAME   HOSPITAL NO.

NAME OF DRUG		TIME	DATE → DOSE ↓					
ADDITIONAL INSTRUCTIONS		08:00						
DATE	ROUTE	12:00						
PRESCRIBER'S SIGNATURE								
		18:00						
PRESCRIBER'S NAME AND BLEEP								
		22:00						

NAME OF DRUG		TIME	DATE → DOSE ↓					
ADDITIONAL INSTRUCTIONS		08:00						
DATE	ROUTE	12:00						
PRESCRIBER'S SIGNATURE								
		18:00						
PRESCRIBER'S NAME AND BLEEP								
		22:00						

NAME OF DRUG		TIME	DATE → DOSE ↓					
ADDITIONAL INSTRUCTIONS		08:00						
DATE	ROUTE	12:00						
PRESCRIBER'S SIGNATURE								
		18:00						
PRESCRIBER'S NAME AND BLEEP								
		22:00						

AS REQUIRED PRESCRIPTIONS

NAME OF DRUG		DATE					
INDICATION/ INSTRUCTION	DOSE	TIME					
FREQUENCY	ROUTE	DOSE					
PRESCRIBER'S SIGNATURE		ROUTE					
PRESCRIBER'S NAME AND BLEEP		GIVEN BY					
START DATE	STOP DATE						

PATIENT NAME   HOSPITAL NO.

NAME OF DRUG		DATE					
INDICATION/ INSTRUCTION	DOSE	TIME					
FREQUENCY	ROUTE	DOSE					
PRESCRIBER'S SIGNATURE		ROUTE					
PRESCRIBER'S NAME AND BLEEP		GIVEN BY					
START DATE	STOP DATE						

INTRAVENOUS FLUIDS

DATE	FLUID	ADDITIVE & DOSE	VOLUME	RATE/ DURATION	PRESCRIBER'S SIGNATURE	GIVEN BY	START TIME	END TIME

Record of signatures. ALL prescribers MUST complete.

DATE	NAME	DESIGNATION	SIGNATURE	BLEEP NUMBER

Step 2: Now check your work overleaf

Answer 6

This routine task allows the admitting doctor to do some anticipatory prescribing. It is best to prescribe postoperative analgesia before the patient has their operation, rather than wait for them to be in pain.

Step 3: Compare your answer to the checklist below and the chart opposite ☑

D Details	Checked patient details Used capital letters throughout Used correct abbreviations	☐
R Regular medications	Prescribed: – simvastatin 20mg nocte – paracetamol 1g q.d.s. PO/IV/PR – codeine 30–60mg q.d.s. – senna 7.5mg o.n.	☐
U Unpleasant reactions	Documented her allergy to penicillin and what form it takes	☐
G Gravid?	No	☐

C Contra-indications	Noted no contraindications	☐
H Hydration	Not required	☐
A Analgesia	Prescribed as required: – Oramorph 5–10mg 2–4 hourly PO – cyclizine 50mg t.d.s. PO/IV/IM	☐
R Renal function	Not required	☐
T Thrombo-prophylaxis	Started 40mg enoxaparin SC, this may continue for weeks post orthopaedic surgery	☐
S Signature box	Signed signature box	☐

Rationale

The principles of the WHO pain ladder have been applied here, prescribing regular paracetamol and codeine, and limiting the use of as-required Oramorph to breakthrough pain. The possible side effects of codeine and Oramorph have to be considered: prescribe senna in anticipation of the constipating effects of opiate medications, and prescribe cyclizine as required in case of opiate-induced nausea. It is prudent to prescribe this early. Ibuprofen has not been prescribed here: prescribing NSAIDs should be avoided postoperatively because they increase the risk of renal injury and increased bleeding. The risk to the kidneys is greater in elderly and dehydrated patients. Some analgesics can be given by multiple routes such as the paracetamol prescribed here. This is especially useful in a patient who is vomiting or strictly nil-by-mouth, because an alternative route can be used. In contrast, some analgesics such as codeine and NSAIDs are most frequently used orally although other formularies are available (e.g. codeine injection, diclofenac suppositories).

The patient's regular aspirin 75mg can be restarted postoperatively, it can be written with a review date after the operation to ensure it is not forgotten. Sometimes patients will forget the names of their medications or bring a list of the boxes with them. If in doubt about the drugs they describe to you, don't prescribe: call the patient's general practitioner for an up-to-date list. In this exercise it was reasonably certain that the cholesterol-lowering drug the patient was describing was simvastatin, a relatively safe drug to prescribe.

KEY POINTS

- Anticipate the need for pain relief and treatment for related side effects
- Prescribe pain relief according to the WHO pain ladder
- Avoid NSAIDs in older patients
- If in doubt about a patient's drug history, do not prescribe: check with their general practitioner

LONGBURY HOSPITAL TRUST

HOSPITAL NUMBER	786665
SURNAME	HAWKINGS
FIRST NAME	EMILY
ADDRESS	120 LYONSDOWN ROAD, LONGBURY LB20 0UV
D.O.B	02/03/YYYY (70 YEARS AGO)

DATE OF ADMISSION	13/05/YYYY	ADMISSION WEIGHT (KG)	67kg	WARD	SURGICAL

ALLERGIES	CONSULTANT	JOSHUA GIBB
PENICILLIN - RASH	CHART NO	1...OF...1

ONCE ONLY PRESCRIPTIONS

DATE	TIME	NAME OF DRUG	DOSE	ROUTE	PRESCRIBER'S SIGNATURE	GIVEN BY	TIME GIVEN

REGULAR MEDICATIONS

NAME OF DRUG SIMVASTATIN	TIME	DATE → DOSE ↓	13/05			
ADDITIONAL INSTRUCTIONS	08:00					
DATE 13/05 ROUTE PO	12:00					
PRESCRIBER'S SIGNATURE ALewis	18:00					
PRESCRIBER'S NAME AND BLEEP ALEX LEWIS 4567	22:00	20mg				

NAME OF DRUG PARACETAMOL	TIME	DATE → DOSE ↓	13/05			
ADDITIONAL INSTRUCTIONS	08:00	1g	X			
DATE 13/05 ROUTE PO/IV/PR	12:00	1g				
PRESCRIBER'S SIGNATURE ALewis	18:00	1g				
PRESCRIBER'S NAME AND BLEEP ALEX LEWIS 4567	22:00	1g				

NAME OF DRUG CODEINE	TIME	DATE → DOSE ↓	13/05			
ADDITIONAL INSTRUCTIONS	08:00	30-60mg	X			
DATE 13/05 ROUTE PO	12:00	30-60mg				
PRESCRIBER'S SIGNATURE ALewis	18:00	30-60mg				
PRESCRIBER'S NAME AND BLEEP ALEX LEWIS 4567	22:00	30-60mg				

PATIENT NAME *EMILY HAWKINGS*　　　　HOSPITAL NO. 786665

NAME OF DRUG *SENNA*	TIME	DATE → DOSE ↓	13/05				
ADDITIONAL INSTRUCTIONS	08:00						
DATE 13/05　ROUTE *PO*	12:00						
PRESCRIBER'S SIGNATURE *ALewis*	18:00						
PRESCRIBER'S NAME AND BLEEP *ALEX LEWIS 4567*	22:00	*T*					

NAME OF DRUG *ENOXAPARIN*	TIME	DATE → DOSE ↓	13/05				
ADDITIONAL INSTRUCTIONS	08:00						
DATE 13/05　ROUTE *S/C*	12:00						
PRESCRIBER'S SIGNATURE *ALewis*	18:00	*40mg*					
PRESCRIBER'S NAME AND BLEEP *ALEX LEWIS 4567*	22:00						

NAME OF DRUG	TIME	DATE → DOSE ↓					
ADDITIONAL INSTRUCTIONS	08:00						
DATE　ROUTE	12:00						
PRESCRIBER'S SIGNATURE	18:00						
PRESCRIBER'S NAME AND BLEEP	22:00						

AS REQUIRED PRESCRIPTIONS

NAME OF DRUG *ORAMORPH*		DATE					
INDICATION/ INSTRUCTION *PAIN*	DOSE *5-10mg*	TIME					
FREQUENCY *2-4 HRLY*	ROUTE *PO*	DOSE					
PRESCRIBER'S SIGNATURE *ALewis*		ROUTE					
PRESCRIBER'S NAME AND BLEEP *ALEX LEWIS 4567*		GIVEN BY					
START DATE *13/05*	STOP DATE						

PATIENT NAME *EMILY HAWKINGS*   HOSPITAL NO.   *786665*

NAME OF DRUG *CYCLIZINE*		DATE						
INDICATION/ INSTRUCTION *NAUSEA*	DOSE *50mg*	TIME						
FREQUENCY *TDS*	ROUTE *PO/IM/IV*	DOSE						
PRESCRIBER'S SIGNATURE *ALewis*		ROUTE						
PRESCRIBER'S NAME AND BLEEP *ALEX LEWIS 4567*		GIVEN BY						
START DATE *13/05*	STOP DATE							

INTRAVENOUS FLUIDS

DATE	FLUID	ADDITIVE & DOSE	VOLUME	RATE/ DURATION	PRESCRIBER'S SIGNATURE	GIVEN BY	START TIME	END TIME

Record of signatures. ALL prescribers MUST complete.

DATE	NAME	DESIGNATION	SIGNATURE	BLEEP NUMBER
13/05	*ALEX LEWIS*	*F1*	*ALewis*	*4567*

Alexander Null (hospital number: 020001, DOB 23/06/YYYY [68 years old], address: 80 Church Street, Longbury LB1 7OA) is under the care of the vascular surgeons. He has just come back from theatre and is experiencing postoperative nausea and vomiting. A colleague has already prescribed cyclizine with no effect. The notes reveal Mr Null has Parkinson's disease.

Your task is to prescribe antiemetic therapy.
It is 11:00 on 9th June.

Notes

LONGBURY HOSPITAL TRUST				HOSPITAL NUMBER	020001	
				SURNAME	NULL	
				FIRST NAME	ALEXANDER	
				ADDRESS	80 CHURCH STREET, LONGBURY LB1 7OA	
				D.O.B	23/06/YYYY (68 YEARS AGO)	
DATE OF ADMISSION	09/06/YYYY	ADMISSION WEIGHT (KG)		78	WARD	SURGICAL
ALLERGIES				CONSULTANT		JOSHUA GIBB
PENICILLIN				CHART NO		1...OF...1

ONCE ONLY PRESCRIPTIONS

DATE	TIME	NAME OF DRUG	DOSE	ROUTE	PRESCRIBER'S SIGNATURE	GIVEN BY	TIME GIVEN

REGULAR MEDICATIONS

NAME OF DRUG PARACETAMOL	TIME	DATE → DOSE ↓	09/06				
ADDITIONAL INSTRUCTIONS	08:00	1g					
DATE 09/06 ROUTE PO	12:00	1g					
PRESCRIBER'S SIGNATURE KCho	18:00	1g					
PRESCRIBER'S NAME AND BLEEP KENNETH CHO 5765	22:00	1g					

NAME OF DRUG SELEGILINE	TIME	DATE → DOSE ↓	09/06				
ADDITIONAL INSTRUCTIONS	08:00	10mg					
DATE 09/06 ROUTE PO	12:00						
PRESCRIBER'S SIGNATURE KCho	18:00						
PRESCRIBER'S NAME AND BLEEP KENNETH CHO 5765	22:00						

NAME OF DRUG MADOPAR 25/100 CAPS	TIME	DATE → DOSE ↓	09/06				
ADDITIONAL INSTRUCTIONS	08:00	$\dot{T}$					
DATE 09/06 ROUTE PO	12:00	$\dot{T}$					
PRESCRIBER'S SIGNATURE KCho	18:00	$\dot{T}$					
PRESCRIBER'S NAME AND BLEEP KENNETH CHO 5765	22:00	$\dot{T}$					

PATIENT NAME ALEXANDER NULL   HOSPITAL NO.   020001

NAME OF DRUG		TIME	DATE → DOSE ↓					
ADDITIONAL INSTRUCTIONS		08:00						
DATE	ROUTE	12:00						
PRESCRIBER'S SIGNATURE								
		18:00						
PRESCRIBER'S NAME AND BLEEP								
		22:00						

NAME OF DRUG		TIME	DATE → DOSE ↓					
ADDITIONAL INSTRUCTIONS		08:00						
DATE	ROUTE	12:00						
PRESCRIBER'S SIGNATURE								
		18:00						
PRESCRIBER'S NAME AND BLEEP								
		22:00						

NAME OF DRUG		TIME	DATE → DOSE ↓					
ADDITIONAL INSTRUCTIONS		08:00						
DATE	ROUTE	12:00						
PRESCRIBER'S SIGNATURE								
		18:00						
PRESCRIBER'S NAME AND BLEEP								
		22:00						

AS REQUIRED PRESCRIPTIONS

NAME OF DRUG CYCLIZINE		DATE	09/06				
INDICATION/ INSTRUCTION NAUSEA	DOSE 50mg	TIME	1000				
FREQUENCY TDS	ROUTE IM/PO/IV	DOSE	50mg				
PRESCRIBER'S SIGNATURE KCho		ROUTE	IM				
PRESCRIBER'S NAME AND BLEEP KENNETH CHO 5765		GIVEN BY	YF				
START DATE 09/06	STOP DATE						

PATIENT NAME ALEXANDER NULL   HOSPITAL NO.   020001

NAME OF DRUG		DATE					
INDICATION/ INSTRUCTION	DOSE	TIME					
FREQUENCY	ROUTE	DOSE					
PRESCRIBER'S SIGNATURE		ROUTE					
PRESCRIBER'S NAME AND BLEEP		GIVEN BY					
START DATE	STOP DATE						

INTRAVENOUS FLUIDS

DATE	FLUID	ADDITIVE & DOSE	VOLUME	RATE/ DURATION	PRESCRIBER'S SIGNATURE	GIVEN BY	START TIME	END TIME

Record of signatures. ALL prescribers MUST complete.

DATE	NAME	DESIGNATION	SIGNATURE	BLEEP NUMBER
09/06	KENNETH CHO	F2	KCho	5765

Step 2: Now check your work overleaf

Answer 7

This exercise tests knowledge of the mode of action of the various antiemetics and their practical uses. When considering postoperative nausea and vomiting (PONV) it is important to exclude a surgical reason before concentrating on pharmacological therapies alone. In this case, prescribe for ineffective antiemetic therapy.

Step 3: Compare your answer to the checklist below and the chart opposite ☑

D Details	Checked patient details Used capital letters throughout Used correct abbreviations	☐
R Regular medications	Continued with anti-Parkinson's medications	☐
U Unpleasant reactions	Carried forward and documented the penicillin allergy	☐
G Gravid?	No	☐

C Contra-indications	Metoclopramide (and prochlorperazine) should be avoided in Parkinson's disease	☐
H Hydration	Prescribed a repeat bag of fluid (optional)	☐
A Analgesia	Continued with paracetamol, changed to IV	☐
R Renal function	Not required	☐
T Thrombo-prophylaxis	Prescribed enoxaparin 40mg	☐
S Signature box	Signed signature box	☐

Rationale

The antiemetic metoclopramide was not prescribed in this case because it is contraindicated in Parkinson's disease. It antagonises D2 receptors in the chemoreceptor trigger zone, worsening Parkinsonian symptoms. Metoclopramide should not be used in suspected small bowel obstruction, due to its prokinetic properties. The prescriber has chosen an antiemetic that is an acceptable choice in Parkinson's disease: a stat dose of the serotonin (5-HT$_3$ receptor subtype) antagonist ondansetron which has been prescribed here. An alternative is domperidone, because it does not significantly cross the blood–brain barrier and avoids extrapyramidal side effects. Cyclizine, an antihistamine, is also safe to prescribe in Parkinson's disease. Remember that antiemetics can be added in on top of each other, much like the analgesic ladder.

Consider whether a vomiting patient is able to take medicines orally; if they are not, prescribe antiemetics via another route, e.g. rectal domperidone or intravenous ondansetron.

Inpatients should receive their normal Parkinson's medication at the same time as they take it at home because disturbances in medication routine can worsen symptoms. As with antiemetics, there are alternative routes of administering Parkinson's medications, such as patches, and it is worth liaising with a pharmacist or senior doctor if the oral route is no longer available. It is important to avoid abrupt withdrawal of Parkinson's medications in order to prevent exacerbation of symptoms.

KEY POINTS

- Different classes of antiemetic have different modes of action
- Beware of using metoclopramide or prochlorperazine in Parkinson's disease
- Antiemetic therapy can be additive, much like the pain ladder

LONGBURY HOSPITAL TRUST			HOSPITAL NUMBER	020001	
			SURNAME	NULL	
			FIRST NAME .	ALEXANDER	
			ADDRESS	80 CHURCH STREET, LONGBURY LB1 7OA	
			D.O.B	23/06/YYYY (68 YEARS AGO)	
DATE OF ADMISSION	09/06/YYYY	ADMISSION WEIGHT (KG)	78	WARD	SURGICAL
ALLERGIES PENICILLIN			CONSULTANT	JOSHUA GIBB	
			CHART NO	1...OF...1	

ONCE ONLY PRESCRIPTIONS

DATE	TIME	NAME OF DRUG	DOSE	ROUTE	PRESCRIBER'S SIGNATURE	GIVEN BY	TIME GIVEN
09/06	STAT	ONDANSETRON	4mg	IV	ALewis		

REGULAR MEDICATIONS

NAME OF DRUG PARACETAMOL	TIME	DATE → DOSE ↓	09/06				
ADDITIONAL INSTRUCTIONS	08:00	1g					
DATE 09/06 ROUTE PO/IV	12:00	1g					
PRESCRIBER'S SIGNATURE KCho, ALewis	18:00	1g					
PRESCRIBER'S NAME AND BLEEP KENNETH CHO 5765	22:00	1g					

NAME OF DRUG SELEGILINE	TIME	DATE → DOSE ↓	09/06				
ADDITIONAL INSTRUCTIONS	08:00	10mg					
DATE 09/06 ROUTE PO	12:00						
PRESCRIBER'S SIGNATURE KCho	18:00						
PRESCRIBER'S NAME AND BLEEP KENNETH CHO 5765	22:00						

NAME OF DRUG MADOPAR 25/100 CAPS	TIME	DATE → DOSE ↓	09/06				
ADDITIONAL INSTRUCTIONS	08:00	⊤					
DATE 09/06 ROUTE PO	12:00	⊤					
PRESCRIBER'S SIGNATURE KCho	18:00	⊤					
PRESCRIBER'S NAME AND BLEEP KENNETH CHO 5765	22:00	⊤					

PATIENT NAME ALEXANDER NULL   HOSPITAL NO. 020001

NAME OF DRUG ENOXAPARIN	TIME	DATE → DOSE ↓	09/06				
ADDITIONAL INSTRUCTIONS	08:00						
DATE 09/06 | ROUTE S/C	12:00						
PRESCRIBER'S SIGNATURE ALewis	18:00		40mg				
PRESCRIBER'S NAME AND BLEEP ALEX LEWIS 4567	22:00						

NAME OF DRUG	TIME	DATE → DOSE ↓					
ADDITIONAL INSTRUCTIONS	08:00						
DATE | ROUTE	12:00						
PRESCRIBER'S SIGNATURE	18:00						
PRESCRIBER'S NAME AND BLEEP	22:00						

NAME OF DRUG	TIME	DATE → DOSE ↓					
ADDITIONAL INSTRUCTIONS	08:00						
DATE | ROUTE	12:00						
PRESCRIBER'S SIGNATURE	18:00						
PRESCRIBER'S NAME AND BLEEP	22:00						

AS REQUIRED PRESCRIPTIONS

NAME OF DRUG CYCLIZINE		DATE	09/06				
INDICATION/ INSTRUCTION NAUSEA	DOSE 50mg	TIME	1000				
FREQUENCY TDS	ROUTE IM/PO/IV	DOSE	50mg				
PRESCRIBER'S SIGNATURE KCho		ROUTE	IM				
PRESCRIBER'S NAME AND BLEEP KENNETH CHO 5765		GIVEN BY	YF				
START DATE 09/06	STOP DATE						

PATIENT NAME ALEXANDER NULL   HOSPITAL NO.   020001

NAME OF DRUG ONDANSETRON		DATE						
INDICATION/ INSTRUCTION NAUSEA	DOSE 4mg	TIME						
FREQUENCY TDS	ROUTE PO/IV	DOSE						
PRESCRIBER'S SIGNATURE ALewis		ROUTE						
PRESCRIBER'S NAME AND BLEEP ALEX LEWIS 4567		GIVEN BY						
START DATE 09/06	STOP DATE							

INTRAVENOUS FLUIDS

DATE	FLUID	ADDITIVE & DOSE	VOLUME	RATE/ DURATION	PRESCRIBER'S SIGNATURE	GIVEN BY	START TIME	END TIME

Record of signatures. ALL prescribers MUST complete.

DATE	NAME	DESIGNATION	SIGNATURE	BLEEP NUMBER
09/06	KENNETH CHO	F2	KCho	5765
09/06	ALEX LEWIS	F1	ALewis	4567

Ravi Shanla (hospital number: 100129, DOB 01/01/YYYY [87 years old], address: 39 Selby Street, Longbury LB9 4RB) has been admitted to the medical assessment ward. He has a background of chronic renal failure. He had a fall at home and was found on the floor by his son the next day. He sustained a painful fracture of his pubic ramus. Chest X-ray and blood tests have confirmed the suspicion that he has a left lower zone pneumonia. He has had an initial dose of piperacillin–tazobactam (Tazocin) in the emergency department and some analgesia.

The registrar instructs that the Tazocin is to be continued, Mr Shanla is to be kept comfortable, and the fracture is to be managed conservatively.

Urea and electrolytes	Now	3 months ago
Sodium	135mmol/L	142mmol/L
Potassium	5.4mmol/L	5.3mmol/L
Urea	30mmol/L	26mmol/L
Creatinine	423µmol/L	389µmol/L
eGFR	15mL/min/1.73m^2	19mL/min/1.73m^2

Your task is to prescribe the antibiotics.
It is 14:00 on 16th September.

Notes

LONGBURY HOSPITAL TRUST		HOSPITAL NUMBER	100129
		SURNAME	SHANLA
		FIRST NAME	RAVI
		ADDRESS	39 SELBY STREET, LONGBURY LB9 4RB
		D.O.B	01/01/YYYY (87 YEARS AGO)

DATE OF ADMISSION	15/09/YYYY	ADMISSION WEIGHT (KG)	71	WARD	MEDICAL ASSESSMENT
ALLERGIES			CONSULTANT		ERIN JOHNSON
NIL			CHART NO		1...OF...1

ONCE ONLY PRESCRIPTIONS

DATE	TIME	NAME OF DRUG	DOSE	ROUTE	PRESCRIBER'S SIGNATURE	GIVEN BY	TIME GIVEN
15/09	2000	TAZOCIN	4.5g	IV	EJones	MR	2010
15/09	2000	ORAMORPH	10mg	PO	EJones	MR	2010

REGULAR MEDICATIONS

NAME OF DRUG PARACETAMOL	TIME	DATE → DOSE ↓	16/09				
ADDITIONAL INSTRUCTIONS	08:00	1g	AD				
DATE 16/09 ROUTE PO/IV	12:00	1g	AD				
PRESCRIBER'S SIGNATURE EJones	18:00	1g					
PRESCRIBER'S NAME AND BLEEP EMMA JONES 4876	22:00	1g					

NAME OF DRUG ENOXAPARIN	TIME	DATE → DOSE ↓	16/09				
ADDITIONAL INSTRUCTIONS	08:00						
DATE 16/09 ROUTE S/C	12:00						
PRESCRIBER'S SIGNATURE EJones	18:00	40mg					
PRESCRIBER'S NAME AND BLEEP EMMA JONES 4876	22:00						

NAME OF DRUG CODEINE	TIME	DATE → DOSE ↓	16/09				
ADDITIONAL INSTRUCTIONS	08:00	30mg	AD				
DATE 16/09 ROUTE PO	12:00	30mg	AD				
PRESCRIBER'S SIGNATURE EJones	18:00	30mg					
PRESCRIBER'S NAME AND BLEEP EMMA JONES 4876	22:00	30mg					

68

PATIENT NAME RAVI SHANLA   HOSPITAL NO.   100129

NAME OF DRUG	TIME	DATE → DOSE ↓				
ADDITIONAL INSTRUCTIONS	08:00					
DATE / ROUTE	12:00					
PRESCRIBER'S SIGNATURE						
	18:00					
PRESCRIBER'S NAME AND BLEEP						
	22:00					

NAME OF DRUG	TIME	DATE → DOSE ↓				
ADDITIONAL INSTRUCTIONS	08:00					
DATE / ROUTE	12:00					
PRESCRIBER'S SIGNATURE						
	18:00					
PRESCRIBER'S NAME AND BLEEP						
	22:00					

NAME OF DRUG	TIME	DATE → DOSE ↓				
ADDITIONAL INSTRUCTIONS	08:00					
DATE / ROUTE	12:00					
PRESCRIBER'S SIGNATURE						
	18:00					
PRESCRIBER'S NAME AND BLEEP						
	22:00					

AS REQUIRED PRESCRIPTIONS

NAME OF DRUG ORAMORPH		DATE	15/09	16/09			
INDICATION/ INSTRUCTION PAIN	DOSE 10mg	TIME	2350	0400			
FREQUENCY 4 HRLY	ROUTE PO	DOSE	10mg	10mg			
PRESCRIBER'S SIGNATURE EJones		ROUTE	PO	PO			
PRESCRIBER'S NAME AND BLEEP EMMA JONES 4876		GIVEN BY	MR	MR			
START DATE 15/09	STOP DATE						

PATIENT NAME RAVI SHANLA   HOSPITAL NO.   100129

NAME OF DRUG		DATE					
INDICATION/INSTRUCTION	DOSE	TIME					
FREQUENCY	ROUTE	DOSE					
PRESCRIBER'S SIGNATURE		ROUTE					
PRESCRIBER'S NAME AND BLEEP		GIVEN BY					
START DATE	STOP DATE						

INTRAVENOUS FLUIDS

DATE	FLUID	ADDITIVE & DOSE	VOLUME	RATE/DURATION	PRESCRIBER'S SIGNATURE	GIVEN BY	START TIME	END TIME

Record of signatures. ALL prescribers MUST complete.

DATE	NAME	DESIGNATION	SIGNATURE	BLEEP NUMBER
15/09	EMMA JONES	F2	EJones	4876

Step 2: Now check your work overleaf

Answer 8

Prescribing in renal failure requires a full assessment of the patient's medication. Many drugs are excreted by the kidneys: if kidney function is impaired then reduced excretion will result in an accumulation of drugs and/or metabolites.

Step 3: Compare your answer to the checklist below and the chart opposite ✔

D Details	Checked patient details Used capital letters throughout Used correct abbreviations	☐
R Regular medications	Stopped codeine and Oramorph	☐
U Unpleasant reactions	Not required	☐
G Gravid?	No	☐

C Contra-indications	Danger: see renal function	☐
H Hydration	The need for fluid restriction will need to be considered	☐
A Analgesia	Continued paracetamol	☐
R Renal function	Withheld codeine and Oramorph, amended enoxaparin, prescribed renal dose Tazocin	☐
T Thrombo-prophylaxis	Changed enoxaparin prescription to 20mg	☐
S Signature box	Signed signature box	☐

Rationale

Consider the drug you have been asked to prescribe. Is it safe in renal failure? What should the adjusted dose be? It is good practice to check this in the formulary. Many antibiotics are renally excreted and require caution in renal failure. Here, Tazocin has been prescribed twice daily instead of the normal t.d.s. regimen. The prescription has been added to the drug chart that was started in the emergency department.

Analgesia is difficult to prescribe in end-stage renal failure. Most opioids, including codeine and tramadol, must be prescribed with caution because their half-lives are prolonged in renal failure. Morphine should be prescribed with care, starting with very small doses and an extended dosage interval. Doses should be reviewed often and carefully titrated to achieve analgesia without causing sedation or respiratory depression. This patient had already received 30mg of morphine in less than 24 hours and it is safest to stop it and seek advice. In end-stage renal failure, the use of analgesics that are either metabolised mainly by the liver or have inactive metabolites is advised: paracetamol is safe as it is metabolised by the liver.

Don't forget that the dose of enoxaparin for this indication should be halved in renal failure, as shown here.

KEY POINTS

- Review all medications prescribed for patients with renal failure even if they were admitted on them
- Many antibiotics are renally excreted and require particular caution in renal failure
- Recognise and stop medications that are nephrotoxic and could be making renal failure worse

LONGBURY HOSPITAL TRUST		HOSPITAL NUMBER	100129
		SURNAME	SHANLA
		FIRST NAME	RAVI
		ADDRESS	39 SELBY STREET, LONGBURY LB9 4RB
		D.O.B	01/01/YYYY (87 YEARS AGO)

DATE OF ADMISSION	15/09/YYYY	ADMISSION WEIGHT (KG)	71	WARD	MEDICAL ASSESSMENT
ALLERGIES			CONSULTANT		ERIN JOHNSON
NIL			CHART NO		1...OF...1

ONCE ONLY PRESCRIPTIONS

DATE	TIME	NAME OF DRUG	DOSE	ROUTE	PRESCRIBER'S SIGNATURE	GIVEN BY	TIME GIVEN
15/09	2000	TAZOCIN	4.5g	IV	EJones	MR	2010
15/09	2000	ORAMORPH	10mg	PO	EJones	MR	2010

REGULAR MEDICATIONS

NAME OF DRUG PARACETAMOL	TIME	DATE → DOSE ↓	16/09				
ADDITIONAL INSTRUCTIONS	08:00	1g	AD				
DATE 16/09 ROUTE PO/IV	12:00	1g	AD				
PRESCRIBER'S SIGNATURE EJones	18:00	1g					
PRESCRIBER'S NAME AND BLEEP EMMA JONES 4876	22:00	1g					

NAME OF DRUG ENOXAPARIN	TIME	DATE → DOSE ↓	16/09				
ADDITIONAL INSTRUCTIONS *CHANGED TO RENAL DOSE*	08:00						
DATE 16/09 ROUTE S/C	12:00				ALewis 16/09		
PRESCRIBER'S SIGNATURE EJones	18:00	~~40mg~~					
PRESCRIBER'S NAME AND BLEEP EMMA JONES 4876	18:00	20mg	X	X	X	X	X
	22:00						

NAME OF DRUG CODEINE	TIME	DATE → DOSE ↓	16/09	STOP	ALewis	16/09	
ADDITIONAL INSTRUCTIONS	08:00	30mg	AD				
DATE 16/09 ROUTE PO	12:00	30mg	AD				
PRESCRIBER'S SIGNATURE EJones	18:00	30mg					
PRESCRIBER'S NAME AND BLEEP EMMA JONES 4876	22:00	30mg					

PATIENT NAME RAVI SHANLA   HOSPITAL NO. 100129

NAME OF DRUG TAZOCIN	TIME	DATE → DOSE ↓	16/09				
							REVIEW
ADDITIONAL INSTRUCTIONS PNEUMONIA	08:00	4.5g	X				
DATE 16/09 ROUTE IV	12:00						
PRESCRIBER'S SIGNATURE ALewis	18:00						
PRESCRIBER'S NAME AND BLEEP ALEX LEWIS 4567	20:00	4.5g					
	22:00						

NAME OF DRUG	TIME	DATE → DOSE ↓					
ADDITIONAL INSTRUCTIONS	08:00						
DATE ROUTE	12:00						
PRESCRIBER'S SIGNATURE	18:00						
PRESCRIBER'S NAME AND BLEEP	22:00						

NAME OF DRUG	TIME	DATE → DOSE ↓					
ADDITIONAL INSTRUCTIONS	08:00						
DATE ROUTE	12:00						
PRESCRIBER'S SIGNATURE	18:00						
PRESCRIBER'S NAME AND BLEEP	22:00						

AS REQUIRED PRESCRIPTIONS

NAME OF DRUG ORAMORPH		DATE	15/09	16/09			
INDICATION/ INSTRUCTION PAIN	DOSE 10mg	TIME	2350	0400		STOP ALewis 16/09	
FREQUENCY 4 HRLY	ROUTE PO	DOSE	10mg	10mg			
PRESCRIBER'S SIGNATURE EJones		ROUTE	PO	PO			
PRESCRIBER'S NAME AND BLEEP EMMA JONES 4876		GIVEN BY	MR	MR			
START DATE 15/09	STOP DATE 16/09						

PATIENT NAME RAVI SHANLA   HOSPITAL NO.   100129

NAME OF DRUG		DATE					
INDICATION/ INSTRUCTION	DOSE	TIME					
FREQUENCY	ROUTE	DOSE					
PRESCRIBER'S SIGNATURE		ROUTE					
PRESCRIBER'S NAME AND BLEEP		GIVEN BY					
START DATE	STOP DATE						

INTRAVENOUS FLUIDS

DATE	FLUID	ADDITIVE & DOSE	VOLUME	RATE/ DURATION	PRESCRIBER'S SIGNATURE	GIVEN BY	START TIME	END TIME

Record of signatures. ALL prescribers MUST complete.

DATE	NAME	DESIGNATION	SIGNATURE	BLEEP NUMBER
15/09	EMMA JONES	F2	EJones	4876
16/09	ALEX LEWIS	F1	ALewis	4567

Baljinder Surpur (hospital number: 237621, DOB 02/09/YYYY [64 years old], address: 77 Cabara Road, Longbury LB3 4GJ), has been admitted to the medical assessment ward. He has had tight central chest pain for the last hour. He reports that the pain has been continuous and was not relieved by the spray the paramedics gave him in the ambulance. Otherwise fit and well, he is on no regular medications and has no significant past medical history or allergies. Mr Surpur's consultant is Dr Erin Johnson.

An ECG performed in the ambulance showed widespread T-wave inversion and no other notable features.

Observations:
Heart rate 105bpm
Blood pressure 145/95mmHg
Respiratory rate 22 breaths/minute
SaO_2 95% on air

Blood test results at presentation:
White cell count 6.3 x 10^9cells/L
Neutrophils 5.5 x 10^9cells/L
Haemoglobin 136g/L
Platelets 350 x 10^9cells/L
Sodium 135mmol/L
Potassium 3.9mmol/L
Creatinine 65μmol/L
Troponin 0.56ng/mL
Glucose 4.4mmol/L

Liver function tests: normal

On examination Mr Surpur is clammy and is clutching at his chest. Both heart sounds are easily heard and his lung bases are clear. There is no evidence of ankle oedema. He weighs 80kg.

Your task is to assess this patient in the medical assessment unit and initiate appropriate treatment.
It is 09:00 on 9th October.

Notes

Step 1: Complete your answers in the drug chart opposite and overleaf

LONGBURY HOSPITAL TRUST				HOSPITAL NUMBER SURNAME FIRST NAME ADDRESS			
				D.O.B			
DATE OF ADMISSION		ADMISSION WEIGHT (KG)				WARD	
ALLERGIES				CONSULTANT			
				CHART NO			...OF...

ONCE ONLY PRESCRIPTIONS

DATE	TIME	NAME OF DRUG	DOSE	ROUTE	PRESCRIBER'S SIGNATURE	GIVEN BY	TIME GIVEN

REGULAR MEDICATIONS

NAME OF DRUG		TIME	DATE → DOSE ↓					
ADDITIONAL INSTRUCTIONS		08:00						
DATE	ROUTE	12:00						
PRESCRIBER'S SIGNATURE								
		18:00						
PRESCRIBER'S NAME AND BLEEP		22:00						

NAME OF DRUG		TIME	DATE → DOSE ↓					
ADDITIONAL INSTRUCTIONS		08:00						
DATE	ROUTE	12:00						
PRESCRIBER'S SIGNATURE								
		18:00						
PRESCRIBER'S NAME AND BLEEP		22:00						

NAME OF DRUG		TIME	DATE → DOSE ↓					
ADDITIONAL INSTRUCTIONS		08:00						
DATE	ROUTE	12:00						
PRESCRIBER'S SIGNATURE								
		18:00						
PRESCRIBER'S NAME AND BLEEP		22:00						

PATIENT NAME   HOSPITAL NO.

NAME OF DRUG		TIME	DATE → DOSE ↓					
ADDITIONAL INSTRUCTIONS		08:00						
DATE	ROUTE	12:00						
PRESCRIBER'S SIGNATURE								
		18:00						
PRESCRIBER'S NAME AND BLEEP		22:00						

NAME OF DRUG		TIME	DATE → DOSE ↓					
ADDITIONAL INSTRUCTIONS		08:00						
DATE	ROUTE	12:00						
PRESCRIBER'S SIGNATURE								
		18:00						
PRESCRIBER'S NAME AND BLEEP		22:00						

NAME OF DRUG		TIME	DATE → DOSE ↓					
ADDITIONAL INSTRUCTIONS		08:00						
DATE	ROUTE	12:00						
PRESCRIBER'S SIGNATURE								
		18:00						
PRESCRIBER'S NAME AND BLEEP		22:00						

AS REQUIRED PRESCRIPTIONS

NAME OF DRUG		DATE					
INDICATION/ INSTRUCTION	DOSE	TIME					
FREQUENCY	ROUTE	DOSE					
PRESCRIBER'S SIGNATURE		ROUTE					
PRESCRIBER'S NAME AND BLEEP							
START DATE	STOP DATE	GIVEN BY					

PATIENT NAME   HOSPITAL NO.

NAME OF DRUG		DATE					
INDICATION/ INSTRUCTION	DOSE	TIME					
FREQUENCY	ROUTE	DOSE					
PRESCRIBER'S SIGNATURE		ROUTE					
PRESCRIBER'S NAME AND BLEEP		GIVEN BY					
START DATE	STOP DATE						

INTRAVENOUS FLUIDS

DATE	FLUID	ADDITIVE & DOSE	VOLUME	RATE/ DURATION	PRESCRIBER'S SIGNATURE	GIVEN BY	START TIME	END TIME

Record of signatures. ALL prescribers MUST complete.

DATE	NAME	DESIGNATION	SIGNATURE	BLEEP NUMBER

Answer 9

Prescribing for common medical emergencies is the mainstay of a junior doctor's work. In this case the patient's condition should be diagnosed correctly and the appropriate medication prescribed. It is worth being familiar with local and national guidance for common acute presentations, such as chest pain.

Step 3: Compare your answer to the checklist below and the chart opposite ☑

D Details	Checked patient details Used capital letters throughout Used correct abbreviations	☐
R Regular medications	Noted there were no regular medications Initiated secondary ACS prevention	☐
U Unpleasant reactions	Not required	☐
G Gravid?	No	☐

C Contra-indications	Noted no serious contraindications	☐
H Hydration	Not required for resuscitation at this stage. Acceptable to have prescribed maintenance fluid but be cautious as the patient may have undiagnosed LVF	☐
A Analgesia	Prescribed GTN spray. Regular analgesia prescribed according to the pain ladder. Avoided NSAIDs	☐
R Renal function	Not required	☐
T Thrombo-prophylaxis	Prescribed STAT fondaparinux	☐
S Signature box	Signed signature box	☐

Rationale

This patient has presented with cardiac chest pain, is clammy and has a raised troponin level. This is in keeping with acute coronary syndrome (ACS). The absence of ST segment elevation on the ECG means this should be managed medically. Although Mr Surpur's troponin was found to be raised on admission, a second sample should be taken 6–12 hours after the onset of his chest pain to establish the degree of myocardial damage. A 12-hour troponin level of 0.4–1.0 ng/mL is consistent with myocyte necrosis and a level above 1ng/mL would be consistent with non-ST elevation myocardial infarction. The management for both is similar.

Patients with ischaemic ECG changes should be given loading one-off doses of aspirin 300mg and clopidogrel 300mg, which are then continued at 75mg o.d. The combination reduces the risk of reinfarction more effectively than either alone. The additional protective effect of clopidogrel stops after 3 months, and it is often discontinued after 12 months. Remember to mention this on discharge letters so general practitioners know when to stop the medication.

Beta-blockers prolong diastole and improve coronary perfusion so are therefore useful antianginal drugs. There is also evidence that in acute coronary syndrome they reduce the risk of progression to infarction in the acute phase. Start with a low dose on admission, as has been done with bisoprolol here (2.5mg o.d.), and titrate upwards according to response.

Secondary prevention is an important consideration following an acute coronary event. Statin therapy is indicated long-term for patients who have had a myocardial infarction or have ischaemic heart disease, as it reduces the likelihood of further coronary events. Statins for secondary prevention are initiated at a dose of simvastatin 40mg (or equivalent); dosage or choice of statin can then be changed according to cholesterol levels. Ensure liver function tests are normal before initiating them.

Post-ACS, angiotensin-converting enzyme (ACE) inhibitors have mortality and morbidity benefits independent of their effect on lowering blood pressure. ACE inhibitors can provoke first-dose hypotension and are initiated at low dose (ramipril 1.25mg o.d. here) and increased thereafter. Check the urea and electrolyte results before prescribing.

In case this patient continues to experience ongoing chest pain, he should be prescribed a GTN spray and shown how to use it. If his chest pain continued he could be started on an intravenous infusion of GTN. Intravenous diamorphine can be used in conjuction with GTN, as it produces coronary artery dilatation and is an analgesic for cardiac chest pain. If the pain still persisted, consider starting an infusion of the glycoprotein IIb/IIIa inhibitor tirofiban or eptifibatide; this would normally take place in a coronary care unit. He may require coronary angiography. The prescriber has noted here that the fondaparinux should be reviewed the next day, to prevent it being given if this is the case.

Common hospital presentations such as ACS often have local prescribing protocols, which specify preferred local drug choices and doses.

KEY POINTS

- Use the once only box to initiate important stat medications
- Be familiar with both national and local guidance for acute medical conditions
- Don't forget secondary preventions in ACS, such as cholesterol and blood pressure control

LONGBURY HOSPITAL TRUST		HOSPITAL NUMBER	237621

LONGBURY HOSPITAL TRUST

HOSPITAL NUMBER 237621
SURNAME SURPUR
FIRST NAME BALJINDER
ADDRESS 77 CABARA ROAD, LONGBURY
LB3 4GJ

D.O.B 02/09/YYYY (64 YEARS AGO)

DATE OF ADMISSION	09/10/YYYY	ADMISSION WEIGHT (KG)	80kg	WARD	MEDICAL ASSESSMENT

ALLERGIES	CONSULTANT	ERIN JOHNSON
NKDA	CHART NO	1...OF...1

ONCE ONLY PRESCRIPTIONS

DATE	TIME	NAME OF DRUG	DOSE	ROUTE	PRESCRIBER'S SIGNATURE	GIVEN BY	TIME GIVEN
09/10	STAT	ASPIRIN	300mg	O	ALewis		
09/10	STAT	CLOPIDOGREL	300mg	O	ALewis		
09/10	STAT	GTN (SPRAY)	ii	S/L	ALewis		
09/10	STAT	FONDAPARINUX	2.5mg	S/C	ALewis		
09/10	STAT	DIAMORPHINE	1.25mg	IV	ALewis		

REGULAR MEDICATIONS

NAME OF DRUG ASPIRIN	TIME	DATE → DOSE ↓	09/10				
ADDITIONAL INSTRUCTIONS	08:00	75mg	———				
DATE 09/10 ROUTE PO	12:00						
PRESCRIBER'S SIGNATURE ALewis	18:00						
PRESCRIBER'S NAME AND BLEEP ALEX LEWIS 4567	22:00						

NAME OF DRUG CLOPIDOGREL	TIME	DATE → DOSE ↓	09/10				
ADDITIONAL INSTRUCTIONS	08:00	75mg	———				
DATE 09/10 ROUTE PO	12:00						
PRESCRIBER'S SIGNATURE ALewis	18:00						
PRESCRIBER'S NAME AND BLEEP ALEX LEWIS 4567	22:00						

NAME OF DRUG FONDAPARINUX	TIME	DATE → DOSE ↓	09/10				
ADDITIONAL INSTRUCTIONS	08:00						
DATE 09/10 ROUTE S/C	12:00			REVIEW			
PRESCRIBER'S SIGNATURE ALewis	18:00	2.5mg	——— [ ]				
PRESCRIBER'S NAME AND BLEEP ALEX LEWIS 4567	22:00						

PATIENT NAME *BALJINDER SURPUR*   HOSPITAL NO.   *237621*

NAME OF DRUG *RAMIPRIL*	TIME	DATE → DOSE ↓	09/10				
ADDITIONAL INSTRUCTIONS	08:00		1.25mg				
DATE 09/10 ROUTE PO	12:00						
PRESCRIBER'S SIGNATURE *ALewis*	18:00						
PRESCRIBER'S NAME AND BLEEP *ALEX LEWIS 4567*	22:00						

NAME OF DRUG *BISOPROLOL*	TIME	DATE → DOSE ↓	09/10				
ADDITIONAL INSTRUCTIONS	08:00		2.5mg				
DATE 09/10 ROUTE PO	12:00						
PRESCRIBER'S SIGNATURE *ALewis*	18:00						
PRESCRIBER'S NAME AND BLEEP *ALEX LEWIS 4567*	22:00						

NAME OF DRUG *SIMVASTATIN*	TIME	DATE → DOSE ↓	09/10				
ADDITIONAL INSTRUCTIONS	08:00						
DATE 09/10 ROUTE PO	12:00						
PRESCRIBER'S SIGNATURE *ALewis*	18:00						
PRESCRIBER'S NAME AND BLEEP *ALEX LEWIS 4567*	22:00	40mg					

AS REQUIRED PRESCRIPTIONS

NAME OF DRUG *GTN SPRAY*		DATE					
INDICATION/ INSTRUCTION *CHEST PAIN*	DOSE *ii*	TIME					
FREQUENCY *PRN*	ROUTE *S/L*	DOSE					
PRESCRIBER'S SIGNATURE *ALewis*		ROUTE					
PRESCRIBER'S NAME AND BLEEP *ALEX LEWIS 4567*		GIVEN BY					
START DATE *09/06*	STOP DATE						

PATIENT NAME _BALJINDER SURPUR_   HOSPITAL NO.   _237621_

NAME OF DRUG		DATE						
INDICATION/ INSTRUCTION	DOSE	TIME						
FREQUENCY	ROUTE	DOSE						
PRESCRIBER'S SIGNATURE		ROUTE						
PRESCRIBER'S NAME AND BLEEP		GIVEN BY						
START DATE	STOP DATE							

INTRAVENOUS FLUIDS

DATE	FLUID	ADDITIVE & DOSE	VOLUME	RATE/ DURATION	PRESCRIBER'S SIGNATURE	GIVEN BY	START TIME	END TIME

Record of signatures. ALL prescribers MUST complete.

DATE	NAME	DESIGNATION	SIGNATURE	BLEEP NUMBER
09/06	ALEX LEWIS	F1	ALewis	4567

Anil Chandrappa (hospital number: 152326, DOB 01/03/YYYY [75 years old], address: 67 Dallas Avenue, Longbury LB17 6LE) is being treated for community-acquired pneumonia. He also has longstanding atrial fibrillation. The nurse has reported he had a minor nose bleed earlier in the day. He has no known drug allergies.

Blood test results:
Haemoglobin 144g/L
White cell count 17.5 x 10^9/L
Sodium 134mmol/L
Potassium 4.3mmol/L
Urea 6.0mmol/L
C-reactive protein 108mg/L
International normalised ratio (INR) 8.2

Your task is to review the chart and alter the prescriptions appropriately.
It is 17:00 on 22nd June.

Notes

Step 1: Complete your answers in the drug chart opposite and overleaf

LONGBURY HOSPITAL TRUST

HOSPITAL NUMBER	152326
SURNAME	CHANDRAPPA
FIRST NAME	ANIL
ADDRESS	67 DALLAS AVENUE, LONGBURY LB17 6LE
D.O.B	01/03/YYYY (75 YEARS AGO)

DATE OF ADMISSION	18/06/YYYY	ADMISSION WEIGHT (KG)	73	WARD MEDICAL ASSESSMENT

ALLERGIES	
NONE	CONSULTANT ERIN JOHNSON
	CHART NO 1...OF...1

ONCE ONLY PRESCRIPTIONS

DATE	TIME	NAME OF DRUG	DOSE	ROUTE	PRESCRIBER'S SIGNATURE	GIVEN BY	TIME GIVEN

REGULAR MEDICATIONS

NAME OF DRUG CLARITHROMYCIN	TIME	DATE → DOSE ↓	19/06	20/06	21/06	22/06	23/06
ADDITIONAL INSTRUCTIONS PNEUMONIA	08:00	500mg	RC	MG	MG	TJ	
DATE 19/06 ROUTE PO	12:00						REVIEW
PRESCRIBER'S SIGNATURE BFord							23/06
	18:00						
PRESCRIBER'S NAME AND BLEEP BEN FORD 1569	22:00	500mg	SS	SS	RC		

NAME OF DRUG SIMVASTATIN	TIME	DATE → DOSE ↓	19/06	20/06	21/06	22/06	23/06
ADDITIONAL INSTRUCTIONS	08:00						
DATE 19/06 ROUTE PO	12:00						
PRESCRIBER'S SIGNATURE BFord							
	18:00						
PRESCRIBER'S NAME AND BLEEP BEN FORD 1569	22:00	20MG	—	—	—	—	
							REVIEW

NAME OF DRUG	TIME	DATE → DOSE ↓					
ADDITIONAL INSTRUCTIONS	08:00						
DATE ROUTE	12:00						
PRESCRIBER'S SIGNATURE							
	18:00						
PRESCRIBER'S NAME AND BLEEP	22:00						

PATIENT NAME ANIL CHANDRAPPA   HOSPITAL NO.   152326

NAME OF DRUG		TIME	DATE → DOSE ↓					
ADDITIONAL INSTRUCTIONS		08:00						
DATE	ROUTE	12:00						
PRESCRIBER'S SIGNATURE								
		18:00						
PRESCRIBER'S NAME AND BLEEP								
		22:00						

NAME OF DRUG		TIME	DATE → DOSE ↓					
ADDITIONAL INSTRUCTIONS		08:00						
DATE	ROUTE	12:00						
PRESCRIBER'S SIGNATURE								
		18:00						
PRESCRIBER'S NAME AND BLEEP								
		22:00						

NAME OF DRUG		TIME	DATE → DOSE ↓					
ADDITIONAL INSTRUCTIONS		08:00						
DATE	ROUTE	12:00						
PRESCRIBER'S SIGNATURE								
		18:00						
PRESCRIBER'S NAME AND BLEEP								
		22:00						

AS REQUIRED PRESCRIPTIONS

NAME OF DRUG PARACETAMOL		DATE	18/06	18/06			
INDICATION/ INSTRUCTION PAIN	DOSE 1g	TIME	1400	2000			
FREQUENCY QDS	ROUTE PO/PR	DOSE	1g	1g			
PRESCRIBER'S SIGNATURE BFord		ROUTE	PO	PO			
PRESCRIBER'S NAME AND BLEEP BEN FORD 1569		GIVEN BY	TJ	JC			
START DATE 18/06	STOP DATE						

PATIENT NAME ANIL CHANDRAPPA   HOSPITAL NO.   152326

NAME OF DRUG		DATE						
INDICATION/ INSTRUCTION	DOSE	TIME						
FREQUENCY	ROUTE	DOSE						
PRESCRIBER'S SIGNATURE		ROUTE						
PRESCRIBER'S NAME AND BLEEP		GIVEN BY						
START DATE	STOP DATE							

INTRAVENOUS FLUIDS

DATE	FLUID	ADDITIVE & DOSE	VOLUME	RATE/ DURATION	PRESCRIBER'S SIGNATURE	GIVEN BY	START TIME	END TIME
22/06	5% DEXTROSE	——————	1l	8°	NShah	TJ	0800	1600
22/06	N. SALINE	20mmol KCl	1l	8°	NShah	TJ	1600	

ANTICOAGULATION CHART

DATE	18/06	19/06	20/06	21/06	22/6	23/06	
INR	2.4	3.2			8.2		
WARFARIN DOSE	3mg	3mg	3mg	3mg	3mg	3mg	
PRESCRIBER'S SIGNATURE	BFord	BFord	BFord	BFord	BFord	BFord	
GIVEN BY	TJ	RC	MG	MG			
TIME	18.00	18.00	18.00	18.00			

Record of signatures. ALL prescribers MUST complete.

DATE	NAME	DESIGNATION	SIGNATURE	BLEEP NUMBER
18/06	BEN FORD	F2	BFord	1569
22/06	NAZIA SHAH	F2	NShah	9761

Step 2: Now check your work overleaf

Answer 10

The management of over-anticoagulation is a core skill for a junior doctor. Warfarin interacts with a wide range of commonly prescribed drugs, resulting in changes to the patient's INR, despite continuing a stable dose. In this case co-administration with clarithomycin has resulted in an increase in the effect of warfarin.

Step 3: Compare your answer to the checklist below and the chart opposite ✔

D	Details	Checked patient details Used capital letters throughout Used correct abbreviations	☐
R	Regular medications	Prescribed amoxicillin in place of clarithromycin	☐
U	Unpleasant reactions	Already documented	☐
G	Gravid?	No	☐

C	Contra-indications	Stopped warfarin: contraindicated as INR=8.2	☐
H	Hydration	Left unchanged or prescribed a continuation	☐
A	Analgesia	Not required	☐
R	Renal function	Not required	☐
T	Thrombo-prophylaxis	Not required	☐
S	Signature box	Signed signature box	☐

Rationale

Clarithromycin is a cytochrome P450 enzyme inhibitor that reduces the metabolism of warfarin and increases its effect. This patient's INR (international normalised ratio) has not been checked since admission and there has been no change in his warfarin dose. This, combined with the prescription of clarithromycin has led to his INR becoming dangerously high. The priority is to prevent the INR from deranging further, putting the patient at risk of haemorrhage. As he is not actively bleeding, he does not require emergency reversal of his warfarin. Partial reversal of the effect is desirable because he has atrial fibrillation and an INR <2.0 would put him at risk of strokes and arterial emboli.

Stopping warfarin for 2–3 days with daily checks of his INR is most likely to resolve the situation. Notice that R/V (review) has been written in the dose box after 24 hours, ensuring that the prescriber checks the patient's INR before restarting warfarin.

A small dose of oral vitamin K (e.g. 1mg) is also helpful here: it is unlikely to cause full reversal but would speed the return to target range. Giving too much vitamin K or giving it intravenously would make would make it difficult to obtain a therapeutic INR on restarting warfarin due to the long half-life of vitamin K. If vitamin K was given intravenously, it would be given slowly to prevent an anaphylactic reaction. A practical tip is to remember that vitamin K is known as phytomenadione, which can cause confusion when looking for it in the drug cupboard in a hurry.

The prescriber has replaced clarithromycin with amoxicillin, which is less likely to increase the effect of warfarin. It is not ideal to switch antibiotics mid-course, and often clarithromycin would be continued and the deranged INR managed concurrently. It is important to stop drugs that are doing more harm than good, until you can get senior help.

The patient's simvastatin was on hold and would be restarted only after senior review. This is because coadministration of statins with macrolide antibiotics (e.g. clarithromycin) carries an increased risk of myopathy. The statin can now be restarted as the macrolide has been changed to penicillin.

KEY POINTS

- Warfarin has many interactions so always monitor INR closely when introducing new drugs
- Be aware of how to reverse a high INR safely; use the formulary
- Stop or replace drugs that are doing more harm than good

		LONGBURY HOSPITAL TRUST			

HOSPITAL NUMBER	152326
SURNAME	CHANDRAPPA
FIRST NAME	ANIL
ADDRESS	67 DALLAS AVENUE, LONGBURY LB17 6LE
D.O.B	01/03/YYYY (75 YEARS AGO)

DATE OF ADMISSION	18/06/YYYY	ADMISSION WEIGHT (KG)	73	WARD	MEDICAL ASSESSMENT

ALLERGIES	CONSULTANT	ERIN JOHNSON
NONE	CHART NO	1...OF...1

ONCE ONLY PRESCRIPTIONS

DATE	TIME	NAME OF DRUG	DOSE	ROUTE	PRESCRIBER'S SIGNATURE	GIVEN BY	TIME GIVEN
22/06	STAT	VITAMIN K	1mg	PO	ALewis		

REGULAR MEDICATIONS

NAME OF DRUG CLARITHROMYCIN	TIME	DATE → DOSE ↓	19/06	20/06	21/06	22/06	23/06
ADDITIONAL INSTRUCTIONS PNEUMONIA	08:00	500 mg	RC	MG	MG	TJ	————
DATE 19/06 ROUTE PO	12:00						REVIEW
PRESCRIBER'S SIGNATURE BFord							23/06
	18:00						STOP
PRESCRIBER'S NAME AND BLEEP BEN FORD 1569						————	ALewis
	22:00	500 MG	SS	SS	RC	————	————
						————	22/06

NAME OF DRUG SIMVASTATIN	TIME	DATE → DOSE ↓	19/06	20/06	21/06	22/06	23/06
ADDITIONAL INSTRUCTIONS	08:00						
DATE 19/06 ROUTE PO	12:00						
PRESCRIBER'S SIGNATURE BFord	18:00						
PRESCRIBER'S NAME AND BLEEP BEN FORD 1569	22:00	20mg	————	————	————	————	
							REVIEW

NAME OF DRUG AMOXICILLIN	TIME	DATE → DOSE ↓			22/06	23/06	24/06
ADDITIONAL INSTRUCTIONS PNEUMONIA REVIEW 26/06	08:00	500mg			X		
DATE 22/06 ROUTE PO	12:00	500mg			X		
PRESCRIBER'S SIGNATURE ALewis	18:00						
PRESCRIBER'S NAME AND BLEEP ALEX LEWIS 4567	22:00	500mg					

PATIENT NAME ANIL CHANDRAPPA   HOSPITAL NO. 152326

NAME OF DRUG		TIME	DATE → DOSE ↓					
ADDITIONAL INSTRUCTIONS		08:00						
DATE	ROUTE	12:00						
PRESCRIBER'S SIGNATURE		18:00						
PRESCRIBER'S NAME AND BLEEP		22:00						

NAME OF DRUG		TIME	DATE → DOSE ↓					
ADDITIONAL INSTRUCTIONS		08:00						
DATE	ROUTE	12:00						
PRESCRIBER'S SIGNATURE		18:00						
PRESCRIBER'S NAME AND BLEEP		22:00						

NAME OF DRUG		TIME	DATE → DOSE ↓					
ADDITIONAL INSTRUCTIONS		08:00						
DATE	ROUTE	12:00						
PRESCRIBER'S SIGNATURE		18:00						
PRESCRIBER'S NAME AND BLEEP		22:00						

AS REQUIRED PRESCRIPTIONS

NAME OF DRUG PARACETAMOL		DATE	18/06	18/06			
INDICATION/ INSTRUCTION PAIN	DOSE 1g	TIME	1400	2000			
FREQUENCY QDS	ROUTE PO/PR	DOSE	1g	1g			
PRESCRIBER'S SIGNATURE BFord		ROUTE	PO	PO			
PRESCRIBER'S NAME AND BLEEP BEN FORD 1569		GIVEN BY	TJ	JC			
START DATE 18/06	STOP DATE						

PATIENT NAME ANIL CHANDRAPPA   HOSPITAL NO.   152326

NAME OF DRUG		DATE					
INDICATION/ INSTRUCTION	DOSE	TIME					
FREQUENCY	ROUTE	DOSE					
PRESCRIBER'S SIGNATURE		ROUTE					
PRESCRIBER'S NAME AND BLEEP		GIVEN BY					
START DATE	STOP DATE						

INTRAVENOUS FLUIDS

DATE	FLUID	ADDITIVE & DOSE	VOLUME	RATE/ DURATION	PRESCRIBER'S SIGNATURE	GIVEN BY	START TIME	END TIME
22/06	5% DEXTROSE	————	1l	8°	NShah	TJ	0800	1600
22/06	N. SALINE	20mmol KCl	1l	8°	NShah	TJ	1600	

ANTICOAGULATION CHART

DATE	18/06	19/06	20/06	21/06	22/6	23/06	24/06	
INR	2.4	3.2			8.2			
WARFARIN DOSE	3mg	3mg	3mg	3mg	3mg	3mg	R/V INR	
PRESCRIBER'S SIGNATURE	BFord	BFord	BFord	BFord	BFord	BFord		
GIVEN BY	TJ	RC	MG	MG	——	——	ALewis	
TIME	18:00	18:00	18:00	18:00				

Record of signatures. ALL prescribers MUST complete.

DATE	NAME	DESIGNATION	SIGNATURE	BLEEP NUMBER
18/06	BEN FORD	F2	BFord	1569
22/06	NAZIA SHAH	F2	NShah	9761
22/06	ALEX LEWIS	F1	ALewis	4567

Gareth Collins (hospital number: 141882, DOB 14/05/YYYY [79 years old], address: 9 Eastway Drive, Longbury LB15 7HM) has developed severe nausea and vomiting secondary to viral gastroenteritis. Ten years ago he had a prosthetic aortic valve replacement. The vomiting is preventing him from eating or taking any medication; clinically he appears dehydrated with dry mucous membranes. His urine output is 20mL/h. He weighs 90kg.

Blood test results:
Haemoglobin 115g/L
Mean cell volume 93fL
White blood cells 15.4 $\times10^9$/L
Neutrophils 8.6 $\times10^9$/L
Platelets 260 $\times10^9$/L
International normalised ratio 1.3
Sodium 141mmol/L
Potassium 3.1mmol/L
Urea 18.0mmol/L
Creatinine 190μmol/L
eGFR 36mL/min/1.73m^2

Observations:
Blood pressure 98/65mmHg
Respiratory rate 26 breaths/minute
SpO_2 98% on air
Pulse 94bpm, regular
Apyrexial

Your task is to prescribe treatment you consider necessary.
It is 07:30 on 23rd June.

Notes

LONGBURY HOSPITAL TRUST				HOSPITAL NUMBER	141882		
				SURNAME	COLLINS		
				FIRST NAME	GARETH		
				ADDRESS	9 EASTWAY DRIVE, LONGBURY LB15 7HM		
				D.O.B	14/05/YYYY (79 YEARS AGO)		
DATE OF ADMISSION	22/06/YYYY	ADMISSION WEIGHT (KG)		90kg	WARD	MEDICAL ASSESSMENT	
ALLERGIES				CONSULTANT		ERIN JOHNSON	
NKDA				CHART NO		1…OF…1	

ONCE ONLY PRESCRIPTIONS

DATE	TIME	NAME OF DRUG	DOSE	ROUTE	PRESCRIBER'S SIGNATURE	GIVEN BY	TIME GIVEN

REGULAR MEDICATIONS

NAME OF DRUG	TIME	DATE → DOSE ↓	23/06				
FUROSEMIDE							
ADDITIONAL INSTRUCTIONS	08:00	40mg					
DATE 23/06 ROUTE PO	12:00						
PRESCRIBER'S SIGNATURE MHughes	18:00						
PRESCRIBER'S NAME AND BLEEP MICHELLE HUGHES 2357	22:00						

NAME OF DRUG	TIME	DATE → DOSE ↓	23/06				
RAMIPRIL							
ADDITIONAL INSTRUCTIONS	08:00	2.5mg					
DATE 23/06 ROUTE PO	12:00						
PRESCRIBER'S SIGNATURE MHughes	18:00						
PRESCRIBER'S NAME AND BLEEP MICHELLE HUGHES 2357	22:00						

NAME OF DRUG	TIME	DATE → DOSE ↓	23/06				
AMLODIPINE							
ADDITIONAL INSTRUCTIONS	08:00	5mg					
DATE 23/06 ROUTE PO	12:00						
PRESCRIBER'S SIGNATURE MHughes	18:00						
PRESCRIBER'S NAME AND BLEEP MICHELLE HUGHES 2357	22:00						

PATIENT NAME GARETH COLLINS   HOSPITAL NO.   141882

NAME OF DRUG		TIME	DATE → DOSE ↓					
ADDITIONAL INSTRUCTIONS		08:00						
DATE	ROUTE	12:00						
PRESCRIBER'S SIGNATURE								
		18:00						
PRESCRIBER'S NAME AND BLEEP								
		22:00						

NAME OF DRUG		TIME	DATE → DOSE ↓					
ADDITIONAL INSTRUCTIONS		08:00						
DATE	ROUTE	12:00						
PRESCRIBER'S SIGNATURE								
		18:00						
PRESCRIBER'S NAME AND BLEEP								
		22:00						

NAME OF DRUG		TIME	DATE → DOSE ↓					
ADDITIONAL INSTRUCTIONS		08:00						
DATE	ROUTE	12:00						
PRESCRIBER'S SIGNATURE								
		18:00						
PRESCRIBER'S NAME AND BLEEP								
		22:00						

AS REQUIRED PRESCRIPTIONS

NAME OF DRUG							
		DATE					
INDICATION/ INSTRUCTION	DOSE	TIME					
FREQUENCY	ROUTE	DOSE					
PRESCRIBER'S SIGNATURE		ROUTE					
PRESCRIBER'S NAME AND BLEEP							
START DATE	STOP DATE	GIVEN BY					

PATIENT NAME GARETH COLLINS   HOSPITAL NO.   141882

NAME OF DRUG		DATE						
INDICATION/ INSTRUCTION	DOSE	TIME						
FREQUENCY	ROUTE	DOSE						
PRESCRIBER'S SIGNATURE		ROUTE						
PRESCRIBER'S NAME AND BLEEP		GIVEN BY						
START DATE	STOP DATE							

INTRAVENOUS FLUIDS

DATE	FLUID	ADDITIVE & DOSE	VOLUME	RATE/ DURATION	PRESCRIBER'S SIGNATURE	GIVEN BY	START TIME	END TIME

ANTICOAGULATION CHART

DATE	22/06	23/06		
INR	1.3			
WARFARIN DOSE	3mg			
PRESCRIBER'S SIGNATURE	MHughes			
GIVEN BY	BN			
TIME	1800			

Record of signatures. ALL prescribers MUST complete.

DATE	NAME	DESIGNATION	SIGNATURE	BLEEP NUMBER
22/06	MICHELLE HUGHES	F2	MHughes	2357

Step 2: Now check your work overleaf

This patient's vomiting is leading to an inability to take his oral medication. Combined with diarrhoea it has also made him become dehydrated and he is at risk of sustaining further acute kidney injury.

This exercise is about treating the patient's condition and reviewing his medication in light of the altered physiology. It is important to ensure the patient's medications have not become harmful and that alternative routes are found for the oral medications that still need to be given.

Step 3: Compare your answer to the checklist below and the chart opposite ☑

D Details	Checked patient details Used capital letters throughout Used correct abbreviations	☐
R Regular medications	Stopped furosemide, ramipril and calcium channel blocker Replaced warfarin with suitable alternative Prescribed an antiemetic	☐
U Unpleasant reactions	None	☐
G Gravid?	No	☐

C Contra-indications	Withheld ACE inhibitors with plan to review once stable	☐
H Hydration	Prescribed fluid challenge: 250mL Hartmann's	☐
A Analgesia	Prescribed IV/PO paracetamol	☐
R Renal function	Moderate AKI likely	☐
T Thrombo-prophylaxis	Changed warfarin to therapeutic enoxaparin Ensure weight is recorded	☐
S Signature box	Signed signature box	☐

Rationale

The patient's INR has become subtherapeutic, which is likely to be due to the vomiting preventing effective absorption of warfarin. He is at risk of suffering a thrombotic event involving his prosthetic heart valve so an alternative route of anticoagulation is required. A frequently used option is 'bridging' therapy, with low molecular weight heparin (LMWH) given at treatment dose. Once the vomiting settles and the patient is able to resume oral medication, the warfarin can be restarted with loading doses and the LMWH only stopped when the INR is back in the correct range. Dosing for therapeutic LMWH is weight-based (in this exercise 1.5mg/kg enoxaparin daily) and is dictated by local hospital policy.

The other oral medications are all antihypertensives. Given this patient's dehydration and acute kidney injury (AKI), it would be prudent to withhold these. They haven't been crossed off indefinitely: writing REVIEW (or R/V) means that they can be restarted when appropriate. It is especially important to withhold angiotensin-converting enzyme (ACE) inhibitors in AKI as they prevent efferent glomerular arteriolar vasoconstriction. The decision to re-start ACE inhibitors requires specialist advice.

It is appropriate to offer this patient an antiemetic; in this case intramuscular/intravenous cyclizine has been prescribed. Intravenous antiemetics such as ondansetron may be used, but if there is only one cannula the priority is fluid. Oral antiemetics are inappropriate given this patient's diarrhoea. Metoclopramide could be used but it has prokinetic properties which could exacerbate this patient's diarrhoea.

A further issue here is the need to correct the patient's fluid loss and electrolyte disturbance. A fluid challenge of 250mL Hartmann's has been prescribed, the volume reflecting the patient's known cardiac problem, and the nature of the fluid lost and the electrolytes that need replacing. Further fluids would be required following the fluid challenge, guided by observations, electrolytes and urine output.

KEY POINTS

- Stop nephrotoxic drugs in AKI
- Patients on warfarin who cannot swallow need bridging anticoagulation with LMWH
- In known cardiac diseases it is safer to give small fluid challenges, review the effect and prescribe further fluid accordingly

LONGBURY HOSPITAL TRUST

HOSPITAL NUMBER	141882
SURNAME	COLLINS
FIRST NAME	GARETH
ADDRESS	9 EASTWAY DRIVE, LONGBURY LB15 7HM
D.O.B	14/05/YYYY (79 YEARS AGO)

DATE OF ADMISSION	22/06/YYYY	ADMISSION WEIGHT (KG)	90kg	WARD	MEDICAL ASSESSMENT

ALLERGIES		CONSULTANT	ERIN JOHNSON
NKDA		CHART NO	1...OF...1

ONCE ONLY PRESCRIPTIONS

DATE	TIME	NAME OF DRUG	DOSE	ROUTE	PRESCRIBER'S SIGNATURE	GIVEN BY	TIME GIVEN

REGULAR MEDICATIONS

NAME OF DRUG FUROSEMIDE	TIME	DATE → DOSE ↓	23/06	24/06			
ADDITIONAL INSTRUCTIONS	08:00	40mg	X				
DATE 23/06 ROUTE PO	12:00			REVIEW			
PRESCRIBER'S SIGNATURE MHughes				ALewis			
	18:00						
PRESCRIBER'S NAME AND BLEEP MICHELLE HUGHES 2357	22:00						

NAME OF DRUG RAMIPRIL	TIME	DATE → DOSE ↓	23/06	24/06			
ADDITIONAL INSTRUCTIONS	08:00	2.5mg	X				
DATE 23/06 ROUTE PO	12:00			REVIEW			
PRESCRIBER'S SIGNATURE MHughes				ALewis			
	18:00						
PRESCRIBER'S NAME AND BLEEP MICHELLE HUGHES 2357	22:00						

NAME OF DRUG AMLODIPINE	TIME	DATE → DOSE ↓	23/06	24/06			
ADDITIONAL INSTRUCTIONS	08:00	5mg	X				
DATE 23/06 ROUTE PO	12:00			REVIEW			
PRESCRIBER'S SIGNATURE MHughes				ALewis			
	18:00						
PRESCRIBER'S NAME AND BLEEP MICHELLE HUGHES 2357	22:00						

PATIENT NAME GARETH COLLINS   HOSPITAL NO. 141882

NAME OF DRUG ENOXAPARIN		TIME	DATE → DOSE ↓	23/06				
ADDITIONAL INSTRUCTIONS		08:00						
DATE 23/06	ROUTE SC	12:00						
PRESCRIBER'S SIGNATURE ALewis		18:00	135mg					
PRESCRIBER'S NAME AND BLEEP ALEX LEWIS 4567		22:00						

NAME OF DRUG		TIME	DATE → DOSE ↓					
ADDITIONAL INSTRUCTIONS		08:00						
DATE	ROUTE	12:00						
PRESCRIBER'S SIGNATURE		18:00						
PRESCRIBER'S NAME AND BLEEP		22:00						

NAME OF DRUG		TIME	DATE → DOSE ↓					
ADDITIONAL INSTRUCTIONS		08:00						
DATE	ROUTE	12:00						
PRESCRIBER'S SIGNATURE		18:00						
PRESCRIBER'S NAME AND BLEEP		22:00						

AS REQUIRED PRESCRIPTIONS

NAME OF DRUG CYCLIZINE		DATE					
INDICATION/ INSTRUCTION NAUSEA	DOSE 50mg	TIME					
FREQUENCY TDS	ROUTE IM/PO/IV	DOSE					
PRESCRIBER'S SIGNATURE ALewis		ROUTE					
PRESCRIBER'S NAME AND BLEEP ALEX LEWIS 4567		GIVEN BY					
START DATE 23/06	STOP DATE						

PATIENT NAME GARETH COLLINS   HOSPITAL NO.   141882

NAME OF DRUG PARACETAMOL		DATE						
INDICATION/ INSTRUCTION PAIN	DOSE 1g	TIME						
FREQUENCY QDS	ROUTE PO/IV	DOSE						
PRESCRIBER'S SIGNATURE ALewis		ROUTE						
PRESCRIBER'S NAME AND BLEEP ALEX LEWIS 4567		GIVEN BY						
START DATE 23/06	STOP DATE							

INTRAVENOUS FLUIDS

DATE	FLUID	ADDITIVE & DOSE	VOLUME	RATE/ DURATION	PRESCRIBER'S SIGNATURE	GIVEN BY	START TIME	END TIME
23/06	HARTMANN'S	——————	250ml	STAT	ALewis			

ANTICOAGULATION CHART

DATE	22/06	23/06			
INR	1.3		STOP		
WARFARIN DOSE	3mg		ALewis		
PRESCRIBER'S SIGNATURE	MHughes		23/06		
GIVEN BY	BN				
TIME	1800				

Record of signatures. ALL prescribers MUST complete.

DATE	NAME	DESIGNATION	SIGNATURE	BLEEP NUMBER
22/06	MICHELLE HUGHES	F2	MHughes	2357
23/06	ALEX LEWIS	F1	ALewis	4567

Veronica Young (hospital number: 719283, DOB 21/07/YYYY [26 years ago], address: 25 Falcare Street, Longbury LB1 8BB) a 26-year-old woman was admitted earlier today for intravenous antibiotics to treat cellulitis affecting her elbow. The nurses have become worried as they have noticed a rash spreading across her chest. She is now struggling to breathe, her tongue is visibly swollen and she has widespread urticaria.

On chest examination Miss Young is found to have widespread wheeze. It has been concluded that she is having an anaphylactic reaction and a call has been made for help.

Observations:
Heart rate 120bpm
Blood pressure 70/50mmHg
Respiratory rate 32 breaths/minute
SaO_2 90% on 15L/min O_2

Your task is to prescribe appropriate immediate treatment (prior to help arriving), and make any necessary changes to the current treatment. She is already receiving oxygen therapy.
It is 08:30 on 7th September.

Notes

Step 1: Complete your answers in the drug chart opposite and overleaf

LONGBURY HOSPITAL TRUST

HOSPITAL NUMBER	719283
SURNAME	YOUNG
FIRST NAME	VERONICA
ADDRESS	25 FALCARE STREET, LONGBURY LB1 8BB
D.O.B	21/07/YYYY (26 YEARS AGO)

DATE OF ADMISSION	07/09/YYYY	ADMISSION WEIGHT (KG)	57kg	WARD	EMERGENCY
ALLERGIES			CONSULTANT		PRADIP CHAND
NKDA			CHART NO		1...OF...1

ONCE ONLY PRESCRIPTIONS

DATE	TIME	NAME OF DRUG	DOSE	ROUTE	PRESCRIBER'S SIGNATURE	GIVEN BY	TIME GIVEN

REGULAR MEDICATIONS

NAME OF DRUG BENZYLPENICILLIN	TIME	DATE → DOSE ↓	07/09				11/09
							REVIEW
ADDITIONAL INSTRUCTIONS CELLULITIS	08:00	1.2g	ZB				
DATE 07/09 ROUTE IV	12:00	1.2g					
PRESCRIBER'S SIGNATURE EJones	18:00	1.2g					
PRESCRIBER'S NAME AND BLEEP EMMA JONES 4876	22:00	1.2g					

NAME OF DRUG FLUCLOXACILLIN	TIME	DATE → DOSE ↓	07/09				11/09
							REVIEW
ADDITIONAL INSTRUCTIONS CELLULITIS	08:00	2g	ZB				
DATE 07/09 ROUTE IV	12:00	2g					
PRESCRIBER'S SIGNATURE EJones	18:00	2g					
PRESCRIBER'S NAME AND BLEEP EMMA JONES 4876	22:00	2g					

NAME OF DRUG	TIME	DATE → DOSE ↓					
ADDITIONAL INSTRUCTIONS	08:00						
DATE ROUTE	12:00						
PRESCRIBER'S SIGNATURE	18:00						
PRESCRIBER'S NAME AND BLEEP	22:00						

PATIENT NAME VERONICA YOUNG   HOSPITAL NO.   719283

NAME OF DRUG		TIME	DATE → DOSE ↓					
ADDITIONAL INSTRUCTIONS		08:00						
DATE	ROUTE	12:00						
PRESCRIBER'S SIGNATURE		18:00						
PRESCRIBER'S NAME AND BLEEP		22:00						

NAME OF DRUG		TIME	DATE → DOSE ↓					
ADDITIONAL INSTRUCTIONS		08:00						
DATE	ROUTE	12:00						
PRESCRIBER'S SIGNATURE		18:00						
PRESCRIBER'S NAME AND BLEEP		22:00						

NAME OF DRUG		TIME	DATE → DOSE ↓					
ADDITIONAL INSTRUCTIONS		08:00						
DATE	ROUTE	12:00						
PRESCRIBER'S SIGNATURE		18:00						
PRESCRIBER'S NAME AND BLEEP		22:00						

AS REQUIRED PRESCRIPTIONS

NAME OF DRUG		DATE					
INDICATION/ INSTRUCTION	DOSE	TIME					
FREQUENCY	ROUTE	DOSE					
PRESCRIBER'S SIGNATURE		ROUTE					
PRESCRIBER'S NAME AND BLEEP							
START DATE	STOP DATE	GIVEN BY					

PATIENT NAME VERONICA YOUNG   HOSPITAL NO.   719283

NAME OF DRUG		DATE					
INDICATION/ INSTRUCTION	DOSE	TIME					
FREQUENCY	ROUTE	DOSE					
PRESCRIBER'S SIGNATURE		ROUTE					
PRESCRIBER'S NAME AND BLEEP		GIVEN BY					
START DATE	STOP DATE						

INTRAVENOUS FLUIDS

DATE	FLUID	ADDITIVE & DOSE	VOLUME	RATE/ DURATION	PRESCRIBER'S SIGNATURE	GIVEN BY	START TIME	END TIME

Record of signatures. ALL prescribers MUST complete.

DATE	NAME	DESIGNATION	SIGNATURE	BLEEP NUMBER
07/09	EMMA JONES	SpR	EJones	4876

Answer 12

This patient is having an anaphylactic reaction, which is likely to be due to an undiagnosed penicillin allergy. Immediate action is required to prevent death or lasting complications. Intramuscular adrenaline must be given as soon as anaphylaxis is suspected.

Step 3: Compare your answer to the checklist below and the chart opposite ☑

D Details	Checked patient details. Used capital letters throughout. Used correct abbreviations	☐
R Regular medications	Prescribed: adrenaline, chlorphenamine, hydrocortisone, salbutamol, fluids	☐
U Unpleasant reactions	Updated allergy box to: penicillin, anaphylaxis. Stopped benzylpenicillin and flucloxacillin	☐
G Gravid?	No	☐

C Contra-indications	None	☐
H Hydration	Prescribed fluid challenge such as Hartmann's or sodium chloride 0.9%	☐
A Analgesia	Not required	☐
R Renal function	Aggressive fluid resuscitation will offset renal injury	☐
T Thrombo-prophylaxis	Not required	☐
S Signature box	Sign signature box	☐

Rationale

Anaphylaxis is a life-threatening emergency and calling for help is essential. Prescribing intramuscular adrenaline is life-saving and should not be delayed. Aside from reversing peripheral vasodilatation and reducing oedema it causes an increase in cardiac contractility and dilates the airway. Adrenaline also has antihistamine and antileukotriene properties, making it a potent tool in combating hypersensitivity reactions. The intramuscular dose is 0.5mL of 1:1000, which can be repeated at 5-minute intervals.

The anaphylactic reaction causes both laryngeal oedema and bronchospasm. Nebulised salbutamol helps to reverse the bronchospasm. Intravenous chlorphenamine (Piriton) and hydrocortisone both prevent relapse of the attack once the effect of the short-acting adrenergic compound has worn off. Hydrocortisone needs to be injected by slow intravenous or intramuscular administration, and care must be taken to avoid inducing further hypotension.

This patient is hypotensive due to vasodilatation and loss of fluid into the extravascular space. A fluid challenge of 500mL Hartmann's has been prescribed to maintain tissue perfusion. This should be repeated as necessary in order to maintain a safe blood pressure. It would also be appropriate to prescribe fluid resuscitation with sodium chloride 0.9%. The 100% oxygen should be continued for as long as the patient is unstable.

Penicillin allergies are common, but not everyone with an allergy will experience anaphylaxis. The offending agents, benzylpenicillin and flucloxacillin, have been stopped on the chart, to prevent the drugs unwittingly being given later. The allergies section of the drug chart has been updated to include penicillin. It also states that the reaction was anaphylactic and not just a simple rash. Ideally, continuing management of this patient will include taking samples to check for mast cell tryptase and a referral to an allergy specialist to confirm the anaphylaxis. Alternative antibiotics will need to be prescribed once the patient recovers from her anaphylaxis.

KEY POINTS

- If anaphylaxis is suspected, call for help and then initiate treatment
- You should know the emergency treatment regimens for anaphylaxis
- If a hypersensitivity reaction is discovered, cross the offending drug off, update the allergies box and detail the nature of the reaction

LONGBURY HOSPITAL TRUST				HOSPITAL NUMBER	719283
				SURNAME	YOUNG
				FIRST NAME	VERONICA
				ADDRESS	25 FALCARE STREET, LONGBURY LB1 8BB
				D.O.B	21/07/YYYY (26 YEARS AGO)

DATE OF ADMISSION	07/09/YYYY	ADMISSION WEIGHT (KG)		57kg	WARD	EMERGENCY
	ALLERGIES ~~NKDA~~	PENICILLIN - ANAPHYLAXIS		CONSULTANT		PRADIP CHAND
				CHART NO		1...OF...1

ONCE ONLY PRESCRIPTIONS

DATE	TIME	NAME OF DRUG	DOSE	ROUTE	PRESCRIBER'S SIGNATURE	GIVEN BY	TIME GIVEN
07/09	STAT	ADRENALINE 1:1000	0.5ml	IM	ALewis		
07/09	STAT	CHLORPHENAMINE	10mg	IV	ALewis		
07/09	STAT	HYDROCORTISONE	200mg	IV	ALewis		
07/09	STAT	SALBUTAMOL	5mg	NEB	ALewis		

REGULAR MEDICATIONS

NAME OF DRUG BENZYLPENICILLIN	TIME	DATE → DOSE ↓	07/09				11/09
							REVIEW
ADDITIONAL INSTRUCTIONS CELLULITIS	08:00	1.2g	ZB				
DATE 07/09 ROUTE IV	12:00	1.2g					
PRESCRIBER'S SIGNATURE EJones	18:00	1.2g				STOP ALewis 07/09	
PRESCRIBER'S NAME AND BLEEP EMMA JONES 4876	22:00	1.2g					

NAME OF DRUG FLUCLOXACILLIN	TIME	DATE → DOSE ↓	07/09				11/09
							REVIEW
ADDITIONAL INSTRUCTIONS CELLULITIS	08:00	2g	ZB				
DATE 07/09 ROUTE IV	12:00	2g					
PRESCRIBER'S SIGNATURE EJones	18:00	2g				STOP ALewis 07/09	
PRESCRIBER'S NAME AND BLEEP EMMA JONES 4876	22:00	2g					

NAME OF DRUG	TIME	DATE → DOSE ↓					
ADDITIONAL INSTRUCTIONS	08:00						
DATE ROUTE	14:00						
PRESCRIBER'S SIGNATURE	18:00						
PRESCRIBER'S NAME AND BLEEP	22:00						

PATIENT NAME VERONICA YOUNG   HOSPITAL NO. 719283

NAME OF DRUG	TIME	DATE → DOSE ↓					
ADDITIONAL INSTRUCTIONS	08:00						
DATE ROUTE	12:00						
PRESCRIBER'S SIGNATURE							
	18:00						
PRESCRIBER'S NAME AND BLEEP							
	22:00						

NAME OF DRUG	TIME	DATE → DOSE ↓					
ADDITIONAL INSTRUCTIONS	08:00						
DATE ROUTE	12:00						
PRESCRIBER'S SIGNATURE							
	18:00						
PRESCRIBER'S NAME AND BLEEP							
	22:00						

NAME OF DRUG	TIME	DATE → DOSE ↓					
ADDITIONAL INSTRUCTIONS	08:00						
DATE ROUTE	12:00						
PRESCRIBER'S SIGNATURE							
	18:00						
PRESCRIBER'S NAME AND BLEEP							
	22:00						

AS REQUIRED PRESCRIPTIONS

NAME OF DRUG		DATE					
INDICATION/ INSTRUCTION	DOSE	TIME					
FREQUENCY	ROUTE	DOSE					
PRESCRIBER'S SIGNATURE		ROUTE					
PRESCRIBER'S NAME AND BLEEP		GIVEN BY					
START DATE	STOP DATE						

PATIENT NAME VERONICA YOUNG   HOSPITAL NO.   719283

NAME OF DRUG		DATE					
INDICATION/ INSTRUCTION	DOSE	TIME					
FREQUENCY	ROUTE	DOSE					
PRESCRIBER'S SIGNATURE		ROUTE					
PRESCRIBER'S NAME AND BLEEP		GIVEN BY					
START DATE	STOP DATE						

INTRAVENOUS FLUIDS

DATE	FLUID	ADDITIVE & DOSE	VOLUME	RATE/ DURATION	PRESCRIBER'S SIGNATURE	GIVEN BY	START TIME	END TIME
07/09	HARTMANN'S		500ml	STAT	ALewis			

Record of signatures. ALL prescribers MUST complete.

DATE	NAME	DESIGNATION	SIGNATURE	BLEEP NUMBER
07/09	EMMA JONES	SpR	EJones	4876
07/09	ALEX LEWIS	F1	ALewis	4567

Robert Branch (hospital number: 197443, DOB 13/04/YYYY [65 years old], address: 14 Globe Avenue, Calder LB12 1DM) has been admitted to the medical assessment ward. He reports a 3-day history of increasing shortness of breath accompanied by a non productive cough. He is known to have chronic obstructive pulmonary disease (COPD), which is well controlled. He has no allergies. He has a history of hypertension and gout. Mr Branch's consultant is Dr Erin Johnson. His weight is 65kg.

Observations:
Heart rate 95bpm
Blood pressure 145/85mmHg
Respiratory rate 32 breaths/minute
SpO_2 90% on air

The current medication is as follows:
Salbutamol inhaler 200 micrograms as required
Tiotropium Handihaler 18 micrograms in the morning
Seretide Accuhaler 500 one dose twice daily
Bendroflumethiazide 2.5mg in the morning
Allopurinol 100mg daily

On chest examination there is a widespread expiratory wheeze with a few scattered crepitations but no focal signs. A chest X-ray shows hyperexpanded lungs with no consolidation.

As the admitting doctor your task is to write out the chart, including any new treatment you feel is necessary.
It is 07:30 on 22nd June.

Notes

LONGBURY HOSPITAL TRUST	HOSPITAL NUMBER SURNAME FIRST NAME ADDRESS D.O.B		
DATE OF ADMISSION	ADMISSION WEIGHT (KG)	WARD	
ALLERGIES	CONSULTANT		
	CHART NO	…OF…	

ONCE ONLY PRESCRIPTIONS

DATE	TIME	NAME OF DRUG	DOSE	ROUTE	PRESCRIBER'S SIGNATURE	GIVEN BY	TIME GIVEN

REGULAR MEDICATIONS

NAME OF DRUG	TIME	DATE → DOSE ↓				
ADDITIONAL INSTRUCTIONS	08:00					
DATE / ROUTE	12:00					
PRESCRIBER'S SIGNATURE						
	18:00					
PRESCRIBER'S NAME AND BLEEP	22:00					

NAME OF DRUG	TIME	DATE → DOSE ↓				
ADDITIONAL INSTRUCTIONS	08:00					
DATE / ROUTE	12:00					
PRESCRIBER'S SIGNATURE						
	18:00					
PRESCRIBER'S NAME AND BLEEP	22:00					

NAME OF DRUG	TIME	DATE → DOSE ↓				
ADDITIONAL INSTRUCTIONS	08:00					
DATE / ROUTE	12:00					
PRESCRIBER'S SIGNATURE						
	18:00					
PRESCRIBER'S NAME AND BLEEP	22:00					

PATIENT NAME

HOSPITAL NO.

NAME OF DRUG		TIME	DATE → DOSE ↓					
ADDITIONAL INSTRUCTIONS		08:00						
DATE	ROUTE	12:00						
PRESCRIBER'S SIGNATURE								
		18:00						
PRESCRIBER'S NAME AND BLEEP		22:00						

NAME OF DRUG		TIME	DATE → DOSE ↓					
ADDITIONAL INSTRUCTIONS		08:00						
DATE	ROUTE	12:00						
PRESCRIBER'S SIGNATURE								
		18:00						
PRESCRIBER'S NAME AND BLEEP		22:00						

NAME OF DRUG		TIME	DATE → DOSE ↓					
ADDITIONAL INSTRUCTIONS		08:00						
DATE	ROUTE	12:00						
PRESCRIBER'S SIGNATURE								
		18:00						
PRESCRIBER'S NAME AND BLEEP		22:00						

AS REQUIRED PRESCRIPTIONS

NAME OF DRUG		DATE					
INDICATION/ INSTRUCTION	DOSE	TIME					
FREQUENCY	ROUTE	DOSE					
PRESCRIBER'S SIGNATURE		ROUTE					
PRESCRIBER'S NAME AND BLEEP							
START DATE	STOP DATE	GIVEN BY					

PATIENT NAME   HOSPITAL NO.

NAME OF DRUG		DATE						
INDICATION/ INSTRUCTION	DOSE	TIME						
FREQUENCY	ROUTE	DOSE						
PRESCRIBER'S SIGNATURE		ROUTE						
PRESCRIBER'S NAME AND BLEEP		GIVEN BY						
START DATE	STOP DATE							

INTRAVENOUS FLUIDS

DATE	FLUID	ADDITIVE & DOSE	VOLUME	RATE/ DURATION	PRESCRIBER'S SIGNATURE	GIVEN BY	START TIME	END TIME

Record of signatures. ALL prescribers MUST complete.

DATE	NAME	DESIGNATION	SIGNATURE	BLEEP NUMBER

This man is experiencing an exacerbation of his COPD. He has no clinical signs of pneumonia and no sputum production, making it unlikely that his symptoms are caused by an infection. This exercise is about learning how to prescribe in cases of exacerbated COPD. It is important to be familiar with the principles of oxygen prescribing in COPD (page 14).

Step 3: Compare your answer to the checklist below and the chart opposite ✔

D	Details	Checked patient details Used capital letters throughout Used correct abbreviations	☐
R	Regular medications	Prescribed: – prednisolone 30mg stat and daily for a defined course – salbutamol nebuliser 2.5mg stat q.d.s. regularly and PRN q.d.s. – ipratropium nebuliser 500 micrograms stat and q.d.s. – Seretide Accuhaler 500 one dose b.d. – bendroflumethiazide 2.5mg morning – allopurinol 100mg daily	☐
U	Unpleasant reactions	Wrote NKDA or equivalent	☐
G	Gravid?	No	☐

C	Contra-indications	Not required	☐
H	Hydration	Wrote maintenance fluid	☐
A	Analgesia	Prescribed p.r.n. paracetamol 1g q.d.s. max.	☐
R	Renal function	N/A	☐
T	Thrombo-prophylaxis	Acceptable to have prescribed enoxaparin 40mg	☐
S	Signature box	Signed signature box	☐

Rationale

The main treatment for non-infective exacerbations of COPD is steroids and nebulised bronchodilators. This patient's salbutamol and tiotropium inhalers have been stopped while he receives the equivalent nebulised forms. Inhalers containing a long-acting beta receptor agonist (e.g. salmeterol) should be continued while on nebulisers. The degree of reversible bronchospasm is lower in COPD than in asthma, therefore salbutamol is given at 2.5mg q.d.s. rather than 5mg q.d.s.

Prednisolone 30mg for 7–14 days is recommended for acute exacerbations of COPD, whether they are infective or not. The aim is to reduce the inflammatory component of the exacerbation. Oral steroids will take hours to work so note the stat nebuliser prescriptions to provide symptomatic relief. There is no benefit to prolonged courses of steroids, their use should be reviewed as the patient's condition improves. Caution must be exercised in patients who have had multiple courses of steroids in the past year: stopping steroids abruptly risks precipitating a hypoadrenal crisis. A standard weaning regimen is to reduce the dose by 5mg every 3 days to zero or to reach the dose the patient was taking as maintenance.

KEY POINTS

- Write NEB to specify nebulised drugs.
- Salbutamol doses are lower in COPD than in asthma
- Ensure appropriate duration of prednisolone course
- Beware of the potential for a hypoadrenal crisis in patients who have had multiple courses of steroids

LONGBURY HOSPITAL TRUST		HOSPITAL NUMBER	197443
		SURNAME	BRANCH
		FIRST NAME	ROBERT
		ADDRESS	14 GLOBE AVENUE, CALDER LB12 1DM
		D.O.B	13/04/YYYY (65 YEARS AGO)

DATE OF ADMISSION	22/06/YYYY	ADMISSION WEIGHT (KG)	65kg	WARD	MEDICAL ASSESSMENT
ALLERGIES			CONSULTANT		ERIN JOHNSON
NKDA			CHART NO		1...OF...1

ONCE ONLY PRESCRIPTIONS

DATE	TIME	NAME OF DRUG	DOSE	ROUTE	PRESCRIBER'S SIGNATURE	GIVEN BY	TIME GIVEN
22/06	STAT	PREDNISOLONE	30mg	PO	ALewis		
22/06	STAT	SALBUTAMOL	2.5mg	NEB	ALewis		
22/06	STAT	IPRATROPIUM BROMIDE	500 micrograms	NEB	ALewis		

REGULAR MEDICATIONS

NAME OF DRUG PREDNISOLONE	TIME	DATE → DOSE ↓	22/06			
ADDITIONAL INSTRUCTIONS REVIEW 29/06	08:00	30mg	X			
DATE 22/06 ROUTE PO	12:00					
PRESCRIBER'S SIGNATURE ALewis	18:00					
PRESCRIBER'S NAME AND BLEEP ALEX LEWIS 4567	22:00					

NAME OF DRUG SALBUTAMOL	TIME	DATE → DOSE ↓	22/06			
ADDITIONAL INSTRUCTIONS	08:00	2.5mg	X			
DATE 22/06 ROUTE NEB	12:00	2.5mg				
PRESCRIBER'S SIGNATURE ALewis	18:00	2.5mg				
PRESCRIBER'S NAME AND BLEEP ALEX LEWIS 4567	22:00	2.5mg				

NAME OF DRUG IPRATROPIUM BROMIDE	TIME	DATE → DOSE ↓	22/06			
ADDITIONAL INSTRUCTIONS	08:00	500micrograms	X			
DATE 22/06 ROUTE NEB	12:00	500micrograms				
PRESCRIBER'S SIGNATURE ALewis	18:00	500micrograms				
PRESCRIBER'S NAME AND BLEEP ALEX LEWIS 4567	22:00	500micrograms				

PATIENT NAME *ROBERT BRANCH*   HOSPITAL NO. *197443*

NAME OF DRUG SERETIDE ACCUHALER 500	TIME	DATE → DOSE ↓	22/06				
ADDITIONAL INSTRUCTIONS	08:00	Ṫ					
DATE 22/06 ROUTE *INH*	12:00						
PRESCRIBER'S SIGNATURE *ALewis*	18:00						
PRESCRIBER'S NAME AND BLEEP *ALEX LEWIS 4567*	22:00	Ṫ					

NAME OF DRUG BENDROFLUMETHIAZIDE	TIME	DATE → DOSE ↓	22/06				
ADDITIONAL INSTRUCTIONS	08:00	2.5mg					
DATE 22/06 ROUTE *PO*	12:00						
PRESCRIBER'S SIGNATURE *ALewis*	18:00						
PRESCRIBER'S NAME AND BLEEP *ALEX LEWIS 4567*	22:00						

NAME OF DRUG ALLOPURINOL	TIME	DATE → DOSE ↓	22/06				
ADDITIONAL INSTRUCTIONS	08:00	100mg					
DATE 22/06 ROUTE *PO*	12:00						
PRESCRIBER'S SIGNATURE *ALewis*	18:00						
PRESCRIBER'S NAME AND BLEEP *ALEX LEWIS 4567*	22:00						

AS REQUIRED PRESCRIPTIONS

NAME OF DRUG SALBUTAMOL		DATE					
INDICATION/ INSTRUCTION SOB	DOSE 2.5mg	TIME					
FREQUENCY PRN MAX QDS	ROUTE NEB	DOSE					
PRESCRIBER'S SIGNATURE *ALewis*		ROUTE					
PRESCRIBER'S NAME AND BLEEP *ALEX LEWIS 4567*		GIVEN BY					
START DATE 22/06	STOP DATE						

PATIENT NAME ROBERT BRANCH   HOSPITAL NO. 197443

NAME OF DRUG PARACETAMOL		DATE						
INDICATION/ INSTRUCTION PAIN	DOSE 1g	TIME						
FREQUENCY QDS	ROUTE PO/IV/PR	DOSE						
PRESCRIBER'S SIGNATURE ALewis		ROUTE						
PRESCRIBER'S NAME AND BLEEP ALEX LEWIS 4567		GIVEN BY						
START DATE 22/06	STOP DATE							

INTRAVENOUS FLUIDS

DATE	FLUID	ADDITIVE & DOSE	VOLUME	RATE/ DURATION	PRESCRIBER'S SIGNATURE	GIVEN BY	START TIME	END TIME
22/06	HARTMANN'S	————	1l	10hrs	ALewis			

Record of signatures. ALL prescribers MUST complete.

DATE	NAME	DESIGNATION	SIGNATURE	BLEEP NUMBER
22/06	ALEX LEWIS	F1	ALewis	4567

Jemima Page (hospital number: 556982, DOB 13/12/YYYY [94 years old], address: 51 Almond Grove, Longbury LB16 9NN) had a hemiarthroplasty yesterday for a fractured neck of femur. The nursing staff report she has not drunk much since her operation and they are concerned because her blood pressure is low.

Mrs Page's blood pressure is 95/75mmHg, compared to her pre-admission 147/98mmHg. She has a heart rate of 105bpm. Her jugular venous pressure is not visible and her mucous membranes are dry. Her operation site is clean and there is no evidence of blood loss. Unfortunately, her notes have been left in theatre and there is no access to her past medical history.

Blood test results from earlier that day:
Haemoglobin 105g/L
Sodium 145mmol/L
Potassium 4.2mmol/L
Urea 8.2mmol/L
Creatinine 137µmol/L

Urine output is recorded as 15mL in the last hour.

Your task is to review the chart and manage the hypotension appropriately.
It is 08:20 on 19th September.

Notes

Step 1: Complete your answers in the drug chart opposite and overleaf

LONGBURY HOSPITAL TRUST		HOSPITAL NUMBER	556982
		SURNAME	PAGE
		FIRST NAME	JEMIMA
		ADDRESS	51 ALMOND GROVE, LONGBURY LB16 9NN
		D.O.B	13/12/YYYY (94 YEARS AGO)

DATE OF ADMISSION	18/09/YYYY	ADMISSION WEIGHT (KG)	60kg	WARD	SURGICAL
ALLERGIES				CONSULTANT	JOSHUA GIBB
NKDA				CHART NO	1...OF...1

ONCE ONLY PRESCRIPTIONS

DATE	TIME	NAME OF DRUG	DOSE	ROUTE	PRESCRIBER'S SIGNATURE	GIVEN BY	TIME GIVEN

REGULAR MEDICATIONS

NAME OF DRUG FUROSEMIDE	TIME	DATE → DOSE ↓	19/09				
ADDITIONAL INSTRUCTIONS	08:00	20mg	DA				
DATE 19/09 ROUTE PO	12:00						
PRESCRIBER'S SIGNATURE KCho	18:00						
PRESCRIBER'S NAME AND BLEEP KENNETH CHO 5765	22:00						

NAME OF DRUG RAMIPRIL	TIME	DATE → DOSE ↓	19/09				
ADDITIONAL INSTRUCTIONS	08:00	5mg	DA				
DATE 19/09 ROUTE PO	12:00						
PRESCRIBER'S SIGNATURE KCho	18:00						
PRESCRIBER'S NAME AND BLEEP KENNETH CHO 5765	22:00						

NAME OF DRUG BISOPROLOL	TIME	DATE → DOSE ↓	19/09				
ADDITIONAL INSTRUCTIONS	08:00	5mg	DA				
DATE 19/09 ROUTE PO	12:00						
PRESCRIBER'S SIGNATURE KCho	18:00						
PRESCRIBER'S NAME AND BLEEP KENNETH CHO 5765	22:00						

PATIENT NAME JEMIMA PAGE   HOSPITAL NO.   556982

NAME OF DRUG ENOXAPARIN	TIME	DATE → DOSE ↓	19/09				
ADDITIONAL INSTRUCTIONS	08:00						
DATE 19/09 ROUTE S/C	12:00						
PRESCRIBER'S SIGNATURE KCho	18:00	40mg					
PRESCRIBER'S NAME AND BLEEP KENNETH CHO 5765	22:00						

NAME OF DRUG	TIME	DATE → DOSE ↓					
ADDITIONAL INSTRUCTIONS	08:00						
DATE ROUTE	12:00						
PRESCRIBER'S SIGNATURE	18:00						
PRESCRIBER'S NAME AND BLEEP	22:00						

NAME OF DRUG	TIME	DATE → DOSE ↓					
ADDITIONAL INSTRUCTIONS	08:00						
DATE ROUTE	12:00						
PRESCRIBER'S SIGNATURE	18:00						
PRESCRIBER'S NAME AND BLEEP	22:00						

AS REQUIRED PRESCRIPTIONS

NAME OF DRUG		DATE					
INDICATION/ INSTRUCTION	DOSE	TIME					
FREQUENCY	ROUTE	DOSE					
PRESCRIBER'S SIGNATURE		ROUTE					
PRESCRIBER'S NAME AND BLEEP							
START DATE	STOP DATE	GIVEN BY					

PATIENT NAME JEMIMA PAGE   HOSPITAL NO.   556982

NAME OF DRUG		DATE					
INDICATION/ INSTRUCTION	DOSE	TIME					
FREQUENCY	ROUTE	DOSE					
PRESCRIBER'S SIGNATURE		ROUTE					
PRESCRIBER'S NAME AND BLEEP		GIVEN BY					
START DATE	STOP DATE						

INTRAVENOUS FLUIDS

DATE	FLUID	ADDITIVE & DOSE	VOLUME	RATE/ DURATION	PRESCRIBER'S SIGNATURE	GIVEN BY	START TIME	END TIME

Record of signatures. ALL prescribers MUST complete.

DATE	NAME	DESIGNATION	SIGNATURE	BLEEP NUMBER
19/09	KENNETH CHO	F1	KCho	5765

Step 2: Now check your work overleaf

Answer 14

Dehydration in the perioperative period is common. This patient's regular medications indicate she may have an underlying heart failure. Attempting to correct the dehydration too quickly can be dangerous.

Step 3: Compare your answer to the checklist below and the chart opposite ✔

D	Details	Checked patient details Used capital letters throughout Used correct abbreviations	☐
R	Regular medications	Witheld furosemide and ramipril (see Renal Function)	☐
U	Unpleasant reactions	Noticed no unpleasant reactions	☐
G	Gravid?	No	☐

C	Contra-indications	Aggressive fluid regimens will overload this patient with heart failure	☐
H	Hydration	Prescribed a fluid challenge. Stopped diuretics	☐
A	Analgesia	Not required	☐
R	Renal function	Withheld ramipril for 2 days to permit the renal function to improve	☐
T	Thrombo-prophylaxis	Noticed enoxaparin already prescribed	☐
S	Signature box	Signed signature box	☐

Rationale

This woman is dehydrated postoperatively, as evidenced by the significant fall in blood pressure since admission, the dry mucous membranes and a low jugular venous pressure. Further signs of dehydration are her poor urine output and deranged serum biochemistry. Raised serum sodium and/or raised urea often point to dehydration.

A response to this scenario is to prescribe a small fluid bolus of 250mL of crystalloid followed by further fluids to treat the dehydration. The fact that this patient is on furosemide, ramipril and bisoprolol should suggest underlying heart failure. Being overly aggressive with fluid resuscitation in a person with heart failure can cause pulmonary oedema.

A fluid challenge should be followed by a reassessment of the situation and can be repeated if it has no effect. Colloids were once commonly used for fluid challenges however recent reviews have shown that there is no benefit over crystalloids. If repeated fluid challenges fail to have an effect then there may be an alternate cause of low blood pressure. It is worth considering that spinal blocks and epidurals used for orthopaedic surgery can cause hypotension: the anaesthetic department will provide advice if this is the case.

The fluid bolus will treat the immediate blood pressure problem but does not address the underlying dehydration, hence a second bag of normal saline was prescribed.

Furosemide and ramipril should be withheld as they can worsen hypotension and renal function in this situation. Cardioselective beta-blockers such as bisoprolol have reduced hypotensive effect compared with non-selective beta-blockers such as propranolol. Therefore, bisoprolol has been continued.

This patient's eGFR has not been given but is worth considering halving the enoxaparin dose if laboratory or calculated results show it to be less than 30mL/min, thereby avoiding the effects of reduced renal clearance.

KEY POINTS

- The patient's medication points to co-morbidities
- When prescribing fluids in heart failure use a small fluid bolus and then repeat if necessary
- Avoid prescribing colloids to dehydrated patients
- Withhold antihypertensives in hypotension

LONGBURY HOSPITAL TRUST			HOSPITAL NUMBER	556982		
			SURNAME	PAGE		
			FIRST NAME	JEMIMA		
			ADDRESS	51 ALMOND GROVE, LONGBURY LB16 9NN		
			D.O.B	13/12/YYYY (94 YEARS AGO)		
DATE OF ADMISSION	18/09/YYYY	ADMISSION WEIGHT (KG)	60kg	WARD	SURGICAL	
ALLERGIES			CONSULTANT		JOSHUA GIBB	
NKDA			CHART NO		1…OF…1	

ONCE ONLY PRESCRIPTIONS

DATE	TIME	NAME OF DRUG	DOSE	ROUTE	PRESCRIBER'S SIGNATURE	GIVEN BY	TIME GIVEN

REGULAR MEDICATIONS

NAME OF DRUG FUROSEMIDE	TIME	DATE → DOSE ↓	19/09				
ADDITIONAL INSTRUCTIONS	08:00	20mg	DA				
DATE 19/09 ROUTE PO	12:00			REVIEW			
PRESCRIBER'S SIGNATURE KCho	18:00						
PRESCRIBER'S NAME AND BLEEP KENNETH CHO 5765	22:00						

NAME OF DRUG RAMIPRIL	TIME	DATE → DOSE ↓	19/09				
ADDITIONAL INSTRUCTIONS	08:00	5mg	DA				
DATE 19/09 ROUTE PO	12:00			REVIEW			
PRESCRIBER'S SIGNATURE KCho	18:00						
PRESCRIBER'S NAME AND BLEEP KENNETH CHO 5765	22:00						

NAME OF DRUG BISOPROLOL	TIME	DATE → DOSE ↓	19/09				
ADDITIONAL INSTRUCTIONS	08:00	5mg	DA				
DATE 19/09 ROUTE PO	12:00						
PRESCRIBER'S SIGNATURE KCho	18:00						
PRESCRIBER'S NAME AND BLEEP KENNETH CHO 5765	22:00						

PATIENT NAME JEMIMA PAGE   HOSPITAL NO. 556982

NAME OF DRUG ENOXAPARIN		TIME	DATE → DOSE ↓	19/09					
ADDITIONAL INSTRUCTIONS		08:00							
DATE 19/09	ROUTE S/C	12:00							
PRESCRIBER'S SIGNATURE KCho		18:00	40mg						
PRESCRIBER'S NAME AND BLEEP KENNETH CHO 5765		22:00							

NAME OF DRUG		TIME	DATE → DOSE ↓						
ADDITIONAL INSTRUCTIONS		08:00							
DATE	ROUTE	12:00							
PRESCRIBER'S SIGNATURE		18:00							
PRESCRIBER'S NAME AND BLEEP		22:00							

NAME OF DRUG		TIME	DATE → DOSE ↓						
ADDITIONAL INSTRUCTIONS		08:00							
DATE	ROUTE	12:00							
PRESCRIBER'S SIGNATURE		18:00							
PRESCRIBER'S NAME AND BLEEP		22:00							

AS REQUIRED PRESCRIPTIONS

NAME OF DRUG		DATE					
INDICATION/ INSTRUCTION	DOSE	TIME					
FREQUENCY	ROUTE	DOSE					
PRESCRIBER'S SIGNATURE		ROUTE					
PRESCRIBER'S NAME AND BLEEP		GIVEN BY					
START DATE	STOP DATE						

PATIENT NAME JEMIMA PAGE   HOSPITAL NO.   556982

NAME OF DRUG		DATE						
INDICATION/ INSTRUCTION	DOSE	TIME						
FREQUENCY	ROUTE	DOSE						
PRESCRIBER'S SIGNATURE		ROUTE						
PRESCRIBER'S NAME AND BLEEP		GIVEN BY						
START DATE	STOP DATE							

INTRAVENOUS FLUIDS

DATE	FLUID	ADDITIVE & DOSE	VOLUME	RATE/ DURATION	PRESCRIBER'S SIGNATURE	GIVEN BY	START TIME	END TIME
19/09	N.SALINE	——	250ml	STAT	ALewis			
19/09	N.SALINE	——	500ml	6hrs	ALewis			

Record of signatures. ALL prescribers MUST complete.

DATE	NAME	DESIGNATION	SIGNATURE	BLEEP NUMBER
19/09	KENNETH CHO	F1	KCho	5765
19/09	ALEX LEWIS	F1	ALewis	4567

Bethany Smith (hospital number: 998997, DOB 12/05/YYYY [2 years old], 1 Latham Avenue, Denby LB14 8JZ) is under the care of the neurosurgical team. She is awaiting an operation to revise a blocked ventriculo-peritoneal shunt that is causing symptoms of raised intracranial pressure. She is first on the operating list tomorrow, and she is to be nil by mouth from midnight. She weighs 14kg.

Observations:
Heart rate 105bpm
Respiratory rate 25 breaths/min
Urinary output 1.5mL/kg/h

Nursing staff have requested prescription of fluids overnight and have asked for the paracetamol prescription to be changed from oral to intravenous. Bethany does not tolerate per rectum analgesia well. She is clinically euvolaemic. A venous blood gas sample showed normal urea and electrolytes.

Your task is to prescribe fluids and paracetamol.
It is 19:00 on 5th May.

Notes

Step 1: Complete your answers in the drug chart opposite and overleaf

LONGBURY HOSPITAL TRUST

HOSPITAL NUMBER	998997
SURNAME	SMITH
FIRST NAME	BETHANY
ADDRESS	1 LATHAM AVENUE, DENBY LB14 8JZ
D.O.B	12/05/YYYY (2 YEARS AGO)

DATE OF ADMISSION	05/05/YYYY	ADMISSION WEIGHT (KG)	14	WARD	PAEDIATRIC

ALLERGIES	CONSULTANT	CAROL WYKE
PENICILLIN - RASH	CHART NO	1...OF...1

ONCE ONLY PRESCRIPTIONS

DATE	TIME	NAME OF DRUG	DOSE	ROUTE	PRESCRIBER'S SIGNATURE	GIVEN BY	TIME GIVEN

REGULAR MEDICATIONS

NAME OF DRUG	TIME	DATE → DOSE ↓	05/05			
PARACETAMOL						
ADDITIONAL INSTRUCTIONS	08:00	250mg	DS			
DATE 05/05 ROUTE PO	12:00	250mg	DS			
PRESCRIBER'S SIGNATURE NShah	18:00	250mg	DS			
PRESCRIBER'S NAME AND BLEEP NAZIA SHAH 9761	22:00	250mg				

NAME OF DRUG	TIME	DATE → DOSE ↓				
ADDITIONAL INSTRUCTIONS	08:00					
DATE ROUTE	12:00					
PRESCRIBER'S SIGNATURE	18:00					
PRESCRIBER'S NAME AND BLEEP	22:00					

NAME OF DRUG	TIME	DATE → DOSE ↓				
ADDITIONAL INSTRUCTIONS	08:00					
DATE ROUTE	12:00					
PRESCRIBER'S SIGNATURE	18:00					
PRESCRIBER'S NAME AND BLEEP	22:00					

124

PATIENT NAME BETHANY SMITH   HOSPITAL NO.   998997

NAME OF DRUG		TIME	DATE →					
			DOSE ↓					
ADDITIONAL INSTRUCTIONS		08:00						
DATE	ROUTE	12:00						
PRESCRIBER'S SIGNATURE								
		18:00						
PRESCRIBER'S NAME AND BLEEP		22:00						

NAME OF DRUG		TIME	DATE →					
			DOSE ↓					
ADDITIONAL INSTRUCTIONS		08:00						
DATE	ROUTE	12:00						
PRESCRIBER'S SIGNATURE								
		18:00						
PRESCRIBER'S NAME AND BLEEP		22:00						

NAME OF DRUG		TIME	DATE →					
			DOSE ↓					
ADDITIONAL INSTRUCTIONS		08:00						
DATE	ROUTE	12:00						
PRESCRIBER'S SIGNATURE								
		18:00						
PRESCRIBER'S NAME AND BLEEP		22:00						

AS REQUIRED PRESCRIPTIONS

NAME OF DRUG		DATE					
INDICATION/ INSTRUCTION	DOSE	TIME					
FREQUENCY	ROUTE	DOSE					
PRESCRIBER'S SIGNATURE		ROUTE					
PRESCRIBER'S NAME AND BLEEP		GIVEN BY					
START DATE	STOP DATE						

PATIENT NAME BETHANY SMITH   HOSPITAL NO.   998997

NAME OF DRUG		DATE					
INDICATION/ INSTRUCTION	DOSE	TIME					
FREQUENCY	ROUTE	DOSE					
PRESCRIBER'S SIGNATURE		ROUTE					
PRESCRIBER'S NAME AND BLEEP		GIVEN BY					
START DATE	STOP DATE						

INTRAVENOUS FLUIDS

DATE	FLUID	ADDITIVE & DOSE	VOLUME	RATE/ DURATION	PRESCRIBER'S SIGNATURE	GIVEN BY	START TIME	END TIME

Record of signatures. ALL prescribers MUST complete.

DATE	NAME	DESIGNATION	SIGNATURE	BLEEP NUMBER
05/05	NAZIA SHAH	ST3	NShah	9761

Answer 15

Prescribing fluids for paediatric patients requires a more precise calculation of requirements than in adult patients and is often a daunting task for junior doctors. In this case the patient has no signs of dehydration so simply requires a maintenance. This exercise is about correctly calculating the fluid requirements for this regimen.

Step 3: Compare your answer to the checklist below and the chart opposite ☑

D Details	Checked patient details Used capital letters throughout Used correct abbreviations	☐
R Regular medications	Stopped oral paracetamol and started IV paracetamol. Did not just change route	☐
U Unpleasant reactions	Crossed off IV times where PO paracetamol has already been given	☐
G Gravid?	No	☐

C Contra-indications	IV paracetamol is lower dose than oral in this case	☐
H Hydration	Prescribed 0.45% sodium chloride + 5% dextrose at 50mL/h	☐
A Analgesia	See regular medications	☐
R Renal function	Not required	☐
T Thrombo-prophylaxis	Not required	☐
S Signature box	Signed signature box	☐

Rationale

The patient's fluid maintenance regimen is calculated as follows:

100mL x 10kg = 1000mL for the first 10kg of the patient's weight

50mL x 4kg = 200mL for the next 4kg of the patient's weight

This gives a total 24-hour fluid requirement of 1200mL. In order to convert this into an hourly rate, divide by 24:

1200mL/24 hours = 50mL/h.

0.45% sodium chloride and 5% dextrose has been prescribed: in children, in order to avoid electrolyte imbalance, this fluid is preferable to sodium chloride 0.9%, because it is closer to children's daily electrolyte requirements. A 500mL bag has been prescribed at 50mL/h, which should last from midnight until the time of the operation.

It would have been acceptable to use the date '06/05' for the fluid prescription, as technically the fluid will be given 'tomorrow': some hospitals allow a fluid prescription to carry forward past midnight.

Remember to check paediatric formularies when prescribing for children. Here, the intravenous dose of paracetamol is slightly different to the oral dose: simply amending the route section of the prescription without rewriting it fully would create an overdose. For this patient, the maximum oral therapy is 250mg q.d.s. The intravenous dose is 15mg/kg/dose, which is equivalent to 210mg q.d.s. To prevent an accidental overdose, don't forget to cross off the time slots where oral paracetamol has already been given during the day.

KEY POINTS

- Check paediatric formularies when prescribing for children
- Calculate fluid requirements before prescribing for children
- Remember that some drugs have different doses by different routes
- Always check the formulary before changing the route of a prescription

LONGBURY HOSPITAL TRUST		HOSPITAL NUMBER	998997	
		SURNAME	SMITH	
		FIRST NAME	BETHANY	
		ADDRESS	1 LATHAM AVENUE, DENBY LB14 8JZ	
		D.O.B	12/05/YYYY (2 YEARS AGO)	

DATE OF ADMISSION	05/05/YYYY	ADMISSION WEIGHT (KG)	14	WARD	PAEDIATRIC
ALLERGIES			CONSULTANT		CAROL WYKE
PENICILLIN - RASH			CHART NO		1...OF...1

ONCE ONLY PRESCRIPTIONS

DATE	TIME	NAME OF DRUG	DOSE	ROUTE	PRESCRIBER'S SIGNATURE	GIVEN BY	TIME GIVEN

REGULAR MEDICATIONS

NAME OF DRUG PARACETAMOL	TIME	DATE → / DOSE ↓	05/05				
ADDITIONAL INSTRUCTIONS	**08:00**	250mg	DS	————			
DATE 05/05 ROUTE PO	**12:00**	250mg	DS	STOP			
PRESCRIBER'S SIGNATURE NShah				05/05			
	18:00	250mg	DS	ALewis			
PRESCRIBER'S NAME AND BLEEP NAZIA SHAH 9761	**22:00**	250mg	————				

NAME OF DRUG PARACETAMOL	TIME	DATE → / DOSE ↓	05/05				
ADDITIONAL INSTRUCTIONS	**08:00**	210mg	————				
DATE 05/05 ROUTE IV	**12:00**	210mg	————				
PRESCRIBER'S SIGNATURE ALewis							
	18:00	210mg	————				
PRESCRIBER'S NAME AND BLEEP ALEX LEWIS 4567	**22:00**	210mg					

NAME OF DRUG	TIME	DATE → / DOSE ↓					
ADDITIONAL INSTRUCTIONS	**08:00**						
DATE ROUTE	**12:00**						
PRESCRIBER'S SIGNATURE							
	18:00						
PRESCRIBER'S NAME AND BLEEP	**22:00**						

PATIENT NAME BETHANY SMITH   HOSPITAL NO. 998997

NAME OF DRUG		TIME	DATE → DOSE ↓					
ADDITIONAL INSTRUCTIONS		08:00						
DATE	ROUTE	12:00						
PRESCRIBER'S SIGNATURE		18:00						
PRESCRIBER'S NAME AND BLEEP		22:00						

NAME OF DRUG		TIME	DATE → DOSE ↓					
ADDITIONAL INSTRUCTIONS		08:00						
DATE	ROUTE	12:00						
PRESCRIBER'S SIGNATURE		18:00						
PRESCRIBER'S NAME AND BLEEP		22:00						

NAME OF DRUG		TIME	DATE → DOSE ↓					
ADDITIONAL INSTRUCTIONS		08:00						
DATE	ROUTE	12:00						
PRESCRIBER'S SIGNATURE		18:00						
PRESCRIBER'S NAME AND BLEEP		22:00						

AS REQUIRED PRESCRIPTIONS

NAME OF DRUG		DATE					
INDICATION/ INSTRUCTION	DOSE	TIME					
FREQUENCY	ROUTE	DOSE					
PRESCRIBER'S SIGNATURE		ROUTE					
PRESCRIBER'S NAME AND BLEEP		GIVEN BY					
START DATE	STOP DATE						

PATIENT NAME BETHANY SMITH   HOSPITAL NO.   998997

NAME OF DRUG		DATE					
INDICATION/ INSTRUCTION	DOSE	TIME					
FREQUENCY	ROUTE	DOSE					
PRESCRIBER'S SIGNATURE		ROUTE					
PRESCRIBER'S NAME AND BLEEP		GIVEN BY					
START DATE	STOP DATE						

INTRAVENOUS FLUIDS

DATE	FLUID	ADDITIVE & DOSE	VOLUME	RATE/ DURATION	PRESCRIBER'S SIGNATURE	GIVEN BY	START TIME	END TIME
05/05	0.45% NaCl +5% DEXTROSE	————	500ml	50ml/hr	A Lewis			

Record of signatures. ALL prescribers MUST complete.

DATE	NAME	DESIGNATION	SIGNATURE	BLEEP NUMBER
05/05	NAZIA SHAH	ST3	NShah	9761
05/05	ALEX LEWIS	F1	ALewis	4567

Frank Lewis (hospital number: 009089, DOB 10/06/YYYY [42 years old], address: 22 Groveham Court, Longbury LB2 4EN) has been admitted to the emergency department. He gives a history of 2 days' continual vomiting associated with severe epigastric pain. He has a history of alcohol dependence, but has no signs of acute withdrawal. He has no known drug allergies. He weighs 64kg. Mr Lewis's consultant is Dr Pradip Chand.

Observations:
Blood pressure 84/53mmHg
Heart rate 122bpm
Respiratory rate 24 breaths/minute
SpO_2 94% on air
Urine output 10mL over last hour

Blood test results:
Haemoglobin 172g/L
Mean cell volume 107.6fL
White blood cells 16 x10^9/L
Neutrophils 13.2 x10^9/L
C-reactive protein 64mg/L
Sodium 146mmol/L
Potassium 2.5mmol/L
Urea 23.4mmol/L
Creatinine 342μmol/L
Amylase 476iU/L

On examination Mr Lewis's jugular venous pressure is not visible, he is tender in the epigastrium with guarding. His chest is clear.

Your task is to prescribe appropriate treatment and fluids.
It is 04:50 on 16th September.

Notes

LONGBURY HOSPITAL TRUST

HOSPITAL NUMBER	
SURNAME	
FIRST NAME	
ADDRESS	
D.O.B	

DATE OF ADMISSION		ADMISSION WEIGHT (KG)		WARD	
ALLERGIES			CONSULTANT		
			CHART NO		...OF...

ONCE ONLY PRESCRIPTIONS

DATE	TIME	NAME OF DRUG	DOSE	ROUTE	PRESCRIBER'S SIGNATURE	GIVEN BY	TIME GIVEN

REGULAR MEDICATIONS

NAME OF DRUG		TIME	DATE → DOSE ↓				
ADDITIONAL INSTRUCTIONS		08:00					
DATE	ROUTE	12:00					
PRESCRIBER'S SIGNATURE		18:00					
PRESCRIBER'S NAME AND BLEEP		22:00					

NAME OF DRUG		TIME	DATE → DOSE ↓				
ADDITIONAL INSTRUCTIONS		08:00					
DATE	ROUTE	12:00					
PRESCRIBER'S SIGNATURE		18:00					
PRESCRIBER'S NAME AND BLEEP		22:00					

NAME OF DRUG		TIME	DATE → DOSE ↓				
ADDITIONAL INSTRUCTIONS		08:00					
DATE	ROUTE	12:00					
PRESCRIBER'S SIGNATURE		18:00					
PRESCRIBER'S NAME AND BLEEP		22:00					

PATIENT NAME   HOSPITAL NO.

NAME OF DRUG		TIME	DATE →					
			DOSE ↓					
ADDITIONAL INSTRUCTIONS		08:00						
DATE	ROUTE	12:00						
PRESCRIBER'S SIGNATURE								
		18:00						
PRESCRIBER'S NAME AND BLEEP		22:00						

NAME OF DRUG		TIME	DATE →					
			DOSE ↓					
ADDITIONAL INSTRUCTIONS		08:00						
DATE	ROUTE	12:00						
PRESCRIBER'S SIGNATURE								
		18:00						
PRESCRIBER'S NAME AND BLEEP		22:00						

NAME OF DRUG		TIME	DATE →					
			DOSE ↓					
ADDITIONAL INSTRUCTIONS		08:00						
DATE	ROUTE	12:00						
PRESCRIBER'S SIGNATURE								
		18:00						
PRESCRIBER'S NAME AND BLEEP		22:00						

AS REQUIRED PRESCRIPTIONS

NAME OF DRUG		DATE					
INDICATION/ INSTRUCTION	DOSE	TIME					
FREQUENCY	ROUTE	DOSE					
PRESCRIBER'S SIGNATURE		ROUTE					
PRESCRIBER'S NAME AND BLEEP		GIVEN BY					
START DATE	STOP DATE						

PATIENT NAME   HOSPITAL NO.

NAME OF DRUG		DATE					
INDICATION/ INSTRUCTION	DOSE	TIME					
FREQUENCY	ROUTE	DOSE					
PRESCRIBER'S SIGNATURE		ROUTE					
PRESCRIBER'S NAME AND BLEEP		GIVEN BY					
START DATE	STOP DATE						

INTRAVENOUS FLUIDS

DATE	FLUID	ADDITIVE & DOSE	VOLUME	RATE/ DURATION	PRESCRIBER'S SIGNATURE	GIVEN BY	START TIME	END TIME

Record of signatures. ALL prescribers MUST complete.

DATE	NAME	DESIGNATION	SIGNATURE	BLEEP NUMBER

Answer 16

Profuse vomiting is a common presentation of acute pancreatitis. In this case the episode has probably been caused by alcohol. Vomiting causes large electrolyte disturbances as well as acid-base imbalance; these need to be carefully corrected.

Step 3: Compare your answer to the checklist below and the chart opposite ✔

D Details	Checked patient details Used capital letters throughout Used correct abbreviation		☐
R Regular medications	Not required		☐
U Unpleasant reactions	NKDA		☐
G Gravid?	No		☐

C Contra-indications	None		☐
H Hydration	Prescribed at least 2 litres of fluid		☐
A Analgesia	Prescribed paracetamol 1g q.d.s, codeine 30–60mg q.d.s, cyclizine 50mg and oramorph 5–10mg		☐
R Renal function	Prescribed aggressive fluid resuscitation to reduce the risk of AKI Monitor opiate use and withhold if renal function worsens		☐
T Thrombo-prophylaxis	Prescribed enoxaparin 20mg		☐
S Signature box	Signed signature box		☐

Rationale

Patients with acute pancreatitis have tremendous fluid deficits due to third-space losses. Excess fluid loss due to vomiting also needs to be taken into account. Aggressive intravenous fluid resuscitation is the mainstay of treatment. Electrolyte abnormalities need to be monitored and corrected.

In this patient, the fluid losses have caused hypotension leading to acute kidney injury, and the vomiting has led to severe hypokalaemia. He should be managed on a cardiac monitor. Evidence as to which type of fluid is best is lacking: because circulatory support is required, dextrose would not be suitable. He is severely volume depleted and needs a large volume to correct his physiology. One litre of crystalloid given stat would be a sensible start followed by fluid at a rate of 500mL/h until his urine output has improved. Remember that an acceptable urine output in adults is >0.5mL/kg/h body weight.

Management of hypokalaemia in this situation is problematic. No more than 10mmol of KCl per hour can be given by peripheral line. In some cases it is necessary to have two lines running; a line for resuscitation in one arm and another for potassium replacement on the other side. When the patient is able to swallow, oral potassium replacement may be added.

Oxygen therapy would be indicated in order to maintain saturation between 94 and 98% as respiratory distress is a frequent complication of acute pancreatitis.

KEY POINTS

- Patients with pancreatitis require aggressive fluid resuscitation
- When choosing fluid consider which compartment you wish the fluid to enter
- Regularly review the effect of your fluid prescriptions in unwell patients

LONGBURY HOSPITAL TRUST		HOSPITAL NUMBER	009089
		SURNAME	LEWIS
		FIRST NAME	FRANK
		ADDRESS	22 GROVEHAM COURT, LONGBURY LB2 4EN
		D.O.B	10/06/YYYY (42 YEARS AGO)

DATE OF ADMISSION	16/09/YYYY	ADMISSION WEIGHT (KG)	64kg	WARD	EMERGENCY
ALLERGIES			CONSULTANT		PRADIP CHAND
NKDA			CHART NO		1...OF...1

ONCE ONLY PRESCRIPTIONS

DATE	TIME	NAME OF DRUG	DOSE	ROUTE	PRESCRIBER'S SIGNATURE	GIVEN BY	TIME GIVEN

REGULAR MEDICATIONS

NAME OF DRUG ENOXAPARIN	TIME	DATE → DOSE ↓	16/09				
ADDITIONAL INSTRUCTIONS	08:00						
DATE 16/09 ROUTE S/C	12:00						
PRESCRIBER'S SIGNATURE ALewis	18:00	20mg					
PRESCRIBER'S NAME AND BLEEP ALEX LEWIS 4567	22:00						

NAME OF DRUG PARACETAMOL	TIME	DATE → DOSE ↓	16/09				
ADDITIONAL INSTRUCTIONS	08:00	1g					
DATE 16/09 ROUTE PO/IV	12:00	1g					
PRESCRIBER'S SIGNATURE ALewis	18:00	1g					
PRESCRIBER'S NAME AND BLEEP ALEX LEWIS 4567	22:00	1g					

NAME OF DRUG CODEINE	TIME	DATE → DOSE ↓	16/09				
ADDITIONAL INSTRUCTIONS	08:00	30-60mg					
DATE 16/09 ROUTE PO	12:00	30-60mg					
PRESCRIBER'S SIGNATURE ALewis	18:00	30-60mg					
PRESCRIBER'S NAME AND BLEEP ALEX LEWIS 4567	22:00	30-60mg					

PATIENT NAME *FRANK LEWIS*　　　　HOSPITAL NO. *009089*

NAME OF DRUG		TIME	DATE → DOSE ↓					
ADDITIONAL INSTRUCTIONS		08:00						
DATE	ROUTE	12:00						
PRESCRIBER'S SIGNATURE		18:00						
PRESCRIBER'S NAME AND BLEEP		22:00						

NAME OF DRUG		TIME	DATE → DOSE ↓					
ADDITIONAL INSTRUCTIONS		08:00						
DATE	ROUTE	12:00						
PRESCRIBER'S SIGNATURE		18:00						
PRESCRIBER'S NAME AND BLEEP		22:00						

NAME OF DRUG		TIME	DATE → DOSE ↓					
ADDITIONAL INSTRUCTIONS		08:00						
DATE	ROUTE	12:00						
PRESCRIBER'S SIGNATURE		18:00						
PRESCRIBER'S NAME AND BLEEP		22:00						

AS REQUIRED PRESCRIPTIONS

NAME OF DRUG *CYCLIZINE*		DATE					
INDICATION/ INSTRUCTION *NAUSEA*	DOSE *50mg*	TIME					
FREQUENCY *8HRLY*	ROUTE *PO/IM/IV*	DOSE					
PRESCRIBER'S SIGNATURE *ALewis*		ROUTE					
PRESCRIBER'S NAME AND BLEEP *ALEX LEWIS 4567*		GIVEN BY					
START DATE *16/09*	STOP DATE						

PATIENT NAME *FRANK LEWIS*   HOSPITAL NO.   *009089*

NAME OF DRUG ORAMORPH		DATE					
INDICATION/ INSTRUCTION PAIN	DOSE 5-10mg	TIME					
FREQUENCY 4HRLY	ROUTE PO	DOSE					
PRESCRIBER'S SIGNATURE ALewis		ROUTE					
PRESCRIBER'S NAME AND BLEEP ALEX LEWIS 4567		GIVEN BY					
START DATE 16/09	STOP DATE						

INTRAVENOUS FLUIDS

DATE	FLUID	ADDITIVE & DOSE	VOLUME	RATE/ DURATION	PRESCRIBER'S SIGNATURE	GIVEN BY	START TIME	END TIME
16/09	HARTMANN'S	————	1l	STAT	ALewis			
16/09	HARTMANN'S	————	1l	2 hours	ALewis			

Record of signatures. ALL prescribers MUST complete.

DATE	NAME	DESIGNATION	SIGNATURE	BLEEP NUMBER
16/09	ALEX LEWIS	F1	ALewis	4567

Olivia McGee (hospital number: 708100, DOB 15/05/YYYY [46 years old], address: 29 Harps Avenue, Longbury LB11 8DS) was admitted today at 07:00 with an upper gastrointestinal bleed. She is known to have alcoholic liver disease and cirrhosis. Oesophageal varices were diagnosed following gastroscopy 6 months ago. She was stable after initial fluid resuscitation and is soon to have an emergency endoscopy. She has already been started on terlipressin to control the bleeding. The consultant has decided she does not need prophylactic antibiotics.

Blood test results:
Haemoglobin 76g/L
Mean cell volume 112fL
Platelets 102 x 10^9/L
International normalised ratio 1.8

First, you would have checked that this woman has already had a 'group and save' sample sent to the transfusion laboratory and would have telephoned the transfusion laboratory to order the blood. They would then do a crossmatch on the saved sample and issue appropriate blood.

Your task is to prescribe two units of blood and two units of fresh frozen plasma (FFP).
It is 13:30 on 12th May.

Notes

Step 1: Complete your answers in the drug chart opposite and overleaf

LONGBURY HOSPITAL TRUST		HOSPITAL NUMBER	708100

		HOSPITAL NUMBER	708100
LONGBURY HOSPITAL TRUST		SURNAME	MCGEE
		FIRST NAME	OLIVIA
		ADDRESS	29 HARPS AVENUE, LONGBURY LB11 8DS
		D.O.B	15/05/YYYY (46 YEARS AGO)
DATE OF ADMISSION	12/05/YYYY	ADMISSION WEIGHT (KG)	62kg	WARD	MEDICAL ASSESSMENT
ALLERGIES			CONSULTANT	ERIN JOHNSON
NKDA			CHART NO	1...OF...1

ONCE ONLY PRESCRIPTIONS

DATE	TIME	NAME OF DRUG	DOSE	ROUTE	PRESCRIBER'S SIGNATURE	GIVEN BY	TIME GIVEN
12/05	08.00	TERLIPRESSIN	2mg	IV	BFord	RN	08.00

REGULAR MEDICATIONS

NAME OF DRUG	TIME	DATE → DOSE ↓	12/05			
TERLIPRESSIN						
ADDITIONAL INSTRUCTIONS 72 HOURS THEN REVIEW	08:00	1mg	X			
DATE 12/05 ROUTE IV	12:00	1mg	RN			
PRESCRIBER'S SIGNATURE BFord						
	18:00	1mg				
PRESCRIBER'S NAME AND BLEEP BEN FORD 1569	22:00	1mg				

NAME OF DRUG	TIME	DATE → DOSE ↓				
ADDITIONAL INSTRUCTIONS	08:00					
DATE ROUTE	12:00					
PRESCRIBER'S SIGNATURE						
	18:00					
PRESCRIBER'S NAME AND BLEEP	22:00					

NAME OF DRUG	TIME	DATE → DOSE ↓				
ADDITIONAL INSTRUCTIONS	08:00					
DATE ROUTE	12:00					
PRESCRIBER'S SIGNATURE						
	18:00					
PRESCRIBER'S NAME AND BLEEP	22:00					

PATIENT NAME OLIVIA MCGEE   HOSPITAL NO.   708100

NAME OF DRUG	TIME	DATE →					
		DOSE ↓					
ADDITIONAL INSTRUCTIONS	08:00						
DATE / ROUTE	12:00						
PRESCRIBER'S SIGNATURE							
	18:00						
PRESCRIBER'S NAME AND BLEEP							
	22:00						

NAME OF DRUG	TIME	DATE →					
		DOSE ↓					
ADDITIONAL INSTRUCTIONS	08:00						
DATE / ROUTE	12:00						
PRESCRIBER'S SIGNATURE							
	18:00						
PRESCRIBER'S NAME AND BLEEP							
	22:00						

NAME OF DRUG	TIME	DATE →					
		DOSE ↓					
ADDITIONAL INSTRUCTIONS	08:00						
DATE / ROUTE	12:00						
PRESCRIBER'S SIGNATURE							
	18:00						
PRESCRIBER'S NAME AND BLEEP							
	22:00						

AS REQUIRED PRESCRIPTIONS

NAME OF DRUG		DATE					
INDICATION/ INSTRUCTION	DOSE	TIME					
FREQUENCY	ROUTE	DOSE					
PRESCRIBER'S SIGNATURE		ROUTE					
PRESCRIBER'S NAME AND BLEEP		GIVEN BY					
START DATE	STOP DATE						

PATIENT NAME OLIVIA MCGEE   HOSPITAL NO.   708100

NAME OF DRUG		DATE						
INDICATION/ INSTRUCTION	DOSE	TIME						
FREQUENCY	ROUTE	DOSE						
PRESCRIBER'S SIGNATURE		ROUTE						
PRESCRIBER'S NAME AND BLEEP		GIVEN BY						
START DATE	STOP DATE							

INTRAVENOUS FLUIDS

DATE	FLUID	ADDITIVE & DOSE	VOLUME	RATE/ DURATION	PRESCRIBER'S SIGNATURE	GIVEN BY	START TIME	END TIME

Record of signatures. ALL prescribers MUST complete.

DATE	NAME	DESIGNATION	SIGNATURE	BLEEP NUMBER
12/05	BEN FORD	F2	BFord	1569

Step 2: Now check your work overleaf

Answer 17

Prescribing blood can be a daunting task when you first start prescribing. In this case underlying liver disease has also caused deranged clotting function.

Step 3: Compare your answer to the checklist below and the chart opposite ☑

D Details	Checked patient details Used capital letters throughout Used correct abbreviations	☐
R Regular medications	Continued terlipressin as prescribed Prescribed 2 units RBC to be given over 2 hours each Prescribed 2 units of FFP to be given over 30 minutes each	☐
U Unpleasant reactions	Not required	☐
G Gravid?	No	☐

C Contra-indications	Not required	☐
H Hydration	Noted that the patient is adequately resuscitated	☐
A Analgesia	Not required	☐
R Renal function	Not required	☐
T Thrombo-prophylaxis	Did not prescribe thromboprophylaxis as it is contraindicated in an acutely bleeding patient	☐
S Signature box	Signed signature box	☐

Rationale

Fresh frozen plasma (FFP) is also a blood product and needs to be requested from the transfusion laboratory. O negative blood is often kept in emergency and surgical departments in case of emergency. Units of blood are supplied as packed red blood cells (RBCs) and are usually prescribed as RBC on a prescription chart. Packed RBCs are usually transfused over 2–3 hours. Blood has a shelf life of 4 hours once out of the fridge and so cannot be given over a period longer than 4 hours. If Mrs McGee was haemodynamically unstable the blood could be given stat; however she is stable and it is safer to give the blood over a 2-hour period. Giving the blood over 2 hours enables monitoring for transfusion reactions.

FFP corrects coagulation abnormalities caused by deficiencies of clotting factors. Patients with liver disease often have deranged clotting due to failure to produce sufficient clotting factors. FFP is usually given over 30 minutes unless there is extensive blood loss due to haemorrhage (exsanguination), in which case it is given stat.

Not all hospitals have a specific chart in which to prescribe blood, like in this exercise. In this case, the most appropriate place to prescribe blood is in the intravenous fluids chart.

KEY POINTS

- Order blood products from the transfusion laboratory
- Packed red cells are usually given over 2 hours if the patient is stable
- Fresh frozen plasma is usually given over 30 minutes if the patient is stable
- O negative blood for emergencies is often kept in emergency and surgical departments

LONGBURY HOSPITAL TRUST

HOSPITAL NUMBER	708100
SURNAME	McGEE
FIRST NAME	OLIVIA
ADDRESS	29 HARPS AVENUE, LONGBURY LB11 8DS
D.O.B	15/05/YYYY (46 YEARS AGO)

DATE OF ADMISSION	12/05/YYYY	ADMISSION WEIGHT (KG)	62kg	WARD	MEDICAL ASSESSMENT
ALLERGIES			CONSULTANT		ERIN JOHNSON
NKDA			CHART NO		1...OF...1

ONCE ONLY PRESCRIPTIONS

DATE	TIME	NAME OF DRUG	DOSE	ROUTE	PRESCRIBER'S SIGNATURE	GIVEN BY	TIME GIVEN
12/05	08.00	TERLIPRESSIN	2mg	IV	BFord	RN	08.00

REGULAR MEDICATIONS

NAME OF DRUG	TIME	DATE → DOSE ↓	12/05				
TERLIPRESSIN							
ADDITIONAL INSTRUCTIONS 72 HOURS THEN REVIEW	08:00	1mg	X				
DATE 12/05 ROUTE IV	12:00	1mg	RN				
PRESCRIBER'S SIGNATURE BFord	18:00	1mg					
PRESCRIBER'S NAME AND BLEEP BEN FORD 1569	22:00	1mg					

NAME OF DRUG	TIME	DATE → DOSE ↓					
ADDITIONAL INSTRUCTIONS	08:00						
DATE ROUTE	12:00						
PRESCRIBER'S SIGNATURE	18:00						
PRESCRIBER'S NAME AND BLEEP	22:00						

NAME OF DRUG	TIME	DATE → DOSE ↓					
ADDITIONAL INSTRUCTIONS	08:00						
DATE ROUTE	12:00						
PRESCRIBER'S SIGNATURE	18:00						
PRESCRIBER'S NAME AND BLEEP	22:00						

PATIENT NAME OLIVIA MCGEE   HOSPITAL NO.   708100

NAME OF DRUG		TIME	DATE → DOSE ↓					
ADDITIONAL INSTRUCTIONS		08:00						
DATE	ROUTE	12:00						
PRESCRIBER'S SIGNATURE								
		18:00						
PRESCRIBER'S NAME AND BLEEP								
		22:00						

NAME OF DRUG		TIME	DATE → DOSE ↓					
ADDITIONAL INSTRUCTIONS		08:00						
DATE	ROUTE	12:00						
PRESCRIBER'S SIGNATURE								
		18:00						
PRESCRIBER'S NAME AND BLEEP								
		22:00						

NAME OF DRUG		TIME	DATE → DOSE ↓					
ADDITIONAL INSTRUCTIONS		08:00						
DATE	ROUTE	12:00						
PRESCRIBER'S SIGNATURE								
		18:00						
PRESCRIBER'S NAME AND BLEEP								
		22:00						

AS REQUIRED PRESCRIPTIONS

NAME OF DRUG			DATE					
INDICATION/ INSTRUCTION	DOSE		TIME					
FREQUENCY	ROUTE		DOSE					
PRESCRIBER'S SIGNATURE			ROUTE					
PRESCRIBER'S NAME AND BLEEP								
START DATE	STOP DATE		GIVEN BY					

PATIENT NAME OLIVIA MCGEE   HOSPITAL NO.   708100

NAME OF DRUG		DATE						
INDICATION/ INSTRUCTION	DOSE	TIME						
FREQUENCY	ROUTE	DOSE						
PRESCRIBER'S SIGNATURE		ROUTE						
PRESCRIBER'S NAME AND BLEEP		GIVEN BY						
START DATE	STOP DATE							

INTRAVENOUS FLUIDS

DATE	FLUID	ADDITIVE & DOSE	VOLUME	RATE/ DURATION	PRESCRIBER'S SIGNATURE	GIVEN BY	START TIME	END TIME
12/05	RBC	————————	1 UNIT	2 hours	ALewis			
12/05	RBC	————————	1 UNIT	2 hours	ALewis			
12/05	FFP	————————	1 UNIT	30 min	ALewis			
12/05	FFP	————————	1 UNIT	30 min	ALewis			

Record of signatures. ALL prescribers MUST complete.

DATE	NAME	DESIGNATION	SIGNATURE	BLEEP NUMBER
12/05	BEN FORD	F2	BFord	1569
12/05	ALEX LEWIS	F1	ALewis	4567

Michael Golding (hospital number: 014325, DOB 10/04/YYYY [59 years old], address: 12 Karatta Drive, Longbury LB14 1ZW) has recently undergone an ileal resection for his Crohn's disease. During the day he has been started on total parenteral nutrition. At handover to the evening shift, the day team have requested that urea and electrolytes are checked and corrected as appropriate. Mr Golding is no longer nil-by-mouth.

Blood test results, at 18.45 on 10th April:
Sodium 143mmol/L
Potassium 3.2mmol/L
Urea 4.2mmol/L
Creatinine 48µmol/L
Magnesium 0.36mmol/L (normal 0.60–0.82mmol/L)
PO_4 0.63mmol/L (normal 0.8–1.5 mmol/L)
Corrected Ca^{2+} 2.12mmol/L (normal 2.05–2.60mmol/L)

Your task is to prescribe appropriate electrolyte replacement.
It is 20:00 on 10th April.

Notes

Step 1: Complete your answers in the drug chart opposite and overleaf

	HOSPITAL NUMBER	014325
LONGBURY HOSPITAL TRUST	SURNAME	GOLDING
	FIRST NAME	MICHAEL
REWRITTEN 08/04	ADDRESS	12 KARATTA DRIVE, LONGBURY LB14 1ZW

			D.O.B	10/04/YYYY (59 YEARS AGO)
DATE OF ADMISSION	03/04/YYYY	ADMISSION WEIGHT (KG)	54kg	WARD	SURGICAL
ALLERGIES			CONSULTANT	JOSHUA GIBB
NKDA			CHART NO	1...OF...1

ONCE ONLY PRESCRIPTIONS

DATE	TIME	NAME OF DRUG	DOSE	ROUTE	PRESCRIBER'S SIGNATURE	GIVEN BY	TIME GIVEN

REGULAR MEDICATIONS

NAME OF DRUG ENOXAPARIN	TIME	DATE → DOSE ↓	08/04	09/04	10/04		
ADDITIONAL INSTRUCTIONS	08:00						
DATE 08/04 ROUTE S/C	12:00						
PRESCRIBER'S SIGNATURE MHughes	18:00	40mg	——	RN	BE		
PRESCRIBER'S NAME AND BLEEP MICHELLE HUGHES 2357	22:00						

NAME OF DRUG CYCLIZINE	TIME	DATE → DOSE ↓	08/04	09/04	10/04		
ADDITIONAL INSTRUCTIONS	08:00	50mg	RN	RN	BE		
DATE 08/04 ROUTE IV	12:00						
PRESCRIBER'S SIGNATURE MHughes	14:00	50mg	RN	RN	BE		
	18:00						
PRESCRIBER'S NAME AND BLEEP MICHELLE HUGHES 2357	22:00	50mg	WP	CB			

NAME OF DRUG PARACETAMOL	TIME	DATE → DOSE ↓	08/04	09/04	10/04		
ADDITIONAL INSTRUCTIONS	08:00	1g	——	——	BE		
DATE 08/04 ROUTE IV	12:00	1g	——	——	BE		
PRESCRIBER'S SIGNATURE MHughes	18:00	1g	——	——	BE		
PRESCRIBER'S NAME AND BLEEP MICHELLE HUGHES 2357	22:00	1g	——	CB			

PATIENT NAME MICHAEL GOLDING   HOSPITAL NO.   014325

NAME OF DRUG	TIME	DATE → DOSE ↓					
ADDITIONAL INSTRUCTIONS	08:00						
DATE	ROUTE	12:00					
PRESCRIBER'S SIGNATURE							
	18:00						
PRESCRIBER'S NAME AND BLEEP	22:00						

NAME OF DRUG	TIME	DATE → DOSE ↓					
ADDITIONAL INSTRUCTIONS	08:00						
DATE	ROUTE	12:00					
PRESCRIBER'S SIGNATURE							
	18:00						
PRESCRIBER'S NAME AND BLEEP	22:00						

NAME OF DRUG	TIME	DATE → DOSE ↓					
ADDITIONAL INSTRUCTIONS	08:00						
DATE	ROUTE	12:00					
PRESCRIBER'S SIGNATURE							
	18:00						
PRESCRIBER'S NAME AND BLEEP	22:00						

AS REQUIRED PRESCRIPTIONS

NAME OF DRUG		DATE					
INDICATION/ INSTRUCTION	DOSE	TIME					
FREQUENCY	ROUTE	DOSE					
PRESCRIBER'S SIGNATURE		ROUTE					
PRESCRIBER'S NAME AND BLEEP		GIVEN BY					
START DATE	STOP DATE						

PATIENT NAME MICHAEL GOLDING   HOSPITAL NO.   014325

NAME OF DRUG		DATE					
INDICATION/ INSTRUCTION	DOSE	TIME					
FREQUENCY	ROUTE	DOSE					
PRESCRIBER'S SIGNATURE		ROUTE					
PRESCRIBER'S NAME AND BLEEP		GIVEN BY					
START DATE	STOP DATE						

INTRAVENOUS FLUIDS

DATE	FLUID	ADDITIVE & DOSE	VOLUME	RATE/ DURATION	PRESCRIBER'S SIGNATURE	GIVEN BY	START TIME	END TIME
09/04	HARTMANN'S	——————	1 l	10hrs	MHughes	CB	2000	0600
10/04	HARTMANN'S	——————	500ml	8 hrs	MHughes	BE	0800	1600

Record of signatures. ALL prescribers MUST complete.

DATE	NAME	DESIGNATION	SIGNATURE	BLEEP NUMBER
08/04	MICHELLE HUGHES	F2	MHughes	2357

This patient has developed refeeding syndrome, a condition characterised by large shifts in electrolytes. Electrolytes must be checked regularly and replaced to avoid complications such as cardiac arrhythmias. Refeeding syndrome usually occurs 24–72 hours after the reintroduction of nutrition in someone who is either chronically malnourished or has had little or no nutritional intake for more than 5 days.

Step 3: Compare your answer to the checklist below and the chart opposite ✔

D Details	Checked patient details Used capital letters throughout Used correct abbreviations	☐
R Regular medications	Continued regular enoxaparin, cyclizine and paracetamol	☐
U Unpleasant reactions	No allergies	☐
G Gravid?	No	☐

C Contra-indications	Not required	☐
H Hydration	There is fluid in the magnesium replacement and in TPN	☐
A Analgesia	Continued paracetamol	☐
R Renal function	Not required	☐
T Thrombo-prophylaxis	Continued enoxaparin	☐
S Signature box	Signed signature box	☐

Rationale

The introduction of parenteral nutrition has triggered the electrolyte disturbances associated with refeeding. During a period of starvation the body's store of phosphate and magnesium becomes depleted. Reintroducing nutrition reignites metabolic activity; the sudden cellular demand for phosphate and magnesium causes serum levels to fall. Both of these should be replaced promptly to prevent cardiac arrhythmias.

Magnesium is poorly absorbed from the gut and is best replaced intravenously. Oral magnesium preparations such as magnesium glycerophosphate are used for supplementation in patients with chronic magnesium losses. Intravenous magnesium replacement has been prescribed as 4g of magnesium sulphate (16mmol of magnesium) at a maximum rate of 2g/h. The magnesium has been diluted in dextrose but it is also safe to use sodium chloride 0.9%. Magnesium infusions can be repeated as needed to keep the serum magnesium level in the normal range. Up to 160mmol of magnesium over up to 5 days may be required to replace the deficit in symptomatic hypomagnesaemia.

Hypokalaemia is difficult to correct in the presence of low magnesium levels because magnesium inhibits renal loss of potassium. Sando-K has been prescribed. Consider checking magnesium levels in any patient with persistently low serum potassium.

The oral route is preferable to intravenous when replacing phosphate: intravenous replacement can cause cardiac arrhythmias and ectopic calcium deposition. There is only one oral phosphate supplement used in the UK: Phosphate-Sandoz is given as 4–6 tablets per day in divided doses, although it is not specifically licensed for hypophosphataemia associated with refeeding syndrome. Oral phosphate replacement can cause diarrhoea. If this occurs, intravenous formulations are available. Hospitals often have their own guidelines for electrolyte replacement, so always check their guidance.

KEY POINTS

- Use of TPN requires robust regular monitoring of renal function and electrolytes
- Monitor serum electrolytes closely in patients being fed after a period of malnutrition
- Check and replace magnesium in patients with intractable hypokalaemia

LONGBURY HOSPITAL TRUST				HOSPITAL NUMBER	014325		
				SURNAME	GOLDING		
REWRITTEN 08/04				FIRST NAME	MICHAEL		
				ADDRESS	12 KARATTA DRIVE, LONGBURY LB14 1ZW		
				D.O.B	10/04/YYYY (59 YEARS AGO)		
DATE OF ADMISSION	03/04/YYYY	ADMISSION WEIGHT (KG)	54kg	WARD	SURGICAL		
ALLERGIES				CONSULTANT	JOSHUA GIBB		
NKDA				CHART NO	1...OF...1		

ONCE ONLY PRESCRIPTIONS

DATE	TIME	NAME OF DRUG	DOSE	ROUTE	PRESCRIBER'S SIGNATURE	GIVEN BY	TIME GIVEN

REGULAR MEDICATIONS

NAME OF DRUG ENOXAPARIN	TIME	DATE → DOSE ↓	08/04	09/04	10/04		
ADDITIONAL INSTRUCTIONS	08:00						
DATE 08/04 ROUTE S/C	12:00						
PRESCRIBER'S SIGNATURE MHughes	18:00	40mg	———	RN	BE		
PRESCRIBER'S NAME AND BLEEP MICHELLE HUGHES 2357	22:00						

NAME OF DRUG CYCLIZINE	TIME	DATE → DOSE ↓	08/04	09/04	10/04		
ADDITIONAL INSTRUCTIONS	08:00	50mg	RN	RN	BE		
DATE 08/04 ROUTE IV	12:00						
PRESCRIBER'S SIGNATURE MHughes	14:00	50mg	RN	RN	BE		
	18:00						
PRESCRIBER'S NAME AND BLEEP MICHELLE HUGHES 2357	22:00	50mg	WP	CB			

NAME OF DRUG PARACETAMOL	TIME	DATE → DOSE ↓	08/04	09/04	10/04		
ADDITIONAL INSTRUCTIONS	08:00	1g	———	———	BE		
DATE 08/04 ROUTE IV	12:00	1g	———	———	BE		
PRESCRIBER'S SIGNATURE MHughes	18:00	1g	———	———	BE		
PRESCRIBER'S NAME AND BLEEP MICHELLE HUGHES 2357	22:00	1g	———	CB			

PATIENT NAME MICHAEL GOLDING   HOSPITAL NO. 014325

NAME OF DRUG PHOSPHATE SANDOZ	TIME	DATE → DOSE ↓			10/04		
ADDITIONAL INSTRUCTIONS	08:00	2 TABLETS			——		
							REVIEW
DATE 10/04 ROUTE PO	12:00						
PRESCRIBER'S SIGNATURE ALewis	18:00	2 TABLETS			——		
PRESCRIBER'S NAME AND BLEEP ALEX LEWIS 4567	22:00	2 TABLETS					

NAME OF DRUG SANDO K	TIME	DATE → DOSE ↓			10/04		
ADDITIONAL INSTRUCTIONS	08:00	2 TABLETS			——		
							REVIEW
DATE 10/04 ROUTE PO	12:00						
PRESCRIBER'S SIGNATURE ALewis	18:00	2 TABLETS			——		
PRESCRIBER'S NAME AND BLEEP ALEX LEWIS 4567	22:00	2 TABLETS					

NAME OF DRUG	TIME	DATE → DOSE ↓					
ADDITIONAL INSTRUCTIONS	08:00						
DATE ROUTE	12:00						
PRESCRIBER'S SIGNATURE	18:00						
PRESCRIBER'S NAME AND BLEEP	22:00						

AS REQUIRED PRESCRIPTIONS

NAME OF DRUG		DATE					
INDICATION/ INSTRUCTION	DOSE	TIME					
FREQUENCY	ROUTE	DOSE					
PRESCRIBER'S SIGNATURE		ROUTE					
PRESCRIBER'S NAME AND BLEEP							
START DATE	STOP DATE	GIVEN BY					

PATIENT NAME MICHAEL GOLDING   HOSPITAL NO.   014325

NAME OF DRUG		DATE						
INDICATION/ INSTRUCTION	DOSE	TIME						
FREQUENCY	ROUTE	DOSE						
PRESCRIBER'S SIGNATURE		ROUTE						
PRESCRIBER'S NAME AND BLEEP		GIVEN BY						
START DATE	STOP DATE							

INTRAVENOUS FLUIDS

DATE	FLUID	ADDITIVE & DOSE	VOLUME	RATE/ DURATION	PRESCRIBER'S SIGNATURE	GIVEN BY	START TIME	END TIME
09/04	HARTMANN'S	————	1 l	10hrs	MHughes	CB	2000	0600
10/04	HARTMANN'S	————	500ml	8 hrs	MHughes	BE	0800	1600
10/04	5% GLUCOSE	4g MAGNESIUM SULPHATE	500ml	2hours	ALewis			

Record of signatures. ALL prescribers MUST complete.

DATE	NAME	DESIGNATION	SIGNATURE	BLEEP NUMBER
08/04	MICHELLE HUGHES	F2	MHughes	2357
10/04	ALEX LEWIS	F1	ALewis	4567

James Gilbert (hospital number: 131986, DOB 19/02/YYYY [71 years old], address: 4 Major Lane, Longbury LB4 4YE) has been under the care of the medical team for a urinary tract infection, although his treatment for this has now finished. He is known to have atrial fibrillation and takes warfarin for this. He now presents with an acute ischaemic arm. The consultant has seen him and confirmed it is an arterial embolus and that Mr Gilbert needs to have an embolectomy in theatre.

The consultant instructs that Mr Gilbert should be started on a heparin infusion.

Your task is to prescribe the heparin infusion.
It is 12:00 on 23rd June.

Notes

Step 1: Complete your answers in the drug chart opposite and overleaf

LONGBURY HOSPITAL TRUST				HOSPITAL NUMBER	131986
				SURNAME	GILBERT
				FIRST NAME	JAMES
				ADDRESS	4 MAJOR LANE, LONGBURY LB4 4YE
				D.O.B	19/02/YYYY (71 YEARS AGO)
DATE OF ADMISSION	18/06/YYYY	ADMISSION WEIGHT (KG)	78kg	WARD	MEDICAL ASSESSMENT
ALLERGIES				CONSULTANT	ERIN JOHNSON
NKDA				CHART NO	1...OF...1

ONCE ONLY PRESCRIPTIONS

DATE	TIME	NAME OF DRUG	DOSE	ROUTE	PRESCRIBER'S SIGNATURE	GIVEN BY	TIME GIVEN

REGULAR MEDICATIONS

NAME OF DRUG		TIME	DATE → DOSE ↓					
ADDITIONAL INSTRUCTIONS		08:00						
DATE	ROUTE	12:00						
PRESCRIBER'S SIGNATURE		18:00						
PRESCRIBER'S NAME AND BLEEP		22:00						

NAME OF DRUG		TIME	DATE → DOSE ↓					
ADDITIONAL INSTRUCTIONS		08:00						
DATE	ROUTE	12:00						
PRESCRIBER'S SIGNATURE		18:00						
PRESCRIBER'S NAME AND BLEEP		22:00						

NAME OF DRUG		TIME	DATE → DOSE ↓					
ADDITIONAL INSTRUCTIONS		08:00						
DATE	ROUTE	12:00						
PRESCRIBER'S SIGNATURE		18:00						
PRESCRIBER'S NAME AND BLEEP		22:00						

PATIENT NAME JAMES GILBERT   HOSPITAL NO.   131986

NAME OF DRUG	TIME	DATE → DOSE ↓					
ADDITIONAL INSTRUCTIONS	08:00						
DATE ROUTE	12:00						
PRESCRIBER'S SIGNATURE							
	18:00						
PRESCRIBER'S NAME AND BLEEP							
	22:00						

NAME OF DRUG	TIME	DATE → DOSE ↓					
ADDITIONAL INSTRUCTIONS	08:00						
DATE ROUTE	12:00						
PRESCRIBER'S SIGNATURE							
	18:00						
PRESCRIBER'S NAME AND BLEEP							
	22:00						

NAME OF DRUG	TIME	DATE → DOSE ↓					
ADDITIONAL INSTRUCTIONS	08:00						
DATE ROUTE	12:00						
PRESCRIBER'S SIGNATURE							
	18:00						
PRESCRIBER'S NAME AND BLEEP							
	22:00						

AS REQUIRED PRESCRIPTIONS

NAME OF DRUG		DATE					
INDICATION/ INSTRUCTION	DOSE	TIME					
FREQUENCY	ROUTE	DOSE					
PRESCRIBER'S SIGNATURE		ROUTE					
PRESCRIBER'S NAME AND BLEEP							
START DATE	STOP DATE	GIVEN BY					

PATIENT NAME JAMES GILBERT   HOSPITAL NO.   131986

NAME OF DRUG		DATE						
INDICATION/ INSTRUCTION	DOSE	TIME						
FREQUENCY	ROUTE	DOSE						
PRESCRIBER'S SIGNATURE		ROUTE						
PRESCRIBER'S NAME AND BLEEP		GIVEN BY						
START DATE	STOP DATE							

ANTICOAGULATION CHART

DATE	18/06	19/06	20/06	21/06	22/06	23/06
INR	1.8	1.4	1.2	1.2	2.1	1.9
WARFARIN DOSE	3mg		3mg	5mg	5mg	
PRESCRIBER'S SIGNATURE	NShah		NShah	EJones	EJones	
GIVEN BY	MK		SS	SS	RC	
TIME	18:00		18:00	18:00	18:00	

INFUSIONS

DATE	DRUG	DILUTION FLUID	TOTAL VOLUME	RATE/ DURATION	PRESCRIBER'S SIGNATURE	GIVEN BY	START TIME	END TIME

Record of signatures. ALL prescribers MUST complete.

DATE	NAME	DESIGNATION	SIGNATURE	BLEEP NUMBER
18/06	NAZIA SHAH	F1	NShah	9761
20/06	EMMA JONES	CT1	EJones	4876

Answer 19

Patients who have atrial fibrillation are at risk of arterial embolism. The risk of an embolism causing stroke is why patients are commonly anticoagulated with warfarin. Unfortunately, this patient's warfarin prescribing has become disorganised, with an unprescribed dose which may represent a missed dose and an attempt to correct his subtherapeutic INR.

Step 3: Compare your answer to the checklist below and the chart opposite ✔

D	Details	Checked patient details Used capital letters throughout Used correct abbreviations	☐
R	Regular medications	Stopped the patient's warfarin Prescribed heparin IV 5000 units loading dose, infusion of 1200 units heparin per hour	☐
U	Unpleasant reactions	None	☐
G	Gravid?	No	☐

C	Contra-indications	Stopped warfarin while the patient is on a heparin infusion	☐
H	Hydration	Not required	☐
A	Analgesia	Not required	☐
R	Renal function	Not required	☐
T	Thrombo-prophylaxis	Noted not required because the patient is taking warfarin/heparin	☐
S	Signature box	Signed signature box	☐

Rationale

This man cannot have surgery while his clotting is deranged by warfarin. Stopping warfarin would require a day's wait for the clotting to return to normal; a full reversal of this man's warfarin to enable the surgery would put him at risk of stroke.

Heparin has a very short half-life and therefore requires continuous infusion to keep the patient anticoagulated. The advantages are that clotting returns to normal around 30 minutes after stopping the infusion and that heparin allows greater control of clotting in patients for whom prevention of clots is essential. The infusion can be stopped just before theatre and restarted immediately after.

A loading dose of heparin was needed before the infusion begins. This was prescribed as a stat dose of 5000 units. The initial dose rate for the infusion is 1200 units per hour. This needs to be adjusted according to the activated partial thromboplastin time (APTT). The APTT should be checked 6 hours after starting the infusion and 6 hours after any change to the infusion rate. Both the initial dose and the dose adjustment should be made according to the hospital protocol for heparin infusions. Pre-mixed heparin bags may be available, e.g. 1000 units/mL.

KEY POINTS

- Begin heparin infusions with a stat dose
- Use the RATE box on an infusion to specify the hourly dose of infusion to administer

LONGBURY HOSPITAL TRUST				HOSPITAL NUMBER	131986			
				SURNAME	GILBERT			
				FIRST NAME	JAMES			
				ADDRESS	4 MAJOR LANE, LONGBURY LB4 4YE			
				D.O.B	19/02/YYYY (71 YEARS AGO)			
DATE OF ADMISSION	18/06/YYYY	ADMISSION WEIGHT (KG)		78kg	WARD	MEDICAL ASSESSMENT		
ALLERGIES				CONSULTANT		ERIN JOHNSON		
NKDA				CHART NO		1...OF...1		

ONCE ONLY PRESCRIPTIONS

DATE	TIME	NAME OF DRUG	DOSE	ROUTE	PRESCRIBER'S SIGNATURE	GIVEN BY	TIME GIVEN
23/06	12:15	HEPARIN	5000 UNITS	IV	ALewis		

REGULAR MEDICATIONS

NAME OF DRUG		TIME	DATE → DOSE ↓					
ADDITIONAL INSTRUCTIONS		**08:00**						
DATE	ROUTE	**12:00**						
PRESCRIBER'S SIGNATURE		**18:00**						
PRESCRIBER'S NAME AND BLEEP		**22:00**						

NAME OF DRUG		TIME	DATE → DOSE ↓					
ADDITIONAL INSTRUCTIONS		**08:00**						
DATE	ROUTE	**12:00**						
PRESCRIBER'S SIGNATURE		**18:00**						
PRESCRIBER'S NAME AND BLEEP		**22:00**						

NAME OF DRUG		TIME	DATE → DOSE ↓					
ADDITIONAL INSTRUCTIONS		**08:00**						
DATE	ROUTE	**12:00**						
PRESCRIBER'S SIGNATURE		**18:00**						
PRESCRIBER'S NAME AND BLEEP		**22:00**						

PATIENT NAME JAMES GILBERT   HOSPITAL NO. 131986

NAME OF DRUG		TIME	DATE → DOSE ↓						
ADDITIONAL INSTRUCTIONS		08:00							
DATE	ROUTE	12:00							
PRESCRIBER'S SIGNATURE		18:00							
PRESCRIBER'S NAME AND BLEEP		22:00							

NAME OF DRUG		TIME	DATE → DOSE ↓						
ADDITIONAL INSTRUCTIONS		08:00							
DATE	ROUTE	12:00							
PRESCRIBER'S SIGNATURE		18:00							
PRESCRIBER'S NAME AND BLEEP		22:00							

NAME OF DRUG		TIME	DATE → DOSE ↓						
ADDITIONAL INSTRUCTIONS		08:00							
DATE	ROUTE	12:00							
PRESCRIBER'S SIGNATURE		18:00							
PRESCRIBER'S NAME AND BLEEP		22:00							

AS REQUIRED PRESCRIPTIONS

NAME OF DRUG		DATE					
INDICATION/ INSTRUCTION	DOSE	TIME					
FREQUENCY	ROUTE	DOSE					
PRESCRIBER'S SIGNATURE		ROUTE					
PRESCRIBER'S NAME AND BLEEP		GIVEN BY					
START DATE	STOP DATE						

PATIENT NAME JAMES GILBERT   HOSPITAL NO.   131986

NAME OF DRUG		DATE						
INDICATION/ INSTRUCTION	DOSE	TIME						
FREQUENCY	ROUTE	DOSE						
PRESCRIBER'S SIGNATURE		ROUTE						
PRESCRIBER'S NAME AND BLEEP		GIVEN BY						
START DATE	STOP DATE							

ANTICOAGULATION CHART

DATE	18/06	19/06	20/06	21/06	22/06	23/06
INR	1.8	1.4	1.2	1.2	2.1	1.9
WARFARIN DOSE	3mg		3mg	5mg	5mg	————
PRESCRIBER'S SIGNATURE	NShah		NShah	EJones	EJones	————
GIVEN BY	MK		SS	SS	RC	ALewis
TIME	18:00		18:00	18:00	18:00	STOP

INFUSIONS

DATE	DRUG	DILUTION FLUID	TOTAL VOLUME	RATE/ DURATION	PRESCRIBER'S SIGNATURE	GIVEN BY	START TIME	END TIME
23/06	HEPARIN	N/A	10ml	1.2ml/h	ALewis			
	1000 units/ml							

Record of signatures. ALL prescribers MUST complete.

DATE	NAME	DESIGNATION	SIGNATURE	BLEEP NUMBER
18/06	NAZIA SHAH	F1	NShah	9761
20/06	EMMA JONES	CT1	EJones	4876
23/06	ALEX LEWIS	F1	ALewis	4567

Christine Jackson (hospital number: 017734, DOB 12/02/YYYY [23 years old], address 2 Macia Park, Longbury LB1 9EI) has been transferred to the medical assessment ward from the emergency department. She is well known to the psychiatry service with a history of anorexia nervosa and self-harm. She takes carbamazepine as a mood stabiliser. She weighs 45kg. She took two boxes of paracetamol 8 hours ago. She is unsure how much paracetamol she swallowed as she vomited once one hour after taking the overdose. Miss Jackson has an allergy to aspirin. Her consultant is Dr Erin Johnson.

Paracetamol level 84mg/L taken one hour ago
Carbamazepine level normal
Pregnancy test negative

**Your task is to see this patient and prescribe treatment you consider necessary.
It is 14:00 on 2nd February.**

Notes

Step 1: Complete your answers in the drug chart opposite and overleaf

LONGBURY HOSPITAL TRUST			HOSPITAL NUMBER SURNAME FIRST NAME ADDRESS D.O.B		
DATE OF ADMISSION		ADMISSION WEIGHT (KG)		WARD	
ALLERGIES			CONSULTANT		
			CHART NO		…OF…

ONCE ONLY PRESCRIPTIONS

DATE	TIME	NAME OF DRUG	DOSE	ROUTE	PRESCRIBER'S SIGNATURE	GIVEN BY	TIME GIVEN

REGULAR MEDICATIONS

NAME OF DRUG	TIME	DATE → DOSE ↓					
ADDITIONAL INSTRUCTIONS	08:00						
DATE / ROUTE	12:00						
PRESCRIBER'S SIGNATURE							
	18:00						
PRESCRIBER'S NAME AND BLEEP							
	22:00						

NAME OF DRUG	TIME	DATE → DOSE ↓					
ADDITIONAL INSTRUCTIONS	08:00						
DATE / ROUTE	12:00						
PRESCRIBER'S SIGNATURE							
	18:00						
PRESCRIBER'S NAME AND BLEEP							
	22:00						

NAME OF DRUG	TIME	DATE → DOSE ↓					
ADDITIONAL INSTRUCTIONS	08:00						
DATE / ROUTE	12:00						
PRESCRIBER'S SIGNATURE							
	18:00						
PRESCRIBER'S NAME AND BLEEP							
	22:00						

PATIENT NAME   HOSPITAL NO.

		DATE →						
NAME OF DRUG	**TIME**	DOSE ↓						
ADDITIONAL INSTRUCTIONS	**08:00**							
DATE / ROUTE	**12:00**							
PRESCRIBER'S SIGNATURE								
	18:00							
PRESCRIBER'S NAME AND BLEEP								
	22:00							

		DATE →						
NAME OF DRUG	**TIME**	DOSE ↓						
ADDITIONAL INSTRUCTIONS	**08:00**							
DATE / ROUTE	**12:00**							
PRESCRIBER'S SIGNATURE								
	18:00							
PRESCRIBER'S NAME AND BLEEP								
	22:00							

		DATE →						
NAME OF DRUG	**TIME**	DOSE ↓						
ADDITIONAL INSTRUCTIONS	**08:00**							
DATE / ROUTE	**12:00**							
PRESCRIBER'S SIGNATURE								
	18:00							
PRESCRIBER'S NAME AND BLEEP								
	22:00							

AS REQUIRED PRESCRIPTIONS

NAME OF DRUG		DATE					
INDICATION/ INSTRUCTION	DOSE	TIME					
FREQUENCY	ROUTE	DOSE					
PRESCRIBER'S SIGNATURE		ROUTE					
PRESCRIBER'S NAME AND BLEEP		GIVEN BY					
START DATE	STOP DATE						

PATIENT NAME   HOSPITAL NO.

NAME OF DRUG		DATE						
INDICATION/ INSTRUCTION	DOSE	TIME						
FREQUENCY	ROUTE	DOSE						
PRESCRIBER'S SIGNATURE		ROUTE						
PRESCRIBER'S NAME AND BLEEP		GIVEN BY						
START DATE	STOP DATE							

INTRAVENOUS FLUIDS

DATE	FLUID	ADDITIVE & DOSE	VOLUME	RATE/ DURATION	PRESCRIBER'S SIGNATURE	GIVEN BY	START TIME	END TIME

Record of signatures. ALL prescribers MUST complete.

DATE	NAME	DESIGNATION	SIGNATURE	BLEEP NUMBER

Answer 20

Overdoses such as this are a common presentation to accident and emergency departments. There are a number of online toxicology databases that provide valuable information for the treatment of overdoses as well as a national poisons helpline.

Step 3: Compare your answer to the checklist below and the chart opposite ☑

D	Details	Checked patient details Used capital letters throughout Used correct abbreviations	☐
R	Regular medications	Prescribed: – 234mL acetylcysteine (NAC) over 1 hour – 512mL NAC over 4 hours – 1023mg NAC over 16 hours	☐
U	Unpleasant reactions	Wrote NKDA or equivalent	☐
G	Gravid?	No	☐

C	Contra-indications	Recognised that this patient is high-risk and requires treatment	☐
H	Hydration	Not required	☐
A	Analgesia	Not required	☐
R	Renal function	N/A	☐
T	Thrombo-prophylaxis	Not prescribed as the patient will not have significantly reduced mobility	☐
S	Signature box	Signed signature box	☐

Rationale

Toxicity is increased if there has been induction of the P450 system via use of drugs such as carbamazepine, rifampicin, phenobarbital, phenytoin and alcohol. Paracetamol overdose is often asymptomatic in the first 24–48 hours, thus prompt treatment is essential even though she may not have any obvious symptoms. Management of paracetamol overdose requires knowledge of the time elapsed since the overdose. Levels should be taken 4–8 hours after ingestion and plotted on a paracetamol poisoning treatment graph (available in formularies). This nomogram is used to decide whether treatment is required. A plasma paracetamol level of 60mg/L at 6 hours after ingestion would not warrant treatment but the same level at 8 hours would be above the treatment line. All patients should be treated as at high-risk of liver damage. Antidote treatment should be started as soon as possible after suspected paracetamol ingestion and should not be delayed while waiting for plasma assay results.

Treatment for paracetamol overdose is with acetylcysteine (NAC) in glucose 5%. Sodium chloride may be used if glucose is unsuitable. NAC is administered intravenously in three infusions of different concentrations over a total of 21 hours. NAC concentrate (200mg/mL) is diluted to create the following infusions based on the patient's body weight of 45kg (see national formulary), as has been prescribed here:
- 1st infusion, 34mL NAC in 200mL 5% glucose over 1 hour then:
- 2nd infusion, 12mL NAC in 500mL 5% glucose over 4 hour then:
- 3rd infusion, 23mL NAC in 1L 5% glucose over 16 hours.

KEY POINTS

- Paracetamol overdose should be treated promptly
- Do not delay antidote treatment while waiting for plasma assay results
- Refer to the treatment graph for thresholds in paracetamol overdose
- Make prescriptions clear when prescribing a volume rather than a dose

LONGBURY HOSPITAL TRUST

HOSPITAL NUMBER	017734
SURNAME	JACKSON
FIRST NAME	CHRISTINE
ADDRESS	2 MACIA PARK, LONGBURY LB1 9EI
D.O.B	12/02/YYYY (23 YEARS AGO)

DATE OF ADMISSION	02/02/YYYY	ADMISSION WEIGHT (KG)	45kg	WARD	MEDICAL ASSESSMENT

ALLERGIES	CONSULTANT	ERIN JOHNSON
ASPIRIN	CHART NO	1...OF...1

ONCE ONLY PRESCRIPTIONS

DATE	TIME	NAME OF DRUG	DOSE	ROUTE	PRESCRIBER'S SIGNATURE	GIVEN BY	TIME GIVEN

REGULAR MEDICATIONS

NAME OF DRUG		TIME	DATE → DOSE ↓				
ADDITIONAL INSTRUCTIONS		08:00					
DATE	ROUTE	12:00					
PRESCRIBER'S SIGNATURE		18:00					
PRESCRIBER'S NAME AND BLEEP		22:00					

NAME OF DRUG		TIME	DATE → DOSE ↓				
ADDITIONAL INSTRUCTIONS		08:00					
DATE	ROUTE	12:00					
PRESCRIBER'S SIGNATURE		18:00					
PRESCRIBER'S NAME AND BLEEP		22:00					

NAME OF DRUG		TIME	DATE → DOSE ↓				
ADDITIONAL INSTRUCTIONS		08:00					
DATE	ROUTE	12:00					
PRESCRIBER'S SIGNATURE		18:00					
PRESCRIBER'S NAME AND BLEEP		22:00					

168

PATIENT NAME *CHRISTINE JACKSON* HOSPITAL NO. *017734*

NAME OF DRUG	TIME	DATE → DOSE ↓					
ADDITIONAL INSTRUCTIONS	08:00						
DATE / ROUTE	12:00						
PRESCRIBER'S SIGNATURE							
	18:00						
PRESCRIBER'S NAME AND BLEEP	22:00						

NAME OF DRUG	TIME	DATE → DOSE ↓					
ADDITIONAL INSTRUCTIONS	08:00						
DATE / ROUTE	12:00						
PRESCRIBER'S SIGNATURE							
	18:00						
PRESCRIBER'S NAME AND BLEEP	22:00						

NAME OF DRUG	TIME	DATE → DOSE ↓					
ADDITIONAL INSTRUCTIONS	08:00						
DATE / ROUTE	12:00						
PRESCRIBER'S SIGNATURE							
	18:00						
PRESCRIBER'S NAME AND BLEEP	22:00						

AS REQUIRED PRESCRIPTIONS

NAME OF DRUG		DATE					
INDICATION/ INSTRUCTION	DOSE	TIME					
FREQUENCY	ROUTE	DOSE					
PRESCRIBER'S SIGNATURE		ROUTE					
PRESCRIBER'S NAME AND BLEEP							
START DATE	STOP DATE	GIVEN BY					

PATIENT NAME *CHRISTINE JACKSON*   HOSPITAL NO. *017734*

NAME OF DRUG		DATE						
INDICATION/ INSTRUCTION	DOSE	TIME						
FREQUENCY	ROUTE	DOSE						
PRESCRIBER'S SIGNATURE		ROUTE						
PRESCRIBER'S NAME AND BLEEP		GIVEN BY						
START DATE	STOP DATE							

INTRAVENOUS FLUIDS

DATE	FLUID	ADDITIVE & DOSE	VOLUME	RATE/ DURATION	PRESCRIBER'S SIGNATURE	GIVEN BY	START TIME	END TIME
02/02	5% GLUCOSE 200ml	ACETYLCYSTEINE 200mg/ml (34ml)	234ml	234 ml/h	ALewis			
02/02	5% GLUCOSE 500ml	ACETYLCYSTEINE 200mg/ml (12ml)	512ml	128 ml/h	ALewis			
02/02	5% GLUCOSE 1000ml	ACETYLCYSTEINE 200mg/ml (23ml)	1023ml	64ml/h	ALewis			

Record of signatures. ALL prescribers MUST complete.

DATE	NAME	DESIGNATION	SIGNATURE	BLEEP NUMBER
02/02	ALEX LEWIS	F1	ALewis	4567

Luke Butcher (hospital number: 145145, DOB 07/05/YYYY [72 years old], address: 88 Forest Street, Longbury LB8 1JY) has been admitted to the medical assessment ward overnight after his neighbours raised the alarm that they hadn't seen him leave the house for a few days. He was confused and unable to provide a history but the ambulance driver brought in his tablets, which were written up by the night doctor. His weight is 54kg. At handover the following jobs were passed on:

- Chase the blood results
- Ring Mr Butcher's general practitioner for a past medical history
- Begin investigating for causes of his presentation

At handover by the night doctor the blood results taken at 04:50 on 5th March were:

Sodium 149mmol/L
Potassium 7.9mmol/L
Urea 42mmol/L
Creatinine 782μmol/L

On further examination Mr Butcher remains confused.

Observations:

Heart rate 115bpm irregular
Respiratory rate 24 breaths/minute
Blood pressure 98/56mmHg
Apyrexial
Urine output 0.2mL/kg/h

ECG: flat P waves, wide QRS complexes and tall T waves

It is concluded that Mr Butcher is suffering severe hyperkalaemia and acute kidney injury (AKI). The registrar is called; she asks for treatment for hyperkalaemia and AKI to be commenced whilst she makes her way to the ward to help.

Your task is to prescribe treatment for hyperkalaemia.
It is 07:30 on 5 March.

Notes

LONGBURY HOSPITAL TRUST		HOSPITAL NUMBER	145145
		SURNAME	BUTCHER
		FIRST NAME	LUKE
		ADDRESS	88 FOREST STREET, LONGBURY LB8 1JY

			D.O.B	07/05/YYYY (72 YEARS AGO)
DATE OF ADMISSION	05/03/YYYY	ADMISSION WEIGHT (KG)	54kg	WARD	MEDICAL ASSESSMENT
ALLERGIES NONE KNOWN			CONSULTANT	ERIN JOHNSON
			CHART NO	1...OF...1

ONCE ONLY PRESCRIPTIONS

DATE	TIME	NAME OF DRUG	DOSE	ROUTE	PRESCRIBER'S SIGNATURE	GIVEN BY	TIME GIVEN

REGULAR MEDICATIONS

NAME OF DRUG: RAMIPRIL	TIME	DATE → DOSE ↓	05/03				
ADDITIONAL INSTRUCTIONS	08:00	10mg					
DATE 05/03 ROUTE PO	12:00						
PRESCRIBER'S SIGNATURE KCho	18:00						
PRESCRIBER'S NAME AND BLEEP KENNETH CHO 5765	22:00						

NAME OF DRUG: FUROSEMIDE	TIME	DATE → DOSE ↓	05/03				
ADDITIONAL INSTRUCTIONS	08:00	40mg					
DATE 05/03 ROUTE PO	12:00						
PRESCRIBER'S SIGNATURE KCho	18:00						
PRESCRIBER'S NAME AND BLEEP KENNETH CHO 5765	22:00						

NAME OF DRUG: SPIRONOLACTONE	TIME	DATE → DOSE ↓	05/03				
ADDITIONAL INSTRUCTIONS	08:00	50mg					
DATE 05/03 ROUTE PO	12:00						
PRESCRIBER'S SIGNATURE KCho	18:00						
PRESCRIBER'S NAME AND BLEEP KENNETH CHO 5765	22:00						

PATIENT NAME LUKE BUTCHER   HOSPITAL NO. 145145

NAME OF DRUG NAPROXEN	TIME	DATE → DOSE ↓	05/03				
ADDITIONAL INSTRUCTIONS	08:00	500mg					
DATE 05/03 ROUTE PO	12:00						
PRESCRIBER'S SIGNATURE KCho	18:00						
PRESCRIBER'S NAME AND BLEEP KENNETH CHO 5765	22:00	500mg					

NAME OF DRUG ENOXAPARIN	TIME	DATE → DOSE ↓	05/03				
ADDITIONAL INSTRUCTIONS	08:00						
DATE 05/03 ROUTE SC	12:00						
PRESCRIBER'S SIGNATURE KCho	18:00	40mg					
PRESCRIBER'S NAME AND BLEEP KENNETH CHO 5765	22:00						

NAME OF DRUG	TIME	DATE → DOSE ↓					
ADDITIONAL INSTRUCTIONS	08:00						
DATE ROUTE	12:00						
PRESCRIBER'S SIGNATURE	18:00						
PRESCRIBER'S NAME AND BLEEP	22:00						

AS REQUIRED PRESCRIPTIONS

NAME OF DRUG		DATE					
INDICATION/ INSTRUCTION	DOSE	TIME					
FREQUENCY	ROUTE	DOSE					
PRESCRIBER'S SIGNATURE		ROUTE					
PRESCRIBER'S NAME AND BLEEP		GIVEN BY					
START DATE	STOP DATE						

PATIENT NAME LUKE BUTCHER   HOSPITAL NO.   145145

NAME OF DRUG		DATE						
INDICATION/ INSTRUCTION	DOSE	TIME						
FREQUENCY	ROUTE	DOSE						
PRESCRIBER'S SIGNATURE		ROUTE						
PRESCRIBER'S NAME AND BLEEP		GIVEN BY						
START DATE	STOP DATE							

INTRAVENOUS FLUIDS

DATE	FLUID	ADDITIVE & DOSE	VOLUME	RATE/ DURATION	PRESCRIBER'S SIGNATURE	GIVEN BY	START TIME	END TIME
05/03	HARTMANN'S	————	500ml	8 hrs	KCho			

Record of signatures. ALL prescribers MUST complete.

DATE	NAME	DESIGNATION	SIGNATURE	BLEEP NUMBER
05/03	KENNETH CHO	F1	KCho	5765

Answer 21

This scenario is an examiner's favourite and requires knowledge of emergency algorithms and their application to specific patients.

Aside from knowing the treatment protocols for hyperkalaemia, it is important to think about potential causes of hyperkalaemia while going through the DRUGCHARTS mnemonic, to help weed out any exacerbating prescriptions (the ramipril, furosemide, spironolactone and naproxen).

Step 3: Compare your answer to the checklist below and the chart opposite ☑

D Details	Checked patient details Used capital letters throughout Used correct abbreviations	☐
R Regular medications	Stopped: ramipril, spironolactone, naproxen, furosemide	☐
U Unpleasant reactions	See contraindications	☐
G Gravid?	No	☐

C Contra-indications	Noticed that ramipril and spironolactone contribute to hyperkalaemia. Naproxen worsens renal failure. Furosemide worsens dehydration	☐
H Hydration	Changed fluid prescription to fluid without potassium	☐
A Analgesia	Not required	☐
R Renal function	See contraindications	☐
T Thrombo-prophylaxis	Reduced enoxaparin dose	☐
S Signature box	Signed signature box	☐

Rationale

Hyperkalaemia >7mmol/L or with evidence of cardiac instability is a medical emergency. Senior help should be sought as early as possible. Initial management aims to stabilise myocardial tissue with calcium gluconate. This has been prescribed in the once only section and is often represcribed at 15 minute intervals up to 5 times (50mL) until ECG activity normalises. The solution has to be given over 2–3 minutes and this must be specified on the prescription chart.

Once steps have been taken to stabilise myocardial tissue, insulin and salbutamol can be used to buy some time by transporting potassium from the extracellular to the intracellular space. Remember that this method is only a temporary solution as it does not eliminate potassium from the body. For this, calcium resonium could be prescribed in an attempt to bind potassium. However, use calcium resonium with caution in patients with renal failure as hypercalcaemia can result.

There is no history for this patient but his regular medications had been written up. They are all contraindicated in his current condition. Angiotensin-converting enzyme inhibitors, e.g. ramipril, and potassium-sparing diuretics, e.g. spironolactone, cause potassium retention. Naproxen is a non-steroidal anti-inflammatory and is contraindicated in renal impairment. The furosemide would, in theory, lower this patient's potassium levels; however, because he is dehydrated and this is likely to be contributing to his acute kidney injury (AKI), it is prudent to withhold furosemide until he has stabilised. The enoxaparin has been reduced to a renal dose and his fluid prescription has been amended to be without potassium.

KEY POINTS

- Omit nephrotoxins in AKI
- Treat the exacerbating factors, e.g. dehydration
- Familiarise yourself with the emergency treatment of hyperkalaemia

LONGBURY HOSPITAL TRUST

HOSPITAL NUMBER	145145
SURNAME	BUTCHER
FIRST NAME	LUKE
ADDRESS	88 FOREST STREET, LONGBURY LB8 1JY
D.O.B	07/05/YYYY (72 YEARS AGO)

DATE OF ADMISSION	05/03/YYYY	ADMISSION WEIGHT (KG)	54kg	WARD	MEDICAL ASSESSMENT

ALLERGIES	CONSULTANT	ERIN JOHNSON
NONE KNOWN	CHART NO	1...OF...1

ONCE ONLY PRESCRIPTIONS

DATE	TIME	NAME OF DRUG	DOSE	ROUTE	PRESCRIBER'S SIGNATURE	GIVEN BY	TIME GIVEN
05/03	STAT	CALCIUM GLUCONATE 10%	10ml OVER 2 MINUTES	IV	ALewis		
05/03	STAT	ACTRAPID 10 UNITS IN 50ml 50% GLUCOSE	GIVE OVER 10 MINS	IV	ALewis		
05/03	STAT	SALBUTAMOL	10mg	NEB	ALewis		

REGULAR MEDICATIONS

NAME OF DRUG RAMIPRIL	TIME	DATE → DOSE ↓	05/03				
ADDITIONAL INSTRUCTIONS	08:00	10mg	▬▬▬ ☐				
DATE 05/03 ROUTE PO	12:00		REVIEW				
PRESCRIBER'S SIGNATURE KCho			05/03				
	18:00		ALewis				
PRESCRIBER'S NAME AND BLEEP KENNETH CHO 5765	22:00						

NAME OF DRUG FUROSEMIDE	TIME	DATE → DOSE ↓	05/03				
ADDITIONAL INSTRUCTIONS	08:00	40mg	▬▬▬ ☐				
DATE 05/03 ROUTE PO	12:00		REVIEW				
PRESCRIBER'S SIGNATURE KCho			05/03				
	18:00		ALewis				
PRESCRIBER'S NAME AND BLEEP KENNETH CHO 5765	22:00						

NAME OF DRUG SPIRONOLACTONE	TIME	DATE → DOSE ↓	05/03				
ADDITIONAL INSTRUCTIONS	08:00	50mg	▬▬▬ ☐				
DATE 05/03 ROUTE PO	12:00		REVIEW				
PRESCRIBER'S SIGNATURE KCho			05/03				
	18:00		ALewis				
PRESCRIBER'S NAME AND BLEEP KENNETH CHO 5765	22:00						

PATIENT NAME LUKE BUTCHER   HOSPITAL NO.   145145

NAME OF DRUG NAPROXEN	TIME	DATE → DOSE ↓	05/03				
			▬ ▬	▬ ▬	▬ ▬	▬ ▬	▬ ▬
ADDITIONAL INSTRUCTIONS	08:00	500mg	▬ ▬	▬ ▬	▬ ▬	▬ ▬	▬ ▬
			▬ ▬	▬ ▬	▬ ▬	▬ ▬	▬ ▬
DATE 05/03 ROUTE PO	12:00		▬ ▬	STOP	▬ ▬	▬ ▬	▬ ▬
PRESCRIBER'S SIGNATURE K Cho			▬ ▬	05/03	▬ ▬	▬ ▬	▬ ▬
	18:00		▬ ▬	ALewis	▬ ▬	▬ ▬	▬ ▬
PRESCRIBER'S NAME AND BLEEP KENNETH CHO 5765	22:00	500mg	▬ ▬	▬ ▬	▬ ▬	▬ ▬	▬ ▬

NAME OF DRUG ENOXAPARIN	TIME	DATE → DOSE ↓	05/03				
ADDITIONAL INSTRUCTIONS	08:00		STOP				
			05/03				
DATE 05/03 ROUTE S/C	12:00		ALewis				
PRESCRIBER'S SIGNATURE KCho							
	18:00	40mg	▬	▬	▬	▬	▬
PRESCRIBER'S NAME AND BLEEP KENNETH CHO 5765C	22:00						

NAME OF DRUG ENOXAPARIN	TIME	DATE → DOSE ↓	05/03				
ADDITIONAL INSTRUCTIONS	08:00						
DATE 05/03 ROUTE S/C	12:00						
PRESCRIBER'S SIGNATURE ALewis							
	18:00	20mg					
PRESCRIBER'S NAME AND BLEEP ALEX LEWIS 4567	22:00						

AS REQUIRED PRESCRIPTIONS

NAME OF DRUG SALBUTAMOL		DATE					
INDICATION/ INSTRUCTION HYPERKALAEMIA ONLY	DOSE 10mg	TIME					
FREQUENCY PRN	ROUTE NEB	DOSE					
PRESCRIBER'S SIGNATURE ALewis		ROUTE					
PRESCRIBER'S NAME AND BLEEP ALEX LEWIS 4567		GIVEN BY					
START DATE 05/03	STOP DATE						

PATIENT NAME LUKE BUTCHER   HOSPITAL NO.   145145

		DATE				
NAME OF DRUG						
INDICATION/ INSTRUCTION	DOSE	TIME				
FREQUENCY	ROUTE	DOSE				
PRESCRIBER'S SIGNATURE		ROUTE				
PRESCRIBER'S NAME AND BLEEP		GIVEN BY				
START DATE	STOP DATE					

INTRAVENOUS FLUIDS

DATE	FLUID	ADDITIVE & DOSE	VOLUME	RATE/ DURATION	PRESCRIBER'S SIGNATURE	GIVEN BY	START TIME	END TIME
05/03	HARTMANN'S	————	500ml	8 hrs	KCho	STOP		
05/03	SODIUM CHLORIDE 0.9%	————	500ml	4 hrs	ALewis			

Record of signatures. ALL prescribers MUST complete.

DATE	NAME	DESIGNATION	SIGNATURE	BLEEP NUMBER
05/03	KENNETH CHO	F1	KCho	5765
05/03	ALEX LEWIS	F1	ALewis	4567

An unknown man (hospital number: UP989707) has been admitted to the emergency department after being found collapsed in an alleyway. In the ambulance he started profusely vomiting blood and has developed signs of hypovolaemic shock.

He is a young man who appears to have been living homeless and smells of alcohol. On examination he is tachycardic with a heart rate of 125bpm, blood pressure 74/63mmHg, respiratory rate 27 breaths/minute and temperature 36.7°C. During the examination he vomits fresh blood again. His Glasgow Coma Scale score is E2V2M5 (9/15) and his blood sugar level is 1.8mmol/L.

Management with oxygen, bilateral wide-bore intravenous access and blood tests are initiated. Two units of O-negative blood are collected from the blood transfusion laboratory and senior help is called for. The consultant for this patient is Dr Pradip Chand.

Your task is to prescribe blood and further supportive treatment.
It is 09:00 on 10th September.

Notes

Step 1: Complete your answers in the drug chart opposite and overleaf

LONGBURY HOSPITAL TRUST				HOSPITAL NUMBER	UP989707		
				SURNAME	UNKNOWN		
				FIRST NAME	UNKNOWN		
				ADDRESS	UNKNOWN		
				D.O.B	UNKNOWN		
DATE OF ADMISSION	10/09/YYYY	ADMISSION WEIGHT (KG)				WARD	EMERGENCY
ALLERGIES				CONSULTANT		PRADIP CHAND	
UNKNOWN				CHART NO		1...OF...1	

ONCE ONLY PRESCRIPTIONS

DATE	TIME	NAME OF DRUG	DOSE	ROUTE	PRESCRIBER'S SIGNATURE	GIVEN BY	TIME GIVEN

REGULAR MEDICATIONS

NAME OF DRUG		**TIME**	DATE → DOSE ↓				
ADDITIONAL INSTRUCTIONS		**08:00**					
DATE	ROUTE	**12:00**					
PRESCRIBER'S SIGNATURE		**18:00**					
PRESCRIBER'S NAME AND BLEEP		**22:00**					

NAME OF DRUG		**TIME**	DATE → DOSE ↓				
ADDITIONAL INSTRUCTIONS		**08:00**					
DATE	ROUTE	**12:00**					
PRESCRIBER'S SIGNATURE		**18:00**					
PRESCRIBER'S NAME AND BLEEP		**22:00**					

NAME OF DRUG		**TIME**	DATE → DOSE ↓				
ADDITIONAL INSTRUCTIONS		**08:00**					
DATE	ROUTE	**12:00**					
PRESCRIBER'S SIGNATURE		**18:00**					
PRESCRIBER'S NAME AND BLEEP		**22:00**					

180

PATIENT NAME UNKNOWN   HOSPITAL NO.   UP989707

NAME OF DRUG	TIME	DATE → DOSE ↓					
ADDITIONAL INSTRUCTIONS	08:00						
DATE	ROUTE	12:00					
PRESCRIBER'S SIGNATURE							
	18:00						
PRESCRIBER'S NAME AND BLEEP	22:00						

NAME OF DRUG	TIME	DATE → DOSE ↓					
ADDITIONAL INSTRUCTIONS	08:00						
DATE	ROUTE	12:00					
PRESCRIBER'S SIGNATURE							
	18:00						
PRESCRIBER'S NAME AND BLEEP	22:00						

NAME OF DRUG	TIME	DATE → DOSE ↓					
ADDITIONAL INSTRUCTIONS	08:00						
DATE	ROUTE	12:00					
PRESCRIBER'S SIGNATURE							
	18:00						
PRESCRIBER'S NAME AND BLEEP	22:00						

AS REQUIRED PRESCRIPTIONS

NAME OF DRUG		DATE					
INDICATION/ INSTRUCTION	DOSE	TIME					
FREQUENCY	ROUTE	DOSE					
PRESCRIBER'S SIGNATURE		ROUTE					
PRESCRIBER'S NAME AND BLEEP		GIVEN BY					
START DATE	STOP DATE						

PATIENT NAME UNKNOWN   HOSPITAL NO.   UP989707

NAME OF DRUG		DATE						
INDICATION/ INSTRUCTION	DOSE	TIME						
FREQUENCY	ROUTE	DOSE						
PRESCRIBER'S SIGNATURE		ROUTE						
PRESCRIBER'S NAME AND BLEEP		GIVEN BY						
START DATE	STOP DATE							

INTRAVENOUS FLUIDS

DATE	FLUID	ADDITIVE & DOSE	VOLUME	RATE/ DURATION	PRESCRIBER'S SIGNATURE	GIVEN BY	START TIME	END TIME

BLOOD PRODUCTS

DATE	FLUID	BATCH NUMBER	VOLUME	RATE/ DURATION	PRESCRIBER'S SIGNATURE	GIVEN BY	START TIME	END TIME

Record of signatures. ALL prescribers MUST complete.

DATE	NAME	DESIGNATION	SIGNATURE	BLEEP NUMBER

Answer 22

This patient presented with hypovolaemic shock secondary to upper gastrointestinal haemorrhage. Likely causes are either a Mallory–Weiss tear or variceal bleeding. The hypoglycaemia may be indicative of liver failure, alcohol-related hypoglycaemia, sepsis, or even the use of another substance in addition to the suspected alcohol use.

Step 3: Compare your answer to the checklist below and the chart opposite ☑

D Details	Checked patient details. Used capital letters throughout. Used correct abbreviations	☐
R Regular medications	Unknown	☐
U Unpleasant reactions	Documented that allergies were unknown	☐
G Gravid?	No	☐

C Contra-indications	Did not prescribe enoxaparin	☐
H Hydration	Prescribed IV fluid and blood for resuscitation	☐
A Analgesia	Witheld analgesia	☐
R Renal function	Unknown	☐
T Thrombo-prophylaxis	Noted that thromboprophylaxis is contraindicated	☐
S Signature box	Signed signature box	☐

Rationale

The priorities are to treat the hypovolaemia and to reverse the hypoglycaemia. The patient may have a low Glasgow Coma Score (GCS) because of shock or hypoglycaemia but once these have been treated other causes such as head injury should be considered. As the patient is young and unlikely to have cardiac pathology, aggressive fluid resuscitation should take place: 1 litre of sodium chloride 0.9% has been prescribed here but it would be appropriate to use other crystalloids. Review the patient after the initial fluid challenge and prescribe accordingly.

As the patient is bleeding, blood also forms an important part of resuscitation. The blood prescription has been written as stat. In elective transfusions, blood is given over 2–3 hours in order to monitor for hypersensitivity. In this exercise there is no time to wait. The blood being used is O negative, which is much less likely to cause a life-threatening reaction. O negative blood is usually kept in fridges near to areas that frequently deal with large haemorrhages. The emergency, surgery and obstetric departments are all likely to have a supply. Further blood products are likely to be required, but the laboratory will have had time to cross match appropriate units once initial resuscitation has taken place.

Glucose is required to correct the hypoglycaemia. In this exercise, 100mL of 20% has been prescribed, although it is acceptable to prescribe 50mL of 50% or 200mL of 10%. Lower concentration solutions are preferable as they are less viscous and less likely to cause thrombophlebitis. Remember to reassess blood sugar levels afterwards.

In this emergency scenario it is likely that further management will involve urgent endoscopy and treatment for end organ damage secondary to hypoperfusion. A full secondary survey will be required to assess for other causes of reduced GCS and shock.

While awaiting blood results it is wise to refrain from any potentially toxic analgesia and especially wise to refrain from giving prophylactic LMWH because the patient is already bleeding.

KEY POINTS

- Prescribe blood STAT in emergencies where haemorrhage is causing haemodynamic compromise
- Hypoglycaemia is life-threatening: check blood sugars regularly even after treatment
- Review the effect of fluid challenges before represcribing

LONGBURY HOSPITAL TRUST			HOSPITAL NUMBER	UP989707	
			SURNAME	UNKNOWN	
			FIRST NAME	UNKNOWN	
			ADDRESS	UNKNOWN	
			D.O.B	UNKNOWN	

DATE OF ADMISSION	10/09/YYYY	ADMISSION WEIGHT (KG)		WARD	EMERGENCY
ALLERGIES			CONSULTANT		PRADIP CHAND
UNKNOWN			CHART NO		1…OF…1

ONCE ONLY PRESCRIPTIONS

DATE	TIME	NAME OF DRUG	DOSE	ROUTE	PRESCRIBER'S SIGNATURE	GIVEN BY	TIME GIVEN
10/09	STAT	20% GLUCOSE	100ml	IV	ALewis		

REGULAR MEDICATIONS

NAME OF DRUG		TIME	DATE → DOSE ↓				
ADDITIONAL INSTRUCTIONS		08:00					
DATE	ROUTE	12:00					
PRESCRIBER'S SIGNATURE		18:00					
PRESCRIBER'S NAME AND BLEEP		22:00					

NAME OF DRUG		TIME	DATE → DOSE ↓				
ADDITIONAL INSTRUCTIONS		08:00					
DATE	ROUTE	12:00					
PRESCRIBER'S SIGNATURE		18:00					
PRESCRIBER'S NAME AND BLEEP		22:00					

NAME OF DRUG		TIME	DATE → DOSE ↓				
ADDITIONAL INSTRUCTIONS		08:00					
DATE	ROUTE	12:00					
PRESCRIBER'S SIGNATURE		18:00					
PRESCRIBER'S NAME AND BLEEP		22:00					

PATIENT NAME UNKNOWN

HOSPITAL NO. UP989707

NAME OF DRUG		TIME	DATE → DOSE ↓					
ADDITIONAL INSTRUCTIONS		08:00						
DATE	ROUTE	12:00						
PRESCRIBER'S SIGNATURE		18:00						
PRESCRIBER'S NAME AND BLEEP		22:00						

NAME OF DRUG		TIME	DATE → DOSE ↓					
ADDITIONAL INSTRUCTIONS		08:00						
DATE	ROUTE	12:00						
PRESCRIBER'S SIGNATURE		18:00						
PRESCRIBER'S NAME AND BLEEP		22:00						

NAME OF DRUG		TIME	DATE → DOSE ↓					
ADDITIONAL INSTRUCTIONS		08:00						
DATE	ROUTE	12:00						
PRESCRIBER'S SIGNATURE		18:00						
PRESCRIBER'S NAME AND BLEEP		22:00						

AS REQUIRED PRESCRIPTIONS

NAME OF DRUG		DATE					
INDICATION/ INSTRUCTION	DOSE	TIME					
FREQUENCY	ROUTE	DOSE					
PRESCRIBER'S SIGNATURE		ROUTE					
PRESCRIBER'S NAME AND BLEEP		GIVEN BY					
START DATE	STOP DATE						

PATIENT NAME UNKNOWN   HOSPITAL NO.   UP989707

NAME OF DRUG		DATE						
INDICATION/ INSTRUCTION	DOSE	TIME						
FREQUENCY	ROUTE	DOSE						
PRESCRIBER'S SIGNATURE		ROUTE						
PRESCRIBER'S NAME AND BLEEP		GIVEN BY						
START DATE	STOP DATE							

INTRAVENOUS FLUIDS

DATE	FLUID	ADDITIVE & DOSE	VOLUME	RATE/ DURATION	PRESCRIBER'S SIGNATURE	GIVEN BY	START TIME	END TIME
10/09	N.SALINE 0.9%	————	1l	STAT	A.Lewis			

BLOOD PRODUCTS

DATE	FLUID	ADDITIVE & DOSE	VOLUME	RATE/ DURATION	PRESCRIBER'S SIGNATURE	GIVEN BY	START TIME	END TIME
10/09	RED BLOOD CELLS	————	1 UNIT	STAT	A.Lewis			
10/09	RED BLOOD CELLS	————	1 UNIT	STAT	A.Lewis			

Record of signatures. ALL prescribers MUST complete.

DATE	NAME	DESIGNATION	SIGNATURE	BLEEP NUMBER
10/09	ALEX LEWIS	F1	A.Lewis	4567

Maureen Lynn (hospital number: 132389, DOB 29/09/YYYY [73 years old], address: 58 Palms Way, Longbury LB16 3WU) has been referred to the surgical team as she has developed a leg haematoma that needs evacuating under general anaesthetic. She suffers from type 2 diabetes. She is scheduled for surgery first thing tomorrow morning.

Preoperative urea and electrolytes at 12:00 19th May:
Sodium 143mmol/L
Potassium 3.4mmol/L
Urea 6.7mmol/L
Creatinine 69μmol/L
Blood glucose 7.8mmol/L

Your task is to preoperatively assess the chart and amend it as needed.
It is 13:15 on 19 May.

Notes

Step 1: Complete your answers in the drug chart opposite and overleaf

LONGBURY HOSPITAL TRUST				HOSPITAL NUMBER	132389		
				SURNAME	LYNN		
				FIRST NAME	MAUREEN		
				ADDRESS	58 PALMS WAY, LONGBURY LB16 3WU		
				D.O.B	29/09/YYYY (73 YEARS AGO)		
DATE OF ADMISSION	18/05/YYYY	ADMISSION WEIGHT (KG)		48kg	WARD	SURGERY	
ALLERGIES				CONSULTANT		JOSHUA GIBB	
NKDA				CHART NO		1...OF...1	

ONCE ONLY PRESCRIPTIONS

DATE	TIME	NAME OF DRUG	DOSE	ROUTE	PRESCRIBER'S SIGNATURE	GIVEN BY	TIME GIVEN

REGULAR MEDICATIONS

NAME OF DRUG	TIME	DATE → / DOSE ↓	18/05	19/05			
GLICLAZIDE							
ADDITIONAL INSTRUCTIONS	08:00	80mg	JC	JC			
DATE 18/05 ROUTE PO	12:00						
PRESCRIBER'S SIGNATURE BFord	18:00						
PRESCRIBER'S NAME AND BLEEP BEN FORD 1569	22:00						

NAME OF DRUG	TIME	DATE → / DOSE ↓	18/05	19/05			
METFORMIN							
ADDITIONAL INSTRUCTIONS	08:00	500mg	JC	JC			
DATE 18/05 ROUTE PO	12:00	500mg	JC	JC			
PRESCRIBER'S SIGNATURE BFord	18:00	500mg	JC				
PRESCRIBER'S NAME AND BLEEP BEN FORD 1569	22:00						

NAME OF DRUG	TIME	DATE → / DOSE ↓	18/05	19/05			
ENOXAPARIN							
ADDITIONAL INSTRUCTIONS	08:00						
DATE 18/05 ROUTE S/C	12:00						
PRESCRIBER'S SIGNATURE BFord	18:00	40mg	JC				
PRESCRIBER'S NAME AND BLEEP BEN FORD 1569	22:00						

PATIENT NAME MAUREEN LYNN   HOSPITAL NO.   132389

NAME OF DRUG PARACETAMOL	TIME	DATE → DOSE ↓	18/05	19/05			
ADDITIONAL INSTRUCTIONS	08:00	1g	JC	JC			
DATE 18/05 ROUTE PO	12:00	1g	JC	JC			
PRESCRIBER'S SIGNATURE BFord	18:00	1g	JC				
PRESCRIBER'S NAME AND BLEEP BEN FORD 1569	22:00	1g	WP				

NAME OF DRUG	TIME	DATE → DOSE ↓					
ADDITIONAL INSTRUCTIONS	08:00						
DATE ROUTE	12:00						
PRESCRIBER'S SIGNATURE	18:00						
PRESCRIBER'S NAME AND BLEEP	22:00						

NAME OF DRUG	TIME	DATE → DOSE ↓					
ADDITIONAL INSTRUCTIONS	08:00						
DATE ROUTE	12:00						
PRESCRIBER'S SIGNATURE	18:00						
PRESCRIBER'S NAME AND BLEEP	22:00						

AS REQUIRED PRESCRIPTIONS

NAME OF DRUG		DATE					
INDICATION/ INSTRUCTION	DOSE	TIME					
FREQUENCY	ROUTE	DOSE					
PRESCRIBER'S SIGNATURE		ROUTE					
PRESCRIBER'S NAME AND BLEEP		GIVEN BY					
START DATE	STOP DATE						

PATIENT NAME MAUREEN LYNN   HOSPITAL NO.   132389

NAME OF DRUG		DATE						
INDICATION/ INSTRUCTION	DOSE	TIME						
FREQUENCY	ROUTE	DOSE						
PRESCRIBER'S SIGNATURE		ROUTE						
PRESCRIBER'S NAME AND BLEEP		GIVEN BY						
START DATE	STOP DATE							

INTRAVENOUS FLUIDS

DATE	FLUID	ADDITIVE & DOSE	VOLUME	RATE/ DURATION	PRESCRIBER'S SIGNATURE	GIVEN BY	START TIME	END TIME

INSULIN SLIDING SCALE

DATE	BLOOD SUGAR LEVEL	FLUID	ADDITIVE & DOSE	VOLUME	PRESCRIBER'S SIGNATURE	START TIME	END TIME

Record of signatures. ALL prescribers MUST complete.

DATE	NAME	DESIGNATION	SIGNATURE	BLEEP NUMBER
18/05	BEN FORD	ST2	BFord	1569

Step 2: Now check your work overleaf

Answer 23

This exercise tests the reader's ability to scan a drug chart and make it safe in the preoperative setting. The main aim in preoperative prescribing is to keep the patient's physiology as stable as possible. This usually means continuing with most regular prescriptions.

Step 3: Compare your answer to the checklist below and the chart opposite ✔

D Details	Checked patient details Used capital letters throughout Used correct abbreviations	☐
R Regular medications	Noticed IV paracetamol overdose in relation to weight	☐
U Unpleasant reactions	NKDA	☐
G Gravid?	No	☐

C Contra-indications	Paracetamol 1g IV q.d.s. contraindicated if bodyweight less than 50kg: calculate at 15mg/kg per dose Sulfonylureas and biguanides are contraindicated on the morning of surgery Metformin contraindicated if GFR <60mL/min	☐
H Hydration	Prescribed slow fluids for nil by mouth period	☐
A Analgesia	Reduced paracetamol and added another analgesic for postoperative period, (maximum paracetamol dose is 720mg but writing 750mg is acceptable)	☐
R Renal function	Not required	☐
T Thrombo-prophylaxis	Stopped enoxaparin for the evening before the operation, and review it postoperatively.	☐
S Signature box	Signed signature box	☐

Rationale

In diabetes, it is preferable to omit oral hypoglycaemic agents during the nil-by-mouth period. For this patient this means omitting the sulfonylurea gliclazide (to prevent hypoglycaemia) and omitting the biguanide metformin (to prevent renal injury), on the day of surgery. Note that ideally metformin should be stopped 48 hours before elective surgery and that here the metformin prescription is for review in the afternoon on the day after operation. Review postoperative renal function and restart metformin if it has returned to baseline. Metformin must be restarted no earlier than 48 hours after surgery.

This patient has been started on a sliding scale (variable rate intravenous insulin infusion) from midnight on the day of the operation, to maintain blood glucose control in the absence of regular medications. Sliding scales are often heavily protocol-driven prescriptions and rarely require the junior doctor to write more than the fluid prescription and the addition of potassium chloride. They are particularly useful for nil-by-mouth diabetic patients already on insulin. The end time has not been fixed but REVIEW has been written; this is because diabetic control can become unpredictable postoperatively as cortisol increases insulin resistance and patients may be slow to regain normal dietary regimens.

Enoxaparin has been stopped on the evening before surgery. LMWH has a plasma half-life of around 4 hours and should be safely metabolised by the time of operation. Restart in accordance with the surgeon's instructions.

Don't forget to check all existing prescriptions on a drug chart. This patient could have received an overdose of intravenous paracetamol if changed from oral to intravenous administration without a dose adjustment, as her body weight is less than 50kg. Halve the intravenous dose to 500mg q.d.s. (or calculate at 15mg/kg per dose) to avoid hepatotoxicity, though the dose can remain at 1g for oral and rectal administration.

KEY POINTS

- Omit sulfonylureas and metformin on the day of surgery. Ideally, omit metformin from 48 hours before surgery
- Use sliding scales (VRIII) for tight diabetic control perioperatively
- Check all prescriptions on a drug chart for potential contraindications and check body weight to avoid overdose

LONGBURY HOSPITAL TRUST				HOSPITAL NUMBER	132389	
				SURNAME	LYNN	
				FIRST NAME	MAUREEN	
				ADDRESS	58 PALMS WAY, LONGBURY LB16 3WU	
				D.O.B	29/09/YYYY (73 YEARS AGO)	
DATE OF ADMISSION	18/05/YYYY	ADMISSION WEIGHT (KG)	48kg	WARD	SURGICAL	
ALLERGIES NKDA			CONSULTANT	JOSHUA GIBB		
			CHART NO	1...OF...1		

ONCE ONLY PRESCRIPTIONS

DATE	TIME	NAME OF DRUG	DOSE	ROUTE	PRESCRIBER'S SIGNATURE	GIVEN BY	TIME GIVEN

REGULAR MEDICATIONS

NAME OF DRUG GLICLAZIDE	TIME	DATE → DOSE ↓	18/05	19/05	20/05	
ADDITIONAL INSTRUCTIONS	08:00	80mg	JC	JC	— [ ] REVIEW	
DATE 18/05 ROUTE PO	12:00				ALewis	
PRESCRIBER'S SIGNATURE BFord	18:00					
PRESCRIBER'S NAME AND BLEEP BEN FORD 1569	22:00					

NAME OF DRUG METFORMIN	TIME	DATE → DOSE ↓	18/05	19/05	20/05	
ADDITIONAL INSTRUCTIONS	08:00	500mg	JC	JC	—	—
DATE 18/055 ROUTE PO	12:00	500mg	JC	JC	—	—
PRESCRIBER'S SIGNATURE BFord	18:00	500mg	JC	—	— REVIEW [ ]	
PRESCRIBER'S NAME AND BLEEP BEN FORD 1569	22:00			ALewis		

NAME OF DRUG ENOXAPARIN	TIME	DATE → DOSE ↓	18/05	19/05	20/05	
ADDITIONAL INSTRUCTIONS	08:00					
DATE 18/05 ROUTE S/C	12:00					
PRESCRIBER'S SIGNATURE BFord	18:00	40mg	JC	— STOP		
PRESCRIBER'S NAME AND BLEEP BEN FORD 1569	22:00			ALewis		

PATIENT NAME MAUREEN LYNN   HOSPITAL NO. 132389

NAME OF DRUG PARACETAMOL	TIME	DATE → DOSE ↓	18/05	19/05			
ADDITIONAL INSTRUCTIONS	08:00	1g	JC	JC	——	——	——
DATE 18/05 ROUTE PO	12:00	1g	JC	JC	——	——	——
PRESCRIBER'S SIGNATURE BFord				STOP ALewis 19/05			
	18:00	1g	JC	——	——	——	——
PRESCRIBER'S NAME AND BLEEP BEN FORD 1569	22:00	1g	WP				

NAME OF DRUG PARACETAMOL	TIME	DATE → DOSE ↓	18/05	19/05	20/05		
ADDITIONAL INSTRUCTIONS	08:00	500mg	——	——			
DATE 19/05 ROUTE IV	12:00	500mg	——	——			
PRESCRIBER'S SIGNATURE ALewis	18:00	500mg	——				
PRESCRIBER'S NAME AND BLEEP ALEX LEWIS 4567	22:00	500mg	——				

NAME OF DRUG CODEINE	TIME	DATE → DOSE ↓	18/05	19/05	20/05		
ADDITIONAL INSTRUCTIONS	08:00	30-60mg	——	——			
DATE 19/05 ROUTE PO	12:00	30-60mg	——	——			
PRESCRIBER'S SIGNATURE ALewis	18:00	30-60mg	——	——			
PRESCRIBER'S NAME AND BLEEP ALEX LEWIS 4567	22:00	30-60mg	——	——			

AS REQUIRED PRESCRIPTIONS

NAME OF DRUG		DATE					
INDICATION/ INSTRUCTION	DOSE	TIME					
FREQUENCY	ROUTE	DOSE					
PRESCRIBER'S SIGNATURE		ROUTE					
PRESCRIBER'S NAME AND BLEEP		GIVEN BY					
START DATE	STOP DATE						

PATIENT NAME MAUREEN LYNN   HOSPITAL NO.   132389

NAME OF DRUG		DATE					
INDICATION/ INSTRUCTION	DOSE	TIME					
FREQUENCY	ROUTE	DOSE					
PRESCRIBER'S SIGNATURE		ROUTE					
PRESCRIBER'S NAME AND BLEEP		GIVEN BY					
START DATE	STOP DATE						

INTRAVENOUS FLUIDS

DATE	FLUID	ADDITIVE & DOSE	VOLUME	RATE/ DURATION	PRESCRIBER'S SIGNATURE	GIVEN BY	START TIME	END TIME
20/05	N.SALINE 0.9%	——————	500ml	8hrs	A.Lewis			

INSULIN SLIDING SCALE

DATE	BLOOD SUGAR LEVEL	FLUID	ADDITIVE & DOSE	VOLUME	PRESCRIBER'S SIGNATURE	START TIME	END TIME
20/05	7.8	5% DEXTROSE	20 mmol KCl	500ml	A.Lewis	00:00hrs	R/V POST OP
			SOLUBLE INSULIN X UNITS AS PER LOCAL PROTOCOL				

Record of signatures. ALL prescribers MUST complete.

DATE	NAME	DESIGNATION	SIGNATURE	BLEEP NUMBER
18/05	BEN FORD	ST2	BFord	1569
19/05	ALEX LEWIS	F1	A.Lewis	4567

Rebecca Fowler (hospital number: 876768, DOB 31/10/YYYY [23 years old], address: 3A Farleigh Place, Longbury LB12 9NE) was admitted to the medical assessment ward with shortness of breath after visiting a pet shop. Pulmonary embolism was excluded by the admitting team and she has been admitted to the medical admissions unit for monitoring and further treatment. She is a non-smoker and works in a local bank. Aside from shortness of breath she is also complaining of a headache.

   On examination Ms Fowler's chest is wheezy and she has a reduced peak flow (48% of predicted), she is struggling to talk in full sentences and is tachycardic. Her blood pressure is normal. Her respiratory rate is 25 breaths/minute and her arterial blood gases are normal except for a mild respiratory alkalosis. She is receiving 0.5L of oxygen via nasal cannulae. Her urine output is 0.38mL/kg/h. She has a positive pregnancy test, and on questioning reveals her last menstrual period was 9 weeks ago. She states that plasters and nickel give her a rash. Ms Fowler's admission weight is 77kg and her consultant is Dr Erin Johnson.

Your task is to prescribe treatment for an exacerbation of asthma.
It is 11:30 on 14th December.

Notes

LONGBURY HOSPITAL TRUST		HOSPITAL NUMBER SURNAME FIRST NAME ADDRESS			
		D.O.B			
DATE OF ADMISSION		ADMISSION WEIGHT (KG)		WARD	
ALLERGIES		CONSULTANT			
		CHART NO		…OF…	

ONCE ONLY PRESCRIPTIONS

DATE	TIME	NAME OF DRUG	DOSE	ROUTE	PRESCRIBER'S SIGNATURE	GIVEN BY	TIME GIVEN

REGULAR MEDICATIONS

NAME OF DRUG		TIME	DATE → DOSE ↓				
ADDITIONAL INSTRUCTIONS		08:00					
DATE	ROUTE	12:00					
PRESCRIBER'S SIGNATURE		18:00					
PRESCRIBER'S NAME AND BLEEP		22:00					

NAME OF DRUG		TIME	DATE → DOSE ↓				
ADDITIONAL INSTRUCTIONS		08:00					
DATE	ROUTE	12:00					
PRESCRIBER'S SIGNATURE		18:00					
PRESCRIBER'S NAME AND BLEEP		22:00					

NAME OF DRUG		TIME	DATE → DOSE ↓				
ADDITIONAL INSTRUCTIONS		08:00					
DATE	ROUTE	12:00					
PRESCRIBER'S SIGNATURE		18:00					
PRESCRIBER'S NAME AND BLEEP		22:00					

PATIENT NAME

HOSPITAL NO.

NAME OF DRUG		TIME	DATE → DOSE ↓						
ADDITIONAL INSTRUCTIONS		08:00							
DATE	ROUTE	12:00							
PRESCRIBER'S SIGNATURE									
		18:00							
PRESCRIBER'S NAME AND BLEEP									
		22:00							

NAME OF DRUG		TIME	DATE → DOSE ↓						
ADDITIONAL INSTRUCTIONS		08:00							
DATE	ROUTE	12:00							
PRESCRIBER'S SIGNATURE									
		18:00							
PRESCRIBER'S NAME AND BLEEP									
		22:00							

NAME OF DRUG		TIME	DATE → DOSE ↓						
ADDITIONAL INSTRUCTIONS		08:00							
DATE	ROUTE	12:00							
PRESCRIBER'S SIGNATURE									
		18:00							
PRESCRIBER'S NAME AND BLEEP									
		22:00							

AS REQUIRED PRESCRIPTIONS

NAME OF DRUG		DATE						
INDICATION/ INSTRUCTION	DOSE	TIME						
FREQUENCY	ROUTE	DOSE						
PRESCRIBER'S SIGNATURE		ROUTE						
PRESCRIBER'S NAME AND BLEEP								
START DATE	STOP DATE	GIVEN BY						

PATIENT NAME   HOSPITAL NO.

NAME OF DRUG		DATE						
INDICATION/ INSTRUCTION	DOSE	TIME						
FREQUENCY	ROUTE	DOSE						
PRESCRIBER'S SIGNATURE		ROUTE						
PRESCRIBER'S NAME AND BLEEP		GIVEN BY						
START DATE	STOP DATE							

INTRAVENOUS FLUIDS

DATE	FLUID	ADDITIVE & DOSE	VOLUME	RATE/ DURATION	PRESCRIBER'S SIGNATURE	GIVEN BY	START TIME	END TIME

Record of signatures. ALL prescribers MUST complete.

DATE	NAME	DESIGNATION	SIGNATURE	BLEEP NUMBER

Step 2: Now check your work overleaf

Answer 24

This woman is suffering from a severe acute asthma attack. Prescribing is complicated by her recent positive pregnancy test. The fact that she is pregnant should prompt you to consider whether this drug safe in pregnancy or not.

Step 3: Compare your answer to the checklist below and the chart opposite ✔

D	Details	Checked patient details Used capital letters throughout Used correct abbreviations	☐	**C**	Contra-indications	None	☐
R	Regular medications	None	☐	**H**	Hydration	Prescribed maintenance fluid as patient is pregnant and oliguric	☐
U	Unpleasant reactions	None	☐	**A**	Analgesia	Prescribed paracetamol according to the pain ladder	☐
G	Gravid?	Yes. Checked the formulary for every medication	☐	**R**	Renal function	Not required	☐
				T	Thrombo-prophylaxis	Not required	☐
				S	Signature box	Signed signature box	☐

Rationale

It is imperative to gain control of this patient's asthma as soon as possible. Once the need for aggressive treatment has been recognised, the next step is to check that the medications you are going to prescribe are safe in pregnancy. The treatment for acute asthma exacerbation is corticosteroids plus inhaled beta-adrenergic agonists and muscarinic antagonists. Inhaled medications are prescribed via the nebulised route, which is considered safe in pregnancy. It is worth noting that prednisolone has been chosen as the corticosteroid: steroids vary in their ability to cross the placenta and approximately 88% of prednisolone is inactivated as it crosses. This makes it a safer choice and the risks of giving it are outweighed by the benefits of improved asthma control.

The nebulisers have been prescribed regularly, as a stat dose and as required. Regular ipratropium nebulisers form part of the treatment of acute severe asthma. In less severe exacerbations they are not required.

Although observations appear normal for this patient it is apparent she is mildly oliguric, with urine output of 0.38mL/kg/h. She is compensating for her mild dehydration at present but this will be at the expense of placental perfusion: therefore fluid resuscitation is indicated.

KEY POINTS

- Check all medications before prescribing in pregnancy
- Tight control of asthma is essential in pregnancy
- Assess the asthma patient fully: is further support required (e.g. fluids)?
- Physiological compensation in pregnancy can come at the expense of placental perfusion: reassess the patient frequently

<table>
<tr><td rowspan="4">**LONGBURY HOSPITAL TRUST**</td><td>HOSPITAL NUMBER</td><td>876768</td></tr>
<tr><td>SURNAME</td><td>FOWLER</td></tr>
<tr><td>FIRST NAME</td><td>REBECCA</td></tr>
<tr><td>ADDRESS</td><td>3A FARLEIGH PLACE, LONGBURY
LB12 9NE</td></tr>
</table>

			D.O.B		31/10/YYYY (23 YEARS AGO)
DATE OF ADMISSION	14/12/YYYY	ADMISSION WEIGHT (KG)	77kg	WARD	MEDICAL ASSESSMENT
ALLERGIES			CONSULTANT		ERIN JOHNSON
PLASTERS - RASH, NICKEL - RASH, ANIMAL FUR?			CHART NO		1...OF...1

ONCE ONLY PRESCRIPTIONS

DATE	TIME	NAME OF DRUG	DOSE	ROUTE	PRESCRIBER'S SIGNATURE	GIVEN BY	TIME GIVEN
14/12	STAT	IPRATROPIUM BROMIDE	500 micrograms	NEB	A Lewis		
14/12	STAT	SALBUTAMOL	5 mg	NEB	A Lewis		
14/12	STAT	PRESNISOLONE	40MG	PO	A Lewis		

REGULAR MEDICATIONS

NAME OF DRUG SALBUTAMOL	TIME	DATE → DOSE ↓	14/12				
ADDITIONAL INSTRUCTIONS	08:00	5mg	X				
DATE 14/12 ROUTE NEB	12:00	5mg					
PRESCRIBER'S SIGNATURE A Lewis	18:00	5mg					
PRESCRIBER'S NAME AND BLEEP ALEX LEWIS 4567	22:00	5mg					

NAME OF DRUG IPRATROPIUM BROMIDE	TIME	DATE → DOSE ↓	14/12				
ADDITIONAL INSTRUCTIONS	08:00	500 micrograms	X				
DATE 14/12 ROUTE NEB	12:00	500 micrograms					
PRESCRIBER'S SIGNATURE A Lewis	18:00	500 micrograms					
PRESCRIBER'S NAME AND BLEEP ALEX LEWIS 4567	22:00	500 micrograms					

NAME OF DRUG PARACETAMOL	TIME	DATE → DOSE ↓	14/12				
ADDITIONAL INSTRUCTIONS	08:00	1g	X				
DATE 14/12 ROUTE PO	12:00	1g					
PRESCRIBER'S SIGNATURE A Lewis	18:00	1g					
PRESCRIBER'S NAME AND BLEEP ALEX LEWIS 4567	22:00	1g					

PATIENT NAME *REBECCA FOWLER* HOSPITAL NO. *876768*

NAME OF DRUG *PREDNISOLONE*	TIME	DATE → DOSE ↓	*14/12*				
ADDITIONAL INSTRUCTIONS	08:00	*40mg*	X				
DATE *14/12* ROUTE *PO*	12:00						*REVIEW (5 DAYS)*
PRESCRIBER'S SIGNATURE *ALewis*	18:00						
PRESCRIBER'S NAME AND BLEEP *ALEX LEWIS 4567*	22:00						

NAME OF DRUG	TIME	DATE → DOSE ↓					
ADDITIONAL INSTRUCTIONS	08:00						
DATE ROUTE	12:00						
PRESCRIBER'S SIGNATURE	18:00						
PRESCRIBER'S NAME AND BLEEP	22:00						

NAME OF DRUG	TIME	DATE → DOSE ↓					
ADDITIONAL INSTRUCTIONS	08:00						
DATE ROUTE	12:00						
PRESCRIBER'S SIGNATURE	18:00						
PRESCRIBER'S NAME AND BLEEP	22:00						

AS REQUIRED PRESCRIPTIONS

NAME OF DRUG *SALBUTAMOL*		DATE					
INDICATION/ INSTRUCTION *BREATHLESSNESS*	DOSE *5mg*	TIME					
FREQUENCY *PRN*	ROUTE *NEB*	DOSE					
PRESCRIBER'S SIGNATURE *ALewis*		ROUTE					
PRESCRIBER'S NAME AND BLEEP *ALEX LEWIS 4567*		GIVEN BY					
START DATE *14/12*	STOP DATE						

PATIENT NAME *REBECCA FOWLER*   HOSPITAL NO. *876768*

NAME OF DRUG *IPRATROPIUM BROMIDE*		DATE						
INDICATION/ INSTRUCTION *BREATHLESSNESS*	DOSE *500 micrograms*	TIME						
FREQUENCY *PRN*	ROUTE *NEB*	DOSE						
PRESCRIBER'S SIGNATURE *ALewis*		ROUTE						
PRESCRIBER'S NAME AND BLEEP *ALEX LEWIS 4567*		GIVEN BY						
START DATE *14/12*	STOP DATE							

INTRAVENOUS FLUIDS

DATE	FLUID	ADDITIVE & DOSE	VOLUME	RATE/ DURATION	PRESCRIBER'S SIGNATURE	GIVEN BY	START TIME	END TIME
14/12	*HARTMANN'S*	————————	*1l*	*8 hrs*	*ALewis*			

Record of signatures. ALL prescribers MUST complete.

DATE	NAME	DESIGNATION	SIGNATURE	BLEEP NUMBER
14/12	*ALEX LEWIS*	*F1*	*ALewis*	*4567*

Joanna May (hospital number: 982567, DOB 14/04/YYYY [31 years old], address: 7 Salina Road, Longbury LB7 6PN) has been admitted to the medical assessment ward after she presented to her general practitioner with breathlessness. She has a past medical history of deep vein thrombosis (DVT) and her general practitioner discovered her to have low oxygen saturation (93% on air) and tachycardia, so decided to refer her to exclude pulmonary embolism. She is a non-smoker who is breastfeeding her second child.

Observations:
SaO_2 on air 94%
Heart rate 94bpm
Respiratory rate 23 breaths/minute
Blood pressure 100/65mmHg

Pregnancy test: negative

Chest X-ray: mild right middle lobe consolidation in keeping with infection

CT pulmonary angiogram: no evidence of pulmonary embolism

The consultant has decided Mrs May should be started on monotherapy with an oral antibiotic and discharged the following morning if she is stable. The hospital's policy is to use amoxicillin or doxycycline for this condition. She does not require fluids.

Your task is to prescribe appropriate antibiotic therapy.
It is 22:00 on 15th July.

Notes

Step 1: Complete your answers in the drug chart opposite and overleaf

LONGBURY HOSPITAL TRUST				HOSPITAL NUMBER	982567		
				SURNAME	MAY		
				FIRST NAME	JOANNA		
				ADDRESS	7 SALINA ROAD, LONGBURY LB7 6PN		
					14/04/YYYY (31 YEARS AGO)		
				D.O.B			
DATE OF ADMISSION	15/07/YYYY	ADMISSION WEIGHT (KG)	65kg	WARD	MEDICAL ASSESSMENT		
ALLERGIES				CONSULTANT	ERIN JOHNSON		
ERYTHROMYCIN - RASH				CHART NO	1...OF...1		

ONCE ONLY PRESCRIPTIONS

DATE	TIME	NAME OF DRUG	DOSE	ROUTE	PRESCRIBER'S SIGNATURE	GIVEN BY	TIME GIVEN
15/07	STAT	PARACETAMOL	1g	PO	MHughes	HJ	2015

REGULAR MEDICATIONS

NAME OF DRUG		TIME	DATE → DOSE ↓				
ADDITIONAL INSTRUCTIONS		08:00					
DATE	ROUTE	12:00					
PRESCRIBER'S SIGNATURE		18:00					
PRESCRIBER'S NAME AND BLEEP		22:00					

NAME OF DRUG		TIME	DATE → DOSE ↓				
ADDITIONAL INSTRUCTIONS		08:00					
DATE	ROUTE	12:00					
PRESCRIBER'S SIGNATURE		18:00					
PRESCRIBER'S NAME AND BLEEP		22:00					

NAME OF DRUG		TIME	DATE → DOSE ↓				
ADDITIONAL INSTRUCTIONS		08:00					
DATE	ROUTE	12:00					
PRESCRIBER'S SIGNATURE		18:00					
PRESCRIBER'S NAME AND BLEEP		22:00					

PATIENT NAME JOANNA MAY   HOSPITAL NO.   982567

NAME OF DRUG		TIME	DATE → DOSE ↓					
ADDITIONAL INSTRUCTIONS		08:00						
DATE	ROUTE	12:00						
PRESCRIBER'S SIGNATURE								
		18:00						
PRESCRIBER'S NAME AND BLEEP								
		22:00						

NAME OF DRUG		TIME	DATE → DOSE ↓					
ADDITIONAL INSTRUCTIONS		08:00						
DATE	ROUTE	12:00						
PRESCRIBER'S SIGNATURE								
		18:00						
PRESCRIBER'S NAME AND BLEEP								
		22:00						

NAME OF DRUG		TIME	DATE → DOSE ↓					
ADDITIONAL INSTRUCTIONS		08:00						
DATE	ROUTE	12:00						
PRESCRIBER'S SIGNATURE								
		18:00						
PRESCRIBER'S NAME AND BLEEP								
		22:00						

AS REQUIRED PRESCRIPTIONS

NAME OF DRUG		DATE					
INDICATION/ INSTRUCTION	DOSE	TIME					
FREQUENCY	ROUTE	DOSE					
PRESCRIBER'S SIGNATURE		ROUTE					
PRESCRIBER'S NAME AND BLEEP							
START DATE	STOP DATE	GIVEN BY					

PATIENT NAME JOANNA MAY   HOSPITAL NO.   982567

NAME OF DRUG			DATE					
INDICATION/ INSTRUCTION	DOSE		TIME					
FREQUENCY	ROUTE		DOSE					
PRESCRIBER'S SIGNATURE			ROUTE					
PRESCRIBER'S NAME AND BLEEP			GIVEN BY					
START DATE	STOP DATE							

INTRAVENOUS FLUIDS

DATE	FLUID	ADDITIVE & DOSE	VOLUME	RATE/ DURATION	PRESCRIBER'S SIGNATURE	GIVEN BY	START TIME	END TIME

Record of signatures. ALL prescribers MUST complete.

DATE	NAME	DESIGNATION	SIGNATURE	BLEEP NUMBER
15/07	MICHELLE HUGHES	F1	MHughes	2357

Answer 25

In this exercise, be alert to the fact the patient is breastfeeding. It is always prudent to check every drug before you prescribe for a breastfeeding woman.

Step 3: Compare your answer to the checklist below and the chart opposite ☑

D Details	Checked patient details	☐
	Used capital letters throughout	
	Used correct abbreviations	
R Regular medications	No regular medications	☐
U Unpleasant reactions	See below	☐
G Gravid?	Recognised that the patient was breastfeeding and reviewed all medications before prescribing	☐

C Contra-indications	Enoxaparin and doxycycline not recommended	☐
H Hydration	Recognised there was no indication to provide fluids IV	☐
A Analgesia	Prescribed paracetamol 1g	☐
R Renal function	Not required	☐
T Thrombo-prophylaxis	Enoxaparin not recommended in breastfeeding Prescribed TED stockings	☐
S Signature box	Signed signature box	☐

Rationale

Amoxicillin has been prescribed rather than doxycycline because it is known to be safe in breastfeeding (there is a risk of tetracyclines causing teeth discolouration in breastfeeding infants).

Despite this patient's history of DVT, enoxaparin has not been prescribed. Some specialist sources advise that LMWHs are safe to use in breastfeeding, so a consideration of the risk/benefit ratio must be made. For a patient with a high risk of DVT the benefit of prescribing enoxaparin would outweigh the risks. However, this patient should be relatively mobile and is likely to be in hospital less than 1 day. Thus, thromboembolic deterrent (TED) stockings have been prescribed instead. Some hospital drug charts have a thromboprophylaxis algorithm with a specific box in which you can prescribe these.

Paracetamol is safe to prescribe in breastfeeding because clinically insignificant amounts are delivered to breast milk.

The amoxicillin prescription has a review date on it: when you write the discharge letter for the general practitioner remember to include this.

KEY POINTS

- Always consider pregnancy/breastfeeding in a woman of child bearing age
- Check every drug in the formulary if the patient is breastfeeding. If unsure, use specialist sources or consult a pharmacist or speciality doctor
- Add a review date when prescribing antibiotics

LONGBURY HOSPITAL TRUST			HOSPITAL NUMBER	982567		
			SURNAME	MAY		
			FIRST NAME	JOANNA		
			ADDRESS	7 SALINA ROAD, LONGBURY LB7 6PN		
			D.O.B	14/04/YYYY (31 YEARS AGO)		
DATE OF ADMISSION	15/07/YYYY	ADMISSION WEIGHT (KG)	65kg	WARD	MEDICAL ASSESSMENT	
ALLERGIES			CONSULTANT		ERIN JOHNSON	
ERYTHROMYCIN - RASH			CHART NO		1...OF...1	

ONCE ONLY PRESCRIPTIONS

DATE	TIME	NAME OF DRUG	DOSE	ROUTE	PRESCRIBER'S SIGNATURE	GIVEN BY	TIME GIVEN
15/07	STAT	PARACETAMOL	1g	PO	MHughes	HJ	2015

REGULAR MEDICATIONS

NAME OF DRUG AMOXICILLIN	TIME	DATE → DOSE ↓	15/07				
ADDITIONAL INSTRUCTIONS CHEST INFECTION	06:00	500mg	X				R/V DAY 5
DATE 15/07 ROUTE PO	12:00						
PRESCRIBER'S SIGNATURE ALewis	14:00	500mg	X				
	18:00						
PRESCRIBER'S NAME AND BLEEP ALEX LEWIS 4567	22:00	500mg					

NAME OF DRUG PARACETAMOL	TIME	DATE → DOSE ↓	15/07				
ADDITIONAL INSTRUCTIONS	08:00	1g	X				
DATE 15/07 ROUTE PO	12:00	1g	X				
PRESCRIBER'S SIGNATURE ALewis	18:00	1g	X				
PRESCRIBER'S NAME AND BLEEP ALEX LEWIS 4567	22:00	1g					

NAME OF DRUG TEDS STOCKINGS	TIME	DATE → DOSE ↓	15/07				
		ALL DAY					
ADDITIONAL INSTRUCTIONS	08:00						
DATE 15/07 ROUTE LEGS	14:00						
PRESCRIBER'S SIGNATURE ALewis	18:00						
PRESCRIBER'S NAME AND BLEEP ALEX LEWIS 4567	22:00						

PATIENT NAME JOANNA MAY   HOSPITAL NO. 982567

NAME OF DRUG		TIME	DATE → DOSE ↓					
ADDITIONAL INSTRUCTIONS		08:00						
DATE	ROUTE	12:00						
PRESCRIBER'S SIGNATURE		18:00						
PRESCRIBER'S NAME AND BLEEP		22:00						

NAME OF DRUG		TIME	DATE → DOSE ↓					
ADDITIONAL INSTRUCTIONS		08:00						
DATE	ROUTE	12:00						
PRESCRIBER'S SIGNATURE		18:00						
PRESCRIBER'S NAME AND BLEEP		22:00						

NAME OF DRUG		TIME	DATE → DOSE ↓					
ADDITIONAL INSTRUCTIONS		08:00						
DATE	ROUTE	12:00						
PRESCRIBER'S SIGNATURE		18:00						
PRESCRIBER'S NAME AND BLEEP		22:00						

AS REQUIRED PRESCRIPTIONS

NAME OF DRUG		DATE					
INDICATION/ INSTRUCTION	DOSE	TIME					
FREQUENCY	ROUTE	DOSE					
PRESCRIBER'S SIGNATURE		ROUTE					
PRESCRIBER'S NAME AND BLEEP		GIVEN BY					
START DATE	STOP DATE						

PATIENT NAME JOANNA MAY   HOSPITAL NO.   982567

NAME OF DRUG		DATE						
INDICATION/ INSTRUCTION	DOSE	TIME						
FREQUENCY	ROUTE	DOSE						
PRESCRIBER'S SIGNATURE		ROUTE						
PRESCRIBER'S NAME AND BLEEP		GIVEN BY						
START DATE	STOP DATE							

INTRAVENOUS FLUIDS

DATE	FLUID	ADDITIVE & DOSE	VOLUME	RATE/ DURATION	PRESCRIBER'S SIGNATURE	GIVEN BY	START TIME	END TIME

Record of signatures. ALL prescribers MUST complete.

DATE	NAME	DESIGNATION	SIGNATURE	BLEEP NUMBER
15/07	MICHELLE HUGHES	F1	MHughes	2357
15/07	ALEX LEWIS	F1	ALewis	4567

Jocelyn Walker (hospital number: 673225, DOB 31/10/YYYY [82 years old], address: 95 Taxus Road, LB1 5LO) has been admitted to the medical assessment ward from her nursing home feeling generally unwell. She suffered a stroke 2 years ago and has since had difficulty swallowing. Her carers have reported that she has been unwell for the last 3 days and has eaten and drunk very little, although she has been taking her regular medications. They have supplied a list of her medications:

Bisoprolol 2.5mg o.d.
Furosemide 40mg b.d.
Ramipril 5mg o.d.
Clopidogrel 75mg o.d.

Mrs Walker is not allergic to any medications.

On examination her jugular venous pressure is not visible and her lips are dry. Her observations are stable and she is apyrexial. Her weight is recorded as 72kg. Mrs Walker's consultant is Dr Erin Johnson.

Her blood test results show:
Sodium 165mmol/L
Potassium 3.6mmol/L
Urea 8.9mmol/L
Creatinine 123µmol/L
eGFR 38mL/min/1.73m^2

Your task is to prescribe the regular medications and any others you consider necessary.
It is 10:00 on 4th July.

Notes

Step 1: Complete your answers in the drug chart opposite and overleaf

LONGBURY HOSPITAL TRUST		HOSPITAL NUMBER SURNAME FIRST NAME ADDRESS				
		D.O.B				
DATE OF ADMISSION		ADMISSION WEIGHT (KG)		WARD		
ALLERGIES		CONSULTANT				
		CHART NO			…OF…	

ONCE ONLY PRESCRIPTIONS

DATE	TIME	NAME OF DRUG	DOSE	ROUTE	PRESCRIBER'S SIGNATURE	GIVEN BY	TIME GIVEN

REGULAR MEDICATIONS

NAME OF DRUG		TIME	DATE → DOSE ↓				
ADDITIONAL INSTRUCTIONS		08:00					
DATE	ROUTE	12:00					
PRESCRIBER'S SIGNATURE		18:00					
PRESCRIBER'S NAME AND BLEEP		22:00					

NAME OF DRUG		TIME	DATE → DOSE ↓				
ADDITIONAL INSTRUCTIONS		08:00					
DATE	ROUTE	12:00					
PRESCRIBER'S SIGNATURE		18:00					
PRESCRIBER'S NAME AND BLEEP		22:00					

NAME OF DRUG		TIME	DATE → DOSE ↓				
ADDITIONAL INSTRUCTIONS		08:00					
DATE	ROUTE	12:00					
PRESCRIBER'S SIGNATURE		18:00					
PRESCRIBER'S NAME AND BLEEP		22:00					

PATIENT NAME   HOSPITAL NO.

NAME OF DRUG		TIME	DATE → DOSE ↓					
ADDITIONAL INSTRUCTIONS		08:00						
DATE	ROUTE	12:00						
PRESCRIBER'S SIGNATURE								
		18:00						
PRESCRIBER'S NAME AND BLEEP								
		22:00						

NAME OF DRUG		TIME	DATE → DOSE ↓					
ADDITIONAL INSTRUCTIONS		08:00						
DATE	ROUTE	12:00						
PRESCRIBER'S SIGNATURE								
		18:00						
PRESCRIBER'S NAME AND BLEEP								
		22:00						

NAME OF DRUG		TIME	DATE → DOSE ↓					
ADDITIONAL INSTRUCTIONS		08:00						
DATE	ROUTE	12:00						
PRESCRIBER'S SIGNATURE								
		18:00						
PRESCRIBER'S NAME AND BLEEP								
		22:00						

AS REQUIRED PRESCRIPTIONS

NAME OF DRUG		DATE					
INDICATION/ INSTRUCTION	DOSE	TIME					
FREQUENCY	ROUTE	DOSE					
PRESCRIBER'S SIGNATURE		ROUTE					
PRESCRIBER'S NAME AND BLEEP		GIVEN BY					
START DATE	STOP DATE						

PATIENT NAME   HOSPITAL NO.

NAME OF DRUG		DATE					
INDICATION/ INSTRUCTION	DOSE	TIME					
FREQUENCY	ROUTE	DOSE					
PRESCRIBER'S SIGNATURE		ROUTE					
PRESCRIBER'S NAME AND BLEEP		GIVEN BY					
START DATE	STOP DATE						

INTRAVENOUS FLUIDS

DATE	FLUID	ADDITIVE & DOSE	VOLUME	RATE/ DURATION	PRESCRIBER'S SIGNATURE	GIVEN BY	START TIME	END TIME

Record of signatures. ALL prescribers MUST complete.

DATE	NAME	DESIGNATION	SIGNATURE	BLEEP NUMBER

Step 2: Now check your work overleaf

Answer 26

This woman has hypernatraemia secondary to dehydration. She has lost more water than sodium causing her serum sodium to rise. The dehydration has occurred due to decreased oral intake in combination with diuretics, forcing renal water loss. Initial treatment involves stopping her furosemide and rehydration using intravenous fluids.

Step 3: Compare your answer to the checklist below and the chart opposite ☑

D Details	Checked patient details Used capital letters throughout Used correct abbreviations	☐
R Regular medications	Prescribed bisoprolol, clopidogrel and ramipril from patient's regular medications and withheld furosemide	☐
U Unpleasant reactions	NKDA	☐
G Gravid?	No	☐

C Contra-indications	Withheld furosemide	☐
H Hydration	Prescribed 2000mL of fluids other than 5% dextrose	☐
A Analgesia	Not required	☐
R Renal function	Ramipril at 5mg is safe for GFR 30–60mL/min and can be continued	☐
T Thrombo-prophylaxis	Prescribed enoxaparin 40mg SC	☐
S Signature box	Signed signature box	☐

Rationale

Correcting hypernatraemia too rapidly is dangerous and leads to complications such as cerebral oedema and seizures. The ideal is to aim for a reduction of no more than 12mmol/L per day. Rehydration with 5% dextrose given too quickly would cause the serum sodium to fall dangerously rapidly. Dextrose–saline (5% dextrose + 0.45% sodium chloride) is a good compromise, rehydrating the patient without causing a rapid drop in serum sodium. If dextrose–saline is not available it would be more appropriate to prescribe a fluid such as sodium chloride 0.9% or Hartmann's especially where the patient needs fluid resuscitation to correct haemodynamic compromise.

When a patient is dehydrated, diuretics such as furosemide need to be withheld as they will exacerbate the situation. Diuretics will force the kidneys to produce urine above the physiological rate, prolonging the patient's dehydration and making any renal injury worse. In this patient's case it is sensible to withhold furosemide for the first 48 hours. It can be reintroduced when the patient is euvolaemic.

KEY POINTS

- Stop diuretics in dehydrated patients
- Do not correct hypernatraemia too quickly: use fluid containing sodium if fluid resuscitation is required

LONGBURY HOSPITAL TRUST							

			HOSPITAL NUMBER	673225			
			SURNAME	WALKER			
			FIRST NAME	JOCELYN			
			ADDRESS	95 TAXUS ROAD, LB1 5LO			
			D.O.B	31/10/YYYY (82 YEARS AGO)			

DATE OF ADMISSION	04/07/YYYY	ADMISSION WEIGHT (KG)	72kg	WARD	MEDICAL ASSESSMENT
ALLERGIES NONE			CONSULTANT	ERIN JOHNSON	
			CHART NO		1...OF...1

ONCE ONLY PRESCRIPTIONS

DATE	TIME	NAME OF DRUG	DOSE	ROUTE	PRESCRIBER'S SIGNATURE	GIVEN BY	TIME GIVEN

REGULAR MEDICATIONS

NAME OF DRUG ENOXAPARIN	TIME	DATE → DOSE ↓	04/07				
ADDITIONAL INSTRUCTIONS	06:00						
DATE 04/07 ROUTE S/C	12:00						
PRESCRIBER'S SIGNATURE A Lewis	18:00	40mg					
PRESCRIBER'S NAME AND BLEEP ALEX LEWIS 4567	22:00						

NAME OF DRUG BISOPROLOL	TIME	DATE → DOSE ↓	04/07				
ADDITIONAL INSTRUCTIONS	08:00	2.5mg	X				
DATE 04/07 ROUTE PO	12:00						
PRESCRIBER'S SIGNATURE A Lewis	18:00						
PRESCRIBER'S NAME AND BLEEP ALEX LEWIS 4567	22:00						

NAME OF DRUG CLOPIDOGREL	TIME	DATE → DOSE ↓	04/07				
ADDITIONAL INSTRUCTIONS	08:00	75mg	X				
DATE 04/07 ROUTE PO	12:00						
PRESCRIBER'S SIGNATURE A Lewis	18:00						
PRESCRIBER'S NAME AND BLEEP ALEX LEWIS 4567	22:00						

PATIENT NAME *JOCELYN WALKER* HOSPITAL NO. 673225

NAME OF DRUG *RAMIPRIL*	TIME	DATE → DOSE ↓	04/07				
ADDITIONAL INSTRUCTIONS	08:00	5mg	X				
DATE *04/07* ROUTE *PO*	12:00						
PRESCRIBER'S SIGNATURE *ALewis*							
	18:00						
PRESCRIBER'S NAME AND BLEEP *ALEX LEWIS 4567*	22:00						

NAME OF DRUG	TIME	DATE → DOSE ↓					
ADDITIONAL INSTRUCTIONS	08:00						
DATE ROUTE	12:00						
PRESCRIBER'S SIGNATURE							
	18:00						
PRESCRIBER'S NAME AND BLEEP	22:00						

NAME OF DRUG	TIME	DATE → DOSE ↓					
ADDITIONAL INSTRUCTIONS	08:00						
DATE ROUTE	12:00						
PRESCRIBER'S SIGNATURE							
	18:00						
PRESCRIBER'S NAME AND BLEEP	22:00						

AS REQUIRED PRESCRIPTIONS

NAME OF DRUG		DATE					
INDICATION/ INSTRUCTION	DOSE	TIME					
FREQUENCY	ROUTE	DOSE					
PRESCRIBER'S SIGNATURE		ROUTE					
PRESCRIBER'S NAME AND BLEEP		GIVEN BY					
START DATE	STOP DATE						

PATIENT NAME *JOCELYN WALKER*   HOSPITAL NO.   673225

NAME OF DRUG		DATE						
INDICATION/INSTRUCTION	DOSE	TIME						
FREQUENCY	ROUTE	DOSE						
PRESCRIBER'S SIGNATURE		ROUTE						
PRESCRIBER'S NAME AND BLEEP		GIVEN BY						
START DATE	STOP DATE							

INTRAVENOUS FLUIDS

DATE	FLUID	ADDITIVE & DOSE	VOLUME	RATE/DURATION	PRESCRIBER'S SIGNATURE	GIVEN BY	START TIME	END TIME
04/07	5% DEXTROSE + 0.45% SODIUM CHLORIDE	————	1000ml	100ml/hr	ALewis			
04/07	5% DEXTROSE +0.45% SODIUM CHLORIDE	————	1000ml	100ml/hr	ALewis			

Record of signatures. ALL prescribers MUST complete.

DATE	NAME	DESIGNATION	SIGNATURE	BLEEP NUMBER
04/07	ALEX LEWIS	F1	ALewis	4567

Jacqueline Adams (hospital number: 401205, DOB 13/12/YYYY [65 years old], address: 72 Rector Drive, Longbury LB18 2CH) has been admitted to the medical assessment ward following referral by her general practitioner. She has a 50-hour history of chest tightness and palpitations but has been otherwise well until today. On examination her pulse is 155bpm, her jugular venous pressure is at the level of the clavicle and her blood pressure is 129/62mmHg. The ECG obtained in the ambulance shows atrial fibrillation with a rapid ventricular response. She is not known to have atrial fibrillation. Her chest X-ray is normal.

The medical registrar has reviewed Mrs Adams and suggests 5mg intravenous metoprolol for rate control and asks for it to be prescribed.

Mrs Adams' regular medications have already been prescribed. Her general practitioner's summary states she is allergic to NSAIDs.

Your task is to prescribe treatment for the atrial fibrillation.
It is 19:00 on 19th November.

Notes

Step 1: Complete your answers in the drug chart opposite and overleaf

LONGBURY HOSPITAL TRUST				HOSPITAL NUMBER	401205		
				SURNAME	ADAMS		
				FIRST NAME	JACQUELINE		
				ADDRESS	72 RECTOR DRIVE, LONGBURY LB18 2CH		
				D.O.B	13/12/YYYY (65 YEARS AGO)		
DATE OF ADMISSION	19/11/YYYY	ADMISSION WEIGHT (KG)	79kg		WARD	MEDICAL ASSESSMENT	
ALLERGIES				CONSULTANT		ERIN JOHNSON	
NSAID				CHART NO		1...OF...1	

ONCE ONLY PRESCRIPTIONS

DATE	TIME	NAME OF DRUG	DOSE	ROUTE	PRESCRIBER'S SIGNATURE	GIVEN BY	TIME GIVEN

REGULAR MEDICATIONS

NAME OF DRUG	TIME	DATE → DOSE ↓	19/11				
ENOXAPARIN							
ADDITIONAL INSTRUCTIONS	08:00						
DATE 19/11 ROUTE S/C	12:00						
PRESCRIBER'S SIGNATURE NShah	18:00	40mg	JD				
PRESCRIBER'S NAME AND BLEEP NAZIA SHAH 9761	22:00						

NAME OF DRUG	TIME	DATE → DOSE ↓	19/11				
SYMBICORT 200/6							
ADDITIONAL INSTRUCTIONS	08:00	TWO	JD				
DATE 19/11 ROUTE INH	12:00						
PRESCRIBER'S SIGNATURE N Shah	18:00						
PRESCRIBER'S NAME AND BLEEP NAZIA SHAH 9761	22:00	TWO					

NAME OF DRUG	TIME	DATE → DOSE ↓					
ADDITIONAL INSTRUCTIONS	08:00						
DATE ROUTE	12:00						
PRESCRIBER'S SIGNATURE	18:00						
PRESCRIBER'S NAME AND BLEEP	22:00						

PATIENT NAME JACQUELINE ADAMS   HOSPITAL NO.   401205

NAME OF DRUG	TIME	DATE → DOSE ↓					
ADDITIONAL INSTRUCTIONS	08:00						
DATE · ROUTE	12:00						
PRESCRIBER'S SIGNATURE	18:00						
PRESCRIBER'S NAME AND BLEEP	22:00						

NAME OF DRUG	TIME	DATE → DOSE ↓					
ADDITIONAL INSTRUCTIONS	08:00						
DATE · ROUTE	12:00						
PRESCRIBER'S SIGNATURE	18:00						
PRESCRIBER'S NAME AND BLEEP	22:00						

NAME OF DRUG	TIME	DATE → DOSE ↓					
ADDITIONAL INSTRUCTIONS	08:00						
DATE · ROUTE	12:00						
PRESCRIBER'S SIGNATURE	18:00						
PRESCRIBER'S NAME AND BLEEP	22:00						

AS REQUIRED PRESCRIPTIONS

NAME OF DRUG SALBUTAMOL		DATE					
INDICATION/ INSTRUCTION WHEEZE	DOSE TWO PUFFS	TIME					
FREQUENCY PRN	ROUTE INH	DOSE					
PRESCRIBER'S SIGNATURE NShah		ROUTE					
PRESCRIBER'S NAME AND BLEEP NAZIA SHAH 9761		GIVEN BY					
START DATE 19/11	STOP DATE						

PATIENT NAME JACQUELINE ADAMS   HOSPITAL NO.   401205

NAME OF DRUG		DATE					
INDICATION/ INSTRUCTION	DOSE	TIME					
FREQUENCY	ROUTE	DOSE					
PRESCRIBER'S SIGNATURE		ROUTE					
PRESCRIBER'S NAME AND BLEEP		GIVEN BY					
START DATE	STOP DATE						

INTRAVENOUS FLUIDS

DATE	FLUID	ADDITIVE & DOSE	VOLUME	RATE/ DURATION	PRESCRIBER'S SIGNATURE	GIVEN BY	START TIME	END TIME

Record of signatures. ALL prescribers MUST complete.

DATE	NAME	DESIGNATION	SIGNATURE	BLEEP NUMBER
19/11	NAZIA SHAH	F1	NShah	9761

Answer 27

This women has new-onset atrial fibrillation (AF). She has a rapid ventricular response that is causing her to become symptomatic.

A key feature of this exercise is to demonstrate that the drug chart can be a clue to a patient's medical history. In this case, it is likely this patient has asthma, which affects your choice of treatment for the atrial fibrillation.

Step 3: Compare your answer to the checklist below and the chart opposite ☑

D Details	Checked patient details Used capital letters throughout Used correct abbreviations	☐
R Regular medications	Recognised that the patient is likely to have a diagnosis of asthma	☐
U Unpleasant reactions	Noticed that NSAIDs had been documented	☐
G Gravid?	No	☐

C Contra-indications	Beta-blockers with asthma	☐
H Hydration	Not required	☐
A Analgesia	Not required	☐
R Renal function	Not required	☐
T Thrombo-prophylaxis	Already prescribed	☐
S Signature box	Signed signature box	☐

Rationale

In most patients with established AF, a fast heart rate is a sign of another disease such as sepsis. Some patients with new AF will have a rapid ventricular response without a precipitating factor. In new AF, control of the ventricular rate is essential and a cardioselective beta-blocker such as metoprolol or bisoprolol is commonly used.

On scanning the drug chart, this patient's NSAIDs allergy and use of a salbutamol inhaler point to a likely underlying diagnosis of asthma. Beta-blockers are contraindicated in asthma as they induce severe bronchospasm. A better choice of medication in asthmatics is a nondihydropyridine calcium channel blocker such as diltiazem or verapamil, but seek senior advice beforehand. Longer-term anticoagulation may also need to be considered.

KEY POINTS

- Beta-blockers are contraindicated in asthma
- The prescription chart is often a clue to a patient's past medical history, check the patient's regular medications before prescribing new ones
- Remember it is your signature on a prescription. Don't prescribe because you were told to, without being sure it is safe yourself

LONGBURY HOSPITAL TRUST				HOSPITAL NUMBER	401205
				SURNAME	ADAMS
				FIRST NAME	JACQUELINE
				ADDRESS	72 RECTOR DRIVE, LONGBURY LB18 2CH
				D.O.B	13/12/YYYY (65 YEARS AGO)
DATE OF ADMISSION	19/11/YYYY	ADMISSION WEIGHT (KG)	79kg	WARD	MEDICAL ASSESSMENT
ALLERGIES				CONSULTANT	ERIN JOHNSON
NSAIDS				CHART NO	1...OF...1

ONCE ONLY PRESCRIPTIONS

DATE	TIME	NAME OF DRUG	DOSE	ROUTE	PRESCRIBER'S SIGNATURE	GIVEN BY	TIME GIVEN

REGULAR MEDICATIONS

NAME OF DRUG / instructions	TIME	DATE → / DOSE ↓	19/11				
NAME OF DRUG ENOXAPARIN	**TIME**	**DOSE ↓**					
ADDITIONAL INSTRUCTIONS	08:00						
DATE 19/11 ROUTE S/C	12:00						
PRESCRIBER'S SIGNATURE NShah	18:00	40mg	JD				
PRESCRIBER'S NAME AND BLEEP NAZIA SHAH 9761	22:00						

NAME OF DRUG / instructions	TIME	DATE → / DOSE ↓	19/11				
NAME OF DRUG SYMBICORT 200/6	**TIME**	**DOSE ↓**					
ADDITIONAL INSTRUCTIONS	08:00	TWO	JD				
DATE 19/11 ROUTE INH	12:00						
PRESCRIBER'S SIGNATURE N Shah	18:00						
PRESCRIBER'S NAME AND BLEEP NAZIA SHAH 9761	22:00	TWO					

NAME OF DRUG / instructions	TIME	DATE → / DOSE ↓	19/11				
NAME OF DRUG VERAPAMIL	**TIME**	**DOSE ↓**					
ADDITIONAL INSTRUCTIONS	08:00	40mg	X				
DATE 19/11 ROUTE PO	12:00						
PRESCRIBER'S SIGNATURE A Lewis	14:00	40mg	X				
	18:00						
PRESCRIBER'S NAME AND BLEEP ALEX LEWIS 4567	22:00	40mg					

PATIENT NAME JACQUELINE ADAMS   HOSPITAL NO. 401205

NAME OF DRUG		TIME	DATE → DOSE ↓					
ADDITIONAL INSTRUCTIONS		08:00						
DATE	ROUTE	12:00						
PRESCRIBER'S SIGNATURE								
		18:00						
PRESCRIBER'S NAME AND BLEEP		22:00						

NAME OF DRUG		TIME	DATE → DOSE ↓					
ADDITIONAL INSTRUCTIONS		08:00						
DATE	ROUTE	12:00						
PRESCRIBER'S SIGNATURE								
		18:00						
PRESCRIBER'S NAME AND BLEEP		22:00						

NAME OF DRUG		TIME	DATE → DOSE ↓					
ADDITIONAL INSTRUCTIONS		08:00						
DATE	ROUTE	12:00						
PRESCRIBER'S SIGNATURE								
		18:00						
PRESCRIBER'S NAME AND BLEEP		22:00						

AS REQUIRED PRESCRIPTIONS

NAME OF DRUG SALBUTAMOL		DATE					
INDICATION/ INSTRUCTION WHEEZE	DOSE TWO PUFFS	TIME					
FREQUENCY PRN	ROUTE INH	DOSE					
PRESCRIBER'S SIGNATURE NShah		ROUTE					
PRESCRIBER'S NAME AND BLEEP NAZIA SHAH 9761		GIVEN BY					
START DATE 19/11	STOP DATE						

PATIENT NAME JACQUELINE ADAMS   HOSPITAL NO.   401205

NAME OF DRUG		DATE						
INDICATION/ INSTRUCTION	DOSE	TIME						
FREQUENCY	ROUTE	DOSE						
PRESCRIBER'S SIGNATURE		ROUTE						
PRESCRIBER'S NAME AND BLEEP		GIVEN BY						
START DATE	STOP DATE							

INTRAVENOUS FLUIDS

DATE	FLUID	ADDITIVE & DOSE	VOLUME	RATE/ DURATION	PRESCRIBER'S SIGNATURE	GIVEN BY	START TIME	END TIME

Record of signatures. ALL prescribers MUST complete.

DATE	NAME	DESIGNATION	SIGNATURE	BLEEP NUMBER
19/11	NAZIA SHAH	F1	NShah	9761
19/11	ALEX LEWIS	F1	ALewis	4567

Francis Hamm (hospital number: 361128, DOB 06/11/YYYY [52 years old], address: 50 Boundary Lane, Longbury LB3 6CM) has been admitted to the emergency department with chest pain due to acute coronary syndrome caused by non-ST elevation myocardial infarction (NSTEMI). He is awaiting transfer to the university hospital for percutaneous coronary intervention. In the last hour his chest pain has returned and is getting worse. His ECG is unchanged from presentation. He has been using his glyceryl trinitrate spray but without benefit.

The nurses have asked for you to review with a view to improving Mr Hamm's symptoms.

Observations:
Heart rate 85bpm
Blood pressure 156/76mmHg
Respiratory rate 22 breaths/minute
SpO_2 97% on 24% O_2

Your task is to prescribe appropriate medication for the chest pain.
It is 10:00 on 20th November.

Notes

Step 1: Complete your answers in the drug chart opposite and overleaf

		LONGBURY HOSPITAL TRUST						

HOSPITAL NUMBER 361128
SURNAME HAMM
FIRST NAME FRANCIS
ADDRESS 50 BOUNDARY LANE, LONGBURY LB3 6CM

D.O.B 06/11/YYYY (52 YEARS AGO)

DATE OF ADMISSION	20/11/YYYY	ADMISSION WEIGHT (KG)	80kg	WARD	EMERGENCY

ALLERGIES
NKDA

CONSULTANT PRADIP CHAND

CHART NO 1...OF...1

ONCE ONLY PRESCRIPTIONS

DATE	TIME	NAME OF DRUG	DOSE	ROUTE	PRESCRIBER'S SIGNATURE	GIVEN BY	TIME GIVEN
20/11	STAT	CLOPIDOGREL	600mg	PO	EJones	HF	0845
20/11	STAT	ASPIRIN	300mg	PO	EJones	HF	0845
20/11	STAT	DIAMORPHINE	2.5mg	IV	EJones	HF	0845
20/11	STAT	FONDAPARINUX	2.5mg	SC	EJones	HF	0845

REGULAR MEDICATIONS

NAME OF DRUG FONDAPARINUX	TIME	DATE → DOSE ↓	20/11	21/11			
ADDITIONAL INSTRUCTIONS	08:00	2.5mg	——				
DATE 20/11 ROUTE S/C	12:00						
PRESCRIBER'S SIGNATURE EJones	18:00						
PRESCRIBER'S NAME AND BLEEP EMMA JONES 4876	22:00						

NAME OF DRUG RAMIPRIL	TIME	DATE → DOSE ↓	20/11				
ADDITIONAL INSTRUCTIONS	08:00	2.5mg	HF				
DATE 20/11 ROUTE PO	12:00						
PRESCRIBER'S SIGNATURE EJones	18:00						
PRESCRIBER'S NAME AND BLEEP EMMA JONES 4876	22:00						

NAME OF DRUG ATORVASTATIN	TIME	DATE → DOSE ↓					
ADDITIONAL INSTRUCTIONS	08:00						
DATE 20/11 ROUTE PO	12:00						
PRESCRIBER'S SIGNATURE EJones	18:00						
PRESCRIBER'S NAME AND BLEEP EMMA JONES 4876	22:00	80mg					

PATIENT NAME FRANCIS HAMM   HOSPITAL NO.   361128

NAME OF DRUG ASPIRIN	TIME	DATE → DOSE ↓	20/11				
ADDITIONAL INSTRUCTIONS	08:00	75mg	————				
DATE 20/11 ROUTE PO	12:00						
PRESCRIBER'S SIGNATURE EJones	18:00						
PRESCRIBER'S NAME AND BLEEP EMMA JONES 4876	22:00						

NAME OF DRUG CLOPIDOGREL	TIME	DATE → DOSE ↓	20/11				
ADDITIONAL INSTRUCTIONS	08:00	75mg	————				
DATE 20/11 ROUTE PO	12:00						
PRESCRIBER'S SIGNATURE EJones	18:00						
PRESCRIBER'S NAME AND BLEEP EMMA JONES 4876	22:00						

NAME OF DRUG	TIME	DATE → DOSE ↓					
ADDITIONAL INSTRUCTIONS	08:00						
DATE ROUTE	12:00						
PRESCRIBER'S SIGNATURE	18:00						
PRESCRIBER'S NAME AND BLEEP	22:00						

AS REQUIRED PRESCRIPTIONS

NAME OF DRUG GTN SPRAY		DATE					
INDICATION/ INSTRUCTION CHEST PAIN	DOSE 2 SPRAYS	TIME					
FREQUENCY PRN	ROUTE S/L	DOSE					
PRESCRIBER'S SIGNATURE EJones		ROUTE					
PRESCRIBER'S NAME AND BLEEP EMMA JONES 4876		GIVEN BY					
START DATE 20/11	STOP DATE						

PATIENT NAME FRANCIS HAMM   HOSPITAL NO.   361128

NAME OF DRUG		DATE						
INDICATION/ INSTRUCTION	DOSE	TIME						
FREQUENCY	ROUTE	DOSE						
PRESCRIBER'S SIGNATURE		ROUTE						
PRESCRIBER'S NAME AND BLEEP		GIVEN BY						
START DATE	STOP DATE							

INTRAVENOUS FLUIDS

DATE	FLUID	ADDITIVE & DOSE	VOLUME	RATE/ DURATION	PRESCRIBER'S SIGNATURE	GIVEN BY	START TIME	END TIME

Record of signatures. ALL prescribers MUST complete.

DATE	NAME	DESIGNATION	SIGNATURE	BLEEP NUMBER
20/11	EMMA JONES	F1	EJones	4876

Step 2: Now check your work overleaf

Answer 28

Ongoing chest pain in a patient with a non-ST segment elevation myocardial infarction (NSTEMI) is a sign that intervention may need to be brought forward. However, it is important to know how to treat the pain effectively.

Step 3: Compare your answer to the checklist below and the chart opposite ☑

D Details	Checked patient details Used capital letters throughout Used correct abbreviations	☐
R Regular medications	Continued ACS treatments	☐
U Unpleasant reactions	NKDA	☐
G Gravid?	No	☐

C Contra-indications	None	☐
H Hydration	Not required	☐
A Analgesia	Prescribed IV diamorphine or morphine and a nitrate infusion to improve analgesia	☐
R Renal function	Not required	☐
T Thrombo-prophylaxis	Already on fondaparinux: no further action required	☐
S Signature box	Signed signature box	☐

Rationale

This man has ongoing ischaemic chest pain due to a non-ST elevation myocardial infarction. Pain relief is achieved by improving myocardial blood supply. Intravenous nitrate infusion is useful in the acute setting because it causes coronary artery dilation improving coronary blood flow. Glyceryl trinitrate (GTN) is the most widely used intravenous nitrate. The infusion has been prescribed as 50mg in 50mL with a variable rate of 1–10mL/h. The intravenous formula is given neat and does not need to be diluted in another fluid. The nurses should be instructed to increase the rate until the patient is pain free. Nitrate infusion will cause the patient's blood pressure to fall. If systolic pressure falls below 100mmHg the rate of infusion should be reduced. There is often a balance between maintaining the patient's blood pressure and keeping them pain free.

Another drug used for ischaemic chest pain is intravenous diamorphine, not only for its analgesic effect but also because it causes coronary vasodilatation and therefore improves the ischaemia. Intravenous doses of 2.5–5.0 mg have been prescribed on the once-only chart and on the as-required chart to allow for follow-up doses to be given. For ongoing pain it may be necessary to refer this patient to the coronary care unit for a senior decision on the use of glycoprotein 2b/3a inhibitors.

Patients with a NSTEMI do not need to have percutaneous coronary intervention as urgently as patients with a STEMI. However, those that have ongoing pain, despite good medical management, should be discussed with the on-call cardiologist for consideration of earlier intervention. If this patient goes for an angiogram his fondaparinux should be withheld on the day of the procedure.

KEY POINTS

- Nitrate infusions can give effective pain relief in cardiac ischaemia
- GTN infusion should be prescribed as a variable dose to allow titration
- Diamorphine has a dual pain relieving effect. Care must be taken with the IV route of administration of opiates

LONGBURY HOSPITAL TRUST		HOSPITAL NUMBER	361128		
		SURNAME	HAMM		
		FIRST NAME	FRANCIS		
		ADDRESS	50 BOUNDARY LANE, LONGBURY LB3 6CM		
		D.O.B	06/11/YYYY (52 YEARS AGO)		

DATE OF ADMISSION	20/11/YYYY	ADMISSION WEIGHT (KG)	80kg	WARD	EMERGENCY
ALLERGIES			CONSULTANT		PRADIP CHAND
NKDA			CHART NO		1...OF...1

ONCE ONLY PRESCRIPTIONS

DATE	TIME	NAME OF DRUG	DOSE	ROUTE	PRESCRIBER'S SIGNATURE	GIVEN BY	TIME GIVEN
20/11	STAT	CLOPIDOGREL	600mg	PO	EJones	HF	0845
20/11	STAT	ASPIRIN	300mg	PO	EJones	HF	0845
20/11	STAT	DIAMORPHINE	2.5mg	IV	EJones	HF	0845
20/11	STAT	FONDAPARINUX	2.5mg	SC	EJones	HF	0845

REGULAR MEDICATIONS

NAME OF DRUG FONDAPARINUX	TIME	DATE → DOSE ↓	20/11	21/11		
ADDITIONAL INSTRUCTIONS	08:00	2.5mg	——			
DATE 20/11 ROUTE S/C	12:00					
PRESCRIBER'S SIGNATURE EJones	18:00					
PRESCRIBER'S NAME AND BLEEP EMMA JONES 4876	22:00					

NAME OF DRUG RAMIPRIL	TIME	DATE → DOSE ↓	20/11			
ADDITIONAL INSTRUCTIONS	08:00	2.5mg	HF			
DATE 20/11 ROUTE PO	12:00					
PRESCRIBER'S SIGNATURE EJones	18:00					
PRESCRIBER'S NAME AND BLEEP EMMA JONES 4876	22:00					

NAME OF DRUG ATORVASTATIN	TIME	DATE → • DOSE ↓				
ADDITIONAL INSTRUCTIONS	08:00					
DATE 20/11 ROUTE PO	12:00					
PRESCRIBER'S SIGNATURE EJones	18:00					
PRESCRIBER'S NAME AND BLEEP EMMA JONES 4876	22:00	80mg				

PATIENT NAME FRANCIS HAMM   HOSPITAL NO. 361128

NAME OF DRUG ASPIRIN	TIME	DATE → DOSE ↓	20/11				
ADDITIONAL INSTRUCTIONS	08:00	75mg	——————				
DATE 20/11 ROUTE PO	12:00						
PRESCRIBER'S SIGNATURE EJones	18:00						
PRESCRIBER'S NAME AND BLEEP EMMA JONES 4876	22:00						

NAME OF DRUG CLOPIDOGREL	TIME	DATE → DOSE ↓	20/11				
ADDITIONAL INSTRUCTIONS	08:00	75mg	——————				
DATE 20/11 ROUTE PO	12:00						
PRESCRIBER'S SIGNATURE EJones	18:00						
PRESCRIBER'S NAME AND BLEEP EMMA JONES 4876	22:00						

NAME OF DRUG	TIME	DATE → DOSE ↓					
ADDITIONAL INSTRUCTIONS	08:00						
DATE ROUTE	12:00						
PRESCRIBER'S SIGNATURE	18:00						
PRESCRIBER'S NAME AND BLEEP	22:00						

AS REQUIRED PRESCRIPTIONS

NAME OF DRUG GTN SPRAY		DATE					
INDICATION/ INSTRUCTION CHEST PAIN	DOSE 2 SPRAYS	TIME					
FREQUENCY PRN	ROUTE S/L	DOSE					
PRESCRIBER'S SIGNATURE EJones		ROUTE					
PRESCRIBER'S NAME AND BLEEP EMMA JONES 4876		GIVEN BY					
START DATE 20/11	STOP DATE						

PATIENT NAME FRANCIS HAMM   HOSPITAL NO.   361128

NAME OF DRUG DIAMORPHINE		DATE						
INDICATION/ INSTRUCTION CHEST PAIN	DOSE 2.5mg	TIME						
FREQUENCY 2 HOURLY	ROUTE IV	DOSE						
PRESCRIBER'S SIGNATURE ALewis		ROUTE						
PRESCRIBER'S NAME AND BLEEP ALEX LEWIS 4567		GIVEN BY						
START DATE 20/11	STOP DATE							

INTRAVENOUS FLUIDS

DATE	FLUID	ADDITIVE & DOSE	VOLUME	RATE/ DURATION	PRESCRIBER'S SIGNATURE	GIVEN BY	START TIME	END TIME
20/11	GLYCERYL TRINITRATE	50mg IN 50ml	50ml	1-10ml/h	ALewis			

Record of signatures. ALL prescribers MUST complete.

DATE	NAME	DESIGNATION	SIGNATURE	BLEEP NUMBER
20/11	EMMA JONES	F1	EJones	4876
20/11	ALEX LEWIS	F1	ALewis	4567

Howard McGill (hospital number: 365789, DOB 14/06/YYYY [74 years old], address: 101 Wicker Street, Longbury LB10 3HQ) was admitted to the medical assessment ward 24 hours ago with epigastric pain and haematemesis. An endoscopy showed oesophageal varices which were bleeding and banded. He has a history of alcoholic liver disease and cirrhosis. The nurses have become concerned because he is agitated and tremulous and is sweating profusely.

Although Mr McGill is agitated, examination confirms that his chest is clear and he has a normal cardiac examination with normal ECG apart from a sinus tachycardia. His blood tests are in keeping with alcoholic liver disease and a recent upper gastrointestinal bleed. Mr McGill has no know allergies. His current weight is 84kg and his consultant is Dr Erin Johnson.

Your task is to prescribe appropriate therapy.
It is 05:00 on 20th November.

Notes

LONGBURY HOSPITAL TRUST				HOSPITAL NUMBER SURNAME FIRST NAME ADDRESS D.O.B		
DATE OF ADMISSION		ADMISSION WEIGHT (KG)			WARD	
ALLERGIES				CONSULTANT		
				CHART NO	...OF...	

ONCE ONLY PRESCRIPTIONS

DATE	TIME	NAME OF DRUG	DOSE	ROUTE	PRESCRIBER'S SIGNATURE	GIVEN BY	TIME GIVEN

REGULAR MEDICATIONS

NAME OF DRUG		TIME	DATE → DOSE ↓					
ADDITIONAL INSTRUCTIONS		08:00						
DATE	ROUTE	12:00						
PRESCRIBER'S SIGNATURE		18:00						
PRESCRIBER'S NAME AND BLEEP		22:00						

NAME OF DRUG		TIME	DATE → DOSE ↓					
ADDITIONAL INSTRUCTIONS		08:00						
DATE	ROUTE	12:00						
PRESCRIBER'S SIGNATURE		18:00						
PRESCRIBER'S NAME AND BLEEP		22:00						

NAME OF DRUG		TIME	DATE → DOSE ↓					
ADDITIONAL INSTRUCTIONS		08:00						
DATE	ROUTE	12:00						
PRESCRIBER'S SIGNATURE		18:00						
PRESCRIBER'S NAME AND BLEEP		22:00						

PATIENT NAME   HOSPITAL NO.

NAME OF DRUG		TIME	DATE → DOSE ↓					
ADDITIONAL INSTRUCTIONS		08:00						
DATE	ROUTE	12:00						
PRESCRIBER'S SIGNATURE								
		18:00						
PRESCRIBER'S NAME AND BLEEP		22:00						

NAME OF DRUG		TIME	DATE → DOSE ↓					
ADDITIONAL INSTRUCTIONS		08:00						
DATE	ROUTE	12:00						
PRESCRIBER'S SIGNATURE								
		18:00						
PRESCRIBER'S NAME AND BLEEP		22:00						

NAME OF DRUG		TIME	DATE → DOSE ↓					
ADDITIONAL INSTRUCTIONS		08:00						
DATE	ROUTE	12:00						
PRESCRIBER'S SIGNATURE								
		18:00						
PRESCRIBER'S NAME AND BLEEP		22:00						

AS REQUIRED PRESCRIPTIONS

NAME OF DRUG		DATE					
INDICATION/ INSTRUCTION	DOSE	TIME					
FREQUENCY	ROUTE	DOSE					
PRESCRIBER'S SIGNATURE		ROUTE					
PRESCRIBER'S NAME AND BLEEP							
START DATE	STOP DATE	GIVEN BY					

PATIENT NAME   HOSPITAL NO.

NAME OF DRUG		DATE					
INDICATION/ INSTRUCTION	DOSE	TIME					
FREQUENCY	ROUTE	DOSE					
PRESCRIBER'S SIGNATURE		ROUTE					
PRESCRIBER'S NAME AND BLEEP		GIVEN BY					
START DATE	STOP DATE						

INTRAVENOUS FLUIDS

DATE	FLUID	ADDITIVE & DOSE	VOLUME	RATE/ DURATION	PRESCRIBER'S SIGNATURE	GIVEN BY	START TIME	END TIME

Record of signatures. ALL prescribers MUST complete.

DATE	NAME	DESIGNATION	SIGNATURE	BLEEP NUMBER

Step 2: Now check your work overleaf

Answer 29

This man is displaying the classic signs of alcohol withdrawal; sweating, tremulousness and agitation. Alcohol withdrawal occurs when the central nervous system becomes tolerant to a continuing exposure to alcohol which is abruptly halted. Typically, symptoms can begin 24–48 hours after the withdrawal of alcohol, which means a patient may already have been clerked and put in a low-dependency unit before a problem arises.

Step 3: Compare your answer to the checklist below and the chart opposite ☑

D Details	Checked patient details / Used capital letters throughout / Used correct abbreviations	☐
R Regular medications	Prescribed Pabrinex and chlordiazepoxide with a reducing dose	☐
U Unpleasant reactions	None	☐
G Gravid?	No	☐

C Contra-indications	Thromboprophylaxis is contraindicated in those with a recent bleed	☐
H Hydration	Not required	☐
A Analgesia	Not required	☐
R Renal function	Not required	☐
T Thrombo-prophylaxis	Recognised that thromboprophylaxis is contraindicated and did not prescribe	☐
S Signature box	Signed signature box	☐

Rationale

In extreme cases alcohol withdrawal can lead to seizures. The benzodiazepine chlordiazepoxide is long-acting and used to treat symptoms and reduce the chance of seizures. Its prescription is normally protocol-driven in hospitals and the regimen is dictated by the patient's normal alcohol intake and symptoms. However, a usual starting dose would be 20mg q.d.s., reduced by 10–20mg per day on a reducing regimen over 5 days so the patient is weaned off. Doses of 10mg–20mg should also be prescribed as required in case the patient develops symptoms despite the regular prescription. Frequent resort to this requires review: consider the dose of your regular prescription, as it may not be enough. Ensure you review PRN use regularly.

Some drug charts have sections for variable doses in which a different dose may be entered for each time the medication is administered. In others it may be necessary to prescribe each day separately. There may be a preprinted chart to allow a common approach within the hospital, which can help in defining appropriate reducing regimens, along with prompting adjuvant therapy, e.g. oral vitamins. The important point is that what is intended must be completely unambiguous to avoid dosing errors.

Alcohol-dependent patients are at risk of serious neurological complications, particularly Wernicke's encephalopathy, as a result of thiamine and vitamin B12 deficiency. Patients with a history of alcohol abuse should be given the intravenous multivitamin Pabrinex over 3–5 days to replenish depleted vitamin stores. The dose prescribed here is prophylactic but serum B vitamins should be checked and, if needed, the Pabrinex uptitrated to 2–3 pairs (ampoules) t.d.s. for 2 days. If this prescription had been started in this exercise, that would be acceptable. Pabrinex is supplied in a pair of ampoules, therefore the prescription is written as 'Pabrinex 1 + 2 - one pair'.

The classic triad of ataxia, confusion and ophthalmoplegia are only seen together in approximately 10% of cases of Wernicke's encephalopathy, so a low threshold is required to recognise and treat this condition. Consider the need for oral vitamin supplementation following parenteral therapy.

KEY POINTS

- Patients with alcohol dependence develop physical withdrawal symptoms around 1–2 days after stopping drinking
- Benzodiazepines treat the withdrawal symptoms. The prescription can be complicated so take care to make it clear
- Most long-term drinkers are vitamin deficient and this should be corrected

LONGBURY HOSPITAL TRUST			HOSPITAL NUMBER	365789		
			SURNAME	MCGILL		
			FIRST NAME	HOWARD		
			ADDRESS	101 WICKER STREET, LONGBURY LB10 3HQ		
			D.O.B	14/06/YYYY (74 YEARS AGO)		

DATE OF ADMISSION	19/11/YYYY	ADMISSION WEIGHT (KG)	84kg	WARD	MEDICAL ASSESSMENT
ALLERGIES NONE			CONSULTANT		ERIN JOHNSON
			CHART NO		1…OF…1

ONCE ONLY PRESCRIPTIONS

DATE	TIME	NAME OF DRUG	DOSE	ROUTE	PRESCRIBER'S SIGNATURE	GIVEN BY	TIME GIVEN

REGULAR MEDICATIONS

NAME OF DRUG PABRINEX 1 + 2	TIME	DATE → DOSE ↓	20/11				
ADDITIONAL INSTRUCTIONS	08:00	1 PAIR					
DATE 20/11 ROUTE IV	12:00						
PRESCRIBER'S SIGNATURE ALewis	18:00						
PRESCRIBER'S NAME AND BLEEP ALEX LEWIS 4567	22:00						

NAME OF DRUG CHLORDIAZEPOXIDE	TIME	DATE → DOSE ↓	20/11	21/11	22/11	23/11	24/11
ADDITIONAL INSTRUCTIONS	08:00	20mg			——	——	——
DATE 20/11 ROUTE PO	12:00	20mg			——	——	——
PRESCRIBER'S SIGNATURE ALewis	18:00	20mg			——	——	——
PRESCRIBER'S NAME AND BLEEP ALEX LEWIS 4567	22:00	20mg			——	——	——

NAME OF DRUG CHLORDIAZEPOXIDE	TIME	DATE → DOSE ↓	20/11	21/11	22/11	23/11	24/11
ADDITIONAL INSTRUCTIONS	08:00	15mg	——		——	——	——
DATE 20/11 ROUTE PO	12:00	15mg	——		——	——	——
PRESCRIBER'S SIGNATURE ALewis	18:00	15mg	——		——	——	——
PRESCRIBER'S NAME AND BLEEP ALEX LEWIS 4567	22:00	15mg	——		——	——	——

PATIENT NAME *HOWARD MCGILL* HOSPITAL NO. *365789*

NAME OF DRUG		TIME	DATE → DOSE ↓					
ADDITIONAL INSTRUCTIONS		08:00						
DATE	ROUTE	12:00						
PRESCRIBER'S SIGNATURE								
		18:00						
PRESCRIBER'S NAME AND BLEEP								
		22:00						

NAME OF DRUG		TIME	DATE → DOSE ↓					
ADDITIONAL INSTRUCTIONS		08:00						
DATE	ROUTE	12:00						
PRESCRIBER'S SIGNATURE								
		18:00						
PRESCRIBER'S NAME AND BLEEP								
		22:00						

NAME OF DRUG		TIME	DATE → DOSE ↓					
ADDITIONAL INSTRUCTIONS		08:00						
DATE	ROUTE	12:00						
PRESCRIBER'S SIGNATURE								
		18:00						
PRESCRIBER'S NAME AND BLEEP								
		22:00						

AS REQUIRED PRESCRIPTIONS

NAME OF DRUG *CHLORDIAZEPOXIDE*		DATE					
INDICATION/ INSTRUCTION *ALCOHOL WITHDRAWAL. BLEEP DOCTOR IF REQUIRED*	DOSE *10mg*	TIME					
FREQUENCY *PRN*	ROUTE *PO*	DOSE					
PRESCRIBER'S SIGNATURE *ALewis*		ROUTE					
PRESCRIBER'S NAME AND BLEEP *ALEX LEWIS 4567*		GIVEN BY					
START DATE *20/11*	STOP DATE						

PATIENT NAME *HOWARD MCGILL*   HOSPITAL NO.   *365789*

NAME OF DRUG		DATE					
INDICATION/ INSTRUCTION	DOSE	TIME					
FREQUENCY	ROUTE	DOSE					
PRESCRIBER'S SIGNATURE		ROUTE					
PRESCRIBER'S NAME AND BLEEP		GIVEN BY					
START DATE	STOP DATE						

INTRAVENOUS FLUIDS

DATE	FLUID	ADDITIVE & DOSE	VOLUME	RATE/ DURATION	PRESCRIBER'S SIGNATURE	GIVEN BY	START TIME	END TIME

Record of signatures. ALL prescribers MUST complete.

DATE	NAME	DESIGNATION	SIGNATURE	BLEEP NUMBER
20/11	ALEX LEWIS	F1	A Lewis	4567

Janice Cox (hospital number: 662107, DOB 28/02/YYYY [68 years old], address: 27 Manor Court, Longbury LB7 2MU) has been admitted to the medical assessment ward where she is under follow up for her bronchiectasis. A sputum sample she gave at her general practitioner's last week has grown *Pseudomonas*. Her consultant, Dr Erin Johnson, would like her to be admitted for intravenous meropenem to treat the infection. She weighs 45kg.

Mrs Cox's past medical history also includes osteoarthritis and hypothyroidism. Mrs Cox is allergic to Elastoplast, which gives her a rash.

Her medications are as follows:

Azithromycin 250mg on Monday, Wednesday and Friday.
Beclomethasone inhaler 400micrograms b.d.
Levothyroxine 125micrograms o.m.
Paracetamol 1g q.d.s.

Blood test results:

Sodium 139mmol/L
Potassium 4.5mmol/L
Urea 4.2mmol/L
Creatinine 115μmol/L
eGFR 40mL/min/1.73m²
Calculated creatinine clearance 29.3mL/min using the Cockcroft–Gault equation

Your task is to write up the chart for this patient's admission.
It is 09:00 on 18th December.

Notes

LONGBURY HOSPITAL TRUST			HOSPITAL NUMBER SURNAME FIRST NAME ADDRESS D.O.B		
DATE OF ADMISSION		ADMISSION WEIGHT (KG)		WARD	
ALLERGIES			CONSULTANT		
			CHART NO		...OF...

ONCE ONLY PRESCRIPTIONS

DATE	TIME	NAME OF DRUG	DOSE	ROUTE	PRESCRIBER'S SIGNATURE	GIVEN BY	TIME GIVEN

REGULAR MEDICATIONS

NAME OF DRUG		TIME	DATE → DOSE ↓				
ADDITIONAL INSTRUCTIONS		08:00					
DATE	ROUTE	12:00					
PRESCRIBER'S SIGNATURE		18:00					
PRESCRIBER'S NAME AND BLEEP		22:00					

NAME OF DRUG		TIME	DATE → DOSE ↓				
ADDITIONAL INSTRUCTIONS		08:00					
DATE	ROUTE	12:00					
PRESCRIBER'S SIGNATURE		18:00					
PRESCRIBER'S NAME AND BLEEP		22:00					

NAME OF DRUG		TIME	DATE → DOSE ↓				
ADDITIONAL INSTRUCTIONS		08:00					
DATE	ROUTE	12:00					
PRESCRIBER'S SIGNATURE		18:00					
PRESCRIBER'S NAME AND BLEEP		22:00					

PATIENT NAME   HOSPITAL NO.

NAME OF DRUG		TIME	DATE → DOSE ↓					
ADDITIONAL INSTRUCTIONS		08:00						
DATE	ROUTE	12:00						
PRESCRIBER'S SIGNATURE								
		18:00						
PRESCRIBER'S NAME AND BLEEP								
		22:00						

NAME OF DRUG		TIME	DATE → DOSE ↓					
ADDITIONAL INSTRUCTIONS		08:00						
DATE	ROUTE	12:00						
PRESCRIBER'S SIGNATURE								
		18:00						
PRESCRIBER'S NAME AND BLEEP								
		22:00						

NAME OF DRUG		TIME	DATE → DOSE ↓					
ADDITIONAL INSTRUCTIONS		08:00						
DATE	ROUTE	12:00						
PRESCRIBER'S SIGNATURE								
		18:00						
PRESCRIBER'S NAME AND BLEEP								
		22:00						

AS REQUIRED PRESCRIPTIONS

NAME OF DRUG		DATE					
INDICATION/ INSTRUCTION	DOSE	TIME					
FREQUENCY	ROUTE	DOSE					
PRESCRIBER'S SIGNATURE		ROUTE					
PRESCRIBER'S NAME AND BLEEP		GIVEN BY					
START DATE	STOP DATE						

PATIENT NAME   HOSPITAL NO.

NAME OF DRUG		DATE					
INDICATION/ INSTRUCTION	DOSE	TIME					
FREQUENCY	ROUTE	DOSE					
PRESCRIBER'S SIGNATURE		ROUTE					
PRESCRIBER'S NAME AND BLEEP		GIVEN BY					
START DATE	STOP DATE						

INTRAVENOUS FLUIDS

DATE	FLUID	ADDITIVE & DOSE	VOLUME	RATE/ DURATION	PRESCRIBER'S SIGNATURE	GIVEN BY	START TIME	END TIME

Record of signatures. ALL prescribers MUST complete.

DATE	NAME	DESIGNATION	SIGNATURE	BLEEP NUMBER

Step 2: Now check your work overleaf

Answer 30

The main focus of this exercise is safe prescribing. The patient is underweight and has borderline renal function: noticing these things should prompt a careful review of what is being prescribed.

Step 3: Compare your answer to the checklist below and the chart opposite ☑

D	Details	Checked patient details Used capital letters throughout Used correct abbreviations	☐
R	Regular medications	Prescribed regular medications Amended IV paracetamol dose in light of body weight	☐
U	Unpleasant reactions	Documented Elastoplast and the symptoms	☐
G	Gravid?	No	☐

C	Contra-indications	Avoided overdosing meropenem and paracetamol	☐
H	Hydration	Not required	☐
A	Analgesia	Reduced intravenous dose of paracetamol to 500mg q.d.s. based on patient's weight	☐
R	Renal function	Impaired	☐
T	Thrombo-prophylaxis	Prescribed enoxaparin 20mg	☐
S	Signature box	Signed signature box	☐

Rationale

This woman has a pseudomonal infection of her bronchiectatic airways. *Pseudomonas* is a gram-negative bacterium which causes respiratory tract infections in people with established airways disease. *Pseudomonas* is usually resistant to all but a handful of antibiotics.

Meropenem requires dose reduction if the patient's GFR is less than 50mL/min/1.73m². In this exercise meropenem was therefore given every 12 hours rather than every 8 hours. The azithromycin the patient takes regularly has been stopped. In general, long-term prophylactic antibiotics should be stopped in any patient being treated with a broad spectrum agent such as meropenem.

The discrepancy between this patient's estimated GFR and calculated creatinine clearance is due to her low body weight. Her creatinine clearance (and therefore renal function) is worse than the estimated GFR, hence prescription of enoxaparin at a low dose.

A hazard which is easily missed is accidental overdosing of intravenous paracetamol. This woman weighs only 45kg therefore the intravenous dose had to be reduced. The recommendation is a maximum of 60mg/kg in 24 hours (equivalent to 15mg/kg/dose), therefore she can safely have no more than 2.7g per day. Thus, 500mg q.d.s. has been prescribed as it is the nearest convenient amount to administer.

Remember to document the sensitivity to Elastoplast and state what the reaction is, in this case a rash. Remember that the beclometasone inhaler should be prescibed by brand name: the different brands are not interchangeable.

KEY POINTS

- Remember to amend prescriptions in renal impairment
- Consider the accuracy of eGFR in patients with low or high body weight. It is sometimes better to calculate the creatinine clearance
- Avoid intravenous paracetamol overdose in low-weight patients

LONGBURY HOSPITAL TRUST				HOSPITAL NUMBER	662107

				SURNAME	COX
				FIRST NAME	JANICE
				ADDRESS	27 MANOR COURT, LONGBURY LB7 2MU
				D.O.B	28/02/YYYY (68 YEARS AGO)
DATE OF ADMISSION	18/12/YYYY	ADMISSION WEIGHT (KG)	45kg	WARD	MEDICAL ASSESSMENT
ALLERGIES				CONSULTANT	ERIN JOHNSON
ELASTOPLAST - RASH				CHART NO	1...OF...1

ONCE ONLY PRESCRIPTIONS

DATE	TIME	NAME OF DRUG	DOSE	ROUTE	PRESCRIBER'S SIGNATURE	GIVEN BY	TIME GIVEN

REGULAR MEDICATIONS

NAME OF DRUG ENOXAPARIN	TIME	DATE → DOSE ↓	18/12				
ADDITIONAL INSTRUCTIONS	06:00						
DATE 18/12 ROUTE S/C	12:00						
PRESCRIBER'S SIGNATURE ALewis	18:00	20mg					
PRESCRIBER'S NAME AND BLEEP ALEX LEWIS 4567	22:00						

NAME OF DRUG MEROPENEM	TIME	DATE → DOSE ↓	18/12			21/12	
						REVIEW	
ADDITIONAL INSTRUCTIONS PSEUDOMONAS INFECTION	08:00	2g					
DATE 18/12 ROUTE IV	12:00						
PRESCRIBER'S SIGNATURE ALewis	18:00						
PRESCRIBER'S NAME AND BLEEP ALEX LEWIS 4567	22:00	2g					

NAME OF DRUG BECLOMETASONE 200 micrograms	TIME	DATE → DOSE ↓	18/12				
ADDITIONAL INSTRUCTIONS CLENIL	08:00	T̈T					
DATE 18/12 ROUTE INH	12:00						
PRESCRIBER'S SIGNATURE ALewis	18:00	T̈T					
PRESCRIBER'S NAME AND BLEEP ALEX LEWIS 4567	22:00						

PATIENT NAME *JANICE COX*   HOSPITAL NO.   *662107*

NAME OF DRUG *LEVOTHYROXINE*		TIME	DATE → DOSE ↓	*18/12*				
ADDITIONAL INSTRUCTIONS		08:00	*125 micrograms*					
DATE *18/12*	ROUTE *PO*	12:00						
PRESCRIBER'S SIGNATURE *A Lewis*		18:00						
PRESCRIBER'S NAME AND BLEEP *ALEX LEWIS 4567*		22:00						

NAME OF DRUG		TIME	DATE → DOSE ↓					
ADDITIONAL INSTRUCTIONS		08:00						
DATE	ROUTE	12:00						
PRESCRIBER'S SIGNATURE		18:00						
PRESCRIBER'S NAME AND BLEEP		22:00						

NAME OF DRUG		TIME	DATE → DOSE ↓					
ADDITIONAL INSTRUCTIONS		08:00						
DATE	ROUTE	12:00						
PRESCRIBER'S SIGNATURE		18:00						
PRESCRIBER'S NAME AND BLEEP		22:00						

AS REQUIRED PRESCRIPTIONS

NAME OF DRUG *PARACETAMOL*		DATE					
INDICATION/ INSTRUCTION *PAIN*	DOSE *500mg*	TIME					
FREQUENCY *QDS*	ROUTE *IV*	DOSE					
PRESCRIBER'S SIGNATURE *A Lewis*		ROUTE					
PRESCRIBER'S NAME AND BLEEP *ALEX LEWIS 4567*		GIVEN BY					
START DATE *18/12*	STOP DATE						

PATIENT NAME *JANICE COX*   HOSPITAL NO. *662107*

NAME OF DRUG		DATE							
INDICATION/ INSTRUCTION	DOSE	TIME							
FREQUENCY	ROUTE	DOSE							
PRESCRIBER'S SIGNATURE		ROUTE							
PRESCRIBER'S NAME AND BLEEP		GIVEN BY							
START DATE	STOP DATE								

INTRAVENOUS FLUIDS

DATE	FLUID	ADDITIVE & DOSE	VOLUME	RATE/ DURATION	PRESCRIBER'S SIGNATURE	GIVEN BY	START TIME	END TIME

Record of signatures. ALL prescribers MUST complete.

DATE	NAME	DESIGNATION	SIGNATURE	BLEEP NUMBER
18/12	ALEX LEWIS	F1	ALewis	4567

Monica Cole (hospital number: 841037, DOB 16/05/YYYY [48 years old], address: 19 Bridge Street, Longbury LB9 2UO) was admitted to the surgical ward yesterday evening with a cervical spine fracture and a left tibial fracture after falling off a horse. She was taken to theatre overnight and a halo brace has been fitted to stabilise her neck. Surgery is planned tomorrow for her tibial fracture. She weighs 64kg. Mrs Cole's consultant is Mr Joshua Gibb.

On the morning ward round the nursing staff have requested that Mrs Cole's regular medication is written up from the list faxed by her general practitioner. Mrs Cole is still in pain; she has no allergies and is not pregnant. The consultant instructs avoidance of thromboprophylaxis until after the tibial surgery.

Prescription history	Issue count	Last issued
Aspirin dispersible 75mg		
90 tablets		
One tablet in the morning	72	Sept, 1 month ago
Citalopram 20mg		
60 tablets		
One tablet in the morning	24	Aug , 3 years ago
Diazepam 5mg		
5 tablets		
One tablet as needed in the evening	10	Aug, 3 years ago
Ramipril 5mg		
90 capsules		
One capsule in the evening	70	Sept, 1 month ago
Simvastatin 40mg		
90 tablets		
One tablet in the evening	84	Sept, 1 month ago
Sodium valproate 500mg		
60 tablets		
Two tablets in the morning	54	Sept, 10 years ago

Your task is to prescribe the regular medications and pain relief.
It is 09:15 on 9th October.

Notes

LONGBURY HOSPITAL TRUST				HOSPITAL NUMBER	841037	
				SURNAME	COLE	
				FIRST NAME	MONICA	
				ADDRESS	19 BRIDGE STREET, LONGBURY, LB9 2UO	
				D.O.B	16/05/YYYY (48 YEARS AGO)	
DATE OF ADMISSION	08/10/YYYY	ADMISSION WEIGHT (KG)	64kg	WARD	SURGICAL	
ALLERGIES				CONSULTANT	JOSHUA GIBB	
NKDA				CHART NO	1...OF...1	

ONCE ONLY PRESCRIPTIONS

DATE	TIME	NAME OF DRUG	DOSE	ROUTE	PRESCRIBER'S SIGNATURE	GIVEN BY	TIME GIVEN

REGULAR MEDICATIONS

NAME OF DRUG PARACETAMOL	TIME	DATE → DOSE ↓	08/10	09/10			
ADDITIONAL INSTRUCTIONS	08:00	1g		WP			
DATE 08/10 ROUTE PO/IV	12:00	1g					
PRESCRIBER'S SIGNATURE EJones	18:00	1g					
PRESCRIBER'S NAME AND BLEEP EMMA JONES 4876	22:00	1g	RN				

NAME OF DRUG CODEINE	TIME	DATE → DOSE ↓	08/10	09/10			
ADDITIONAL INSTRUCTIONS	08:00	30-60mg		WP			
DATE 08/10 ROUTE PO	12:00	30-60mg					
PRESCRIBER'S SIGNATURE EJones	18:00	30-60mg					
PRESCRIBER'S NAME AND BLEEP EMMA JONES 4876	22:00	30-60mg	RN				

NAME OF DRUG	TIME	DATE → DOSE ↓					
ADDITIONAL INSTRUCTIONS	08:00						
DATE ROUTE	12:00						
PRESCRIBER'S SIGNATURE	18:00						
PRESCRIBER'S NAME AND BLEEP	22:00						

PATIENT NAME MONICA COLE   HOSPITAL NO.   841037

NAME OF DRUG		TIME	DATE → DOSE ↓						
ADDITIONAL INSTRUCTIONS		08:00							
DATE	ROUTE	12:00							
PRESCRIBER'S SIGNATURE									
		18:00							
PRESCRIBER'S NAME AND BLEEP									
		22:00							

NAME OF DRUG		TIME	DATE → DOSE ↓						
ADDITIONAL INSTRUCTIONS		08:00							
DATE	ROUTE	12:00							
PRESCRIBER'S SIGNATURE									
		18:00							
PRESCRIBER'S NAME AND BLEEP									
		22:00							

NAME OF DRUG		TIME	DATE → DOSE ↓						
ADDITIONAL INSTRUCTIONS		08:00							
DATE	ROUTE	12:00							
PRESCRIBER'S SIGNATURE									
		18:00							
PRESCRIBER'S NAME AND BLEEP									
		22:00							

AS REQUIRED PRESCRIPTIONS

NAME OF DRUG		DATE						
INDICATION/ INSTRUCTION	DOSE	TIME						
FREQUENCY	ROUTE	DOSE						
PRESCRIBER'S SIGNATURE		ROUTE						
PRESCRIBER'S NAME AND BLEEP		GIVEN BY						
START DATE	STOP DATE							

PATIENT NAME MONICA COLE   HOSPITAL NO.   841037

NAME OF DRUG			DATE						
INDICATION/ INSTRUCTION	DOSE		TIME						
FREQUENCY	ROUTE		DOSE						
PRESCRIBER'S SIGNATURE			ROUTE						
PRESCRIBER'S NAME AND BLEEP			GIVEN BY						
START DATE	STOP DATE								

INTRAVENOUS FLUIDS

DATE	FLUID	ADDITIVE & DOSE	VOLUME	RATE/ DURATION	PRESCRIBER'S SIGNATURE	GIVEN BY	START TIME	END TIME

Record of signatures. ALL prescribers MUST complete.

DATE	NAME	DESIGNATION	SIGNATURE	BLEEP NUMBER
08/10	EMMA JONES	F2	EJones	4876

Answer 31

Care must be taken when prescribing a patient's pre-existing regular medications. Often the temptation is to simply copy whatever list is handed over. In this exercise, the list sent by the general practitioner is a list of all prescriptions ever made to this patient and not a simple list of repeat prescriptions. Therefore the drugs must be checked and interpreted by the prescribing doctor.

Step 3: Compare your answer to the checklist below and the chart opposite ✔

D	Details	Checked patient details Used capital letters throughout Used correct abbreviations	☐
R	Regular medications	Prescribed: ramipril, simvastatin Omitted: diazepam, citalopram, sodium valproate Delayed: aspirin	☐
U	Unpleasant reactions	NKDA	☐
G	Gravid?	No	☐

C	Contra-indications	Did not restart old prescriptions	☐
H	Hydration	Prescribed at least 1L over 8–10 hours. Patient unlikely to maintain adequate oral intake if in bed with halo collar and will be NBM tonight	☐
A	Analgesia	Prescribed according to pain ladder. Considered laxatives with opiates	☐
R	Renal function	Assumed renal function OK	☐
T	Thrombo-prophylaxis	Did not prescribe until after the operation	☐
S	Signature box	Signed signature box	☐

Rationale

Aspirin, ramipril and simvastatin are all drugs that the patient has been using very recently, so these are likely to represent the current regular medications. Looking at the dates, diazepam, citalopram and sodium valproate have not been issued in years, therefore these should not be prescribed. This avoids unintentionally reinitiating a potentially harmful medication.

Another consideration is whether to prescribe aspirin, given that this patient is being prepared for orthopaedic surgery. The irreversible inactivating effect of aspirin on platelets will persist for 7 days after it is stopped, which is long after this patient will have had her operation, so there is little to gain from stopping the aspirin alone. However, in case the surgeon decides that the patient needs a platelet transfusion preoperatively, it would be prudent to ensure that the patient does not then receive aspirin afterwards. Accordingly, in this exercise the prescriber has not restarted aspirin until after the tibial operation.

Pain relief has been prescribed according to the principles of the analgesic ladder (page 6), here, Oramorph 5–10mg and cyclizine 50mg. The patient has been prescribed fluids as she is already recovering from one general anaesthetic and is due to be nil by mouth again shortly.

KEY POINTS

- Check all medication lists carefully
- Look out for notes from the pharmacist, as he or she will also review a patient's drug history

LONGBURY HOSPITAL TRUST				HOSPITAL NUMBER	841037
				SURNAME	COLE
				FIRST NAME	MONICA
				ADDRESS	19 BRIDGE STREET, LONGBURY LB9 2UO
				D.O.B	16/05/YYYY (48 YEARS AGO)
DATE OF ADMISSION	08/10/YYYY	ADMISSION WEIGHT (KG)	64kg	WARD	SURGICAL
ALLERGIES				CONSULTANT	JOSHUA GIBB
NKDA				CHART NO	1…OF…1

ONCE ONLY PRESCRIPTIONS

DATE	TIME	NAME OF DRUG	DOSE	ROUTE	PRESCRIBER'S SIGNATURE	GIVEN BY	TIME GIVEN

REGULAR MEDICATIONS

NAME OF DRUG PARACETAMOL	TIME	DATE → DOSE ↓	08/10	09/10			
ADDITIONAL INSTRUCTIONS	08:00	1g		WP			
DATE 08/10 ROUTE PO/IV	12:00	1g					
PRESCRIBER'S SIGNATURE EJones	18:00	1g					
PRESCRIBER'S NAME AND BLEEP EMMA JONES 4876	22:00	1g	RN				

NAME OF DRUG CODEINE	TIME	DATE → DOSE ↓	08/10	09/10			
ADDITIONAL INSTRUCTIONS	08:00	30-60mg		WP			
DATE 08/10 ROUTE PO	12:00	30-60mg					
PRESCRIBER'S SIGNATURE EJones	18:00	30-60mg					
PRESCRIBER'S NAME AND BLEEP EMMA JONES 4876	22:00	30-60mg	RN				

NAME OF DRUG RAMIPRIL	TIME	DATE → DOSE ↓		09/10			
ADDITIONAL INSTRUCTIONS	06:00						
DATE 09/10 ROUTE PO	12:00						
PRESCRIBER'S SIGNATURE ALewis	18:00						
PRESCRIBER'S NAME AND BLEEP ALEX LEWIS 4567	22:00	5mg					

PATIENT NAME MONICA COLE HOSPITAL NO. 841037

NAME OF DRUG SIMVASTATIN	TIME	DATE → DOSE ↓	09/10			
ADDITIONAL INSTRUCTIONS	08:00					
DATE 09/10 ROUTE PO	12:00					
PRESCRIBER'S SIGNATURE ALewis	18:00					
PRESCRIBER'S NAME AND BLEEP ALEX LEWIS 4567	22:00	40mg				

NAME OF DRUG ASPIRIN DISPERSIBLE	TIME	DATE → DOSE ↓	09/10	10/10	11/10	
ADDITIONAL INSTRUCTIONS	08:00	75mg	———	———		
DATE 09/10 ROUTE PO	12:00					
PRESCRIBER'S SIGNATURE ALewis	18:00					
PRESCRIBER'S NAME AND BLEEP ALEX LEWIS 4567	22:00					

NAME OF DRUG	TIME	DATE → DOSE ↓				
ADDITIONAL INSTRUCTIONS	08:00					
DATE ROUTE	12:00					
PRESCRIBER'S SIGNATURE	18:00					
PRESCRIBER'S NAME AND BLEEP	22:00					

AS REQUIRED PRESCRIPTIONS

NAME OF DRUG ORAMORPH		DATE				
INDICATION/ INSTRUCTION PAIN	DOSE 5-10mg	TIME				
FREQUENCY 2-4 HOURLY	ROUTE PO	DOSE				
PRESCRIBER'S SIGNATURE ALewis		ROUTE				
PRESCRIBER'S NAME AND BLEEP ALEX LEWIS 4567		GIVEN BY				
START DATE 09/10	STOP DATE					

PATIENT NAME MONICA COLE   HOSPITAL NO.   841037

NAME OF DRUG CYCLIZINE		DATE						
INDICATION/ INSTRUCTION NAUSEA	DOSE 50mg	TIME						
FREQUENCY TDS	ROUTE PO/IV/IM	DOSE						
PRESCRIBER'S SIGNATURE ALewis		ROUTE						
PRESCRIBER'S NAME AND BLEEP ALEX LEWIS 4567		GIVEN BY						
START DATE 09/10	STOP DATE							

INTRAVENOUS FLUIDS

DATE	FLUID	ADDITIVE & DOSE	VOLUME	RATE/ DURATION	PRESCRIBER'S SIGNATURE	GIVEN BY	START TIME	END TIME
09/10	HARTMANN'S	————————	1l	100ml/h	ALewis			

Record of signatures. ALL prescribers MUST complete.

DATE	NAME	DESIGNATION	SIGNATURE	BLEEP NUMBER
08/10	EMMA JONES	F2	EJones	4876
09/10	ALEX LEWIS	F1	ALewis	4567

James Rothstein (hospital number: 178412, DOB 04/05/YYYY [62 years old], address: 89 Barrington Avenue, Longbury LB22 9HL) has Parkinson's disease. He was admitted following a fall and was diagnosed with a urinary tract infection sensitive to trimethoprim and co-amoxiclav. Overnight he started vomiting profusely and an abdominal X-ray has shown small bowel obstruction. The surgeons have advised that he be kept nil by mouth until they can review him.

At the start of the ward round, the nurses have asked for review of Mr Rothstein's medications and prescription of an antiemetic for the vomiting.

Your task is to review the medications and prescribe the appropriate treatment.
It is 09:00 on 6th March.

Notes

Step 1: Complete your answers in the drug chart opposite and overleaf

LONGBURY HOSPITAL TRUST

HOSPITAL NUMBER	178412
SURNAME	ROTHSTEIN
FIRST NAME	JAMES
ADDRESS	89 BARRINGTON AVENUE, LONGBURY LB22 9HL
D.O.B	04/05/YYYY (62 YEARS AGO)

DATE OF ADMISSION	04/03/YYYY	ADMISSION WEIGHT (KG)	71kg	WARD	MEDICAL ASSESSMENT

ALLERGIES	CONSULTANT	ERIN JOHNSON
NKDA	CHART NO	1...OF...1

ONCE ONLY PRESCRIPTIONS

DATE	TIME	NAME OF DRUG	DOSE	ROUTE	PRESCRIBER'S SIGNATURE	GIVEN BY	TIME GIVEN

REGULAR MEDICATIONS

NAME OF DRUG ENOXAPARIN	TIME	DOSE ↓	04/03	05/03	06/03		
ADDITIONAL INSTRUCTIONS	08:00						
DATE 04/03 ROUTE SC	12:00						
PRESCRIBER'S SIGNATURE KCho	18:00	40mg	RN	RN			
PRESCRIBER'S NAME AND BLEEP KENNETH CHO 5765	22:00						

NAME OF DRUG MADOPAR (CO-BENELDOPA)	TIME	DOSE ↓	04/03	05/03	06/03		
ADDITIONAL INSTRUCTIONS	08:00	125mg	RN	RN	WITHHELD		
DATE 04/03 ROUTE PO	12:00						
PRESCRIBER'S SIGNATURE KCho	14:00	125mg	RN	RN			
	18:00						
PRESCRIBER'S NAME AND BLEEP KENNETH CHO 5765	22:00	125mg	TJ	WITHHELD			

NAME OF DRUG TRIMETHOPRIM	TIME	DOSE ↓	04/03	05/03	06/03		
ADDITIONAL INSTRUCTIONS UTI 5 DAYS	08:00	200mg	RN	RN	WITHHELD		
DATE 04/03 ROUTE PO	12:00						
PRESCRIBER'S SIGNATURE KCho	18:00						
PRESCRIBER'S NAME AND BLEEP KENNETH CHO 5765	22:00	200mg	TJ	WITHHELD			

PATIENT NAME JAMES ROTHSTEIN   HOSPITAL NO.   178412

NAME OF DRUG	TIME	DATE → / DOSE ↓					
ADDITIONAL INSTRUCTIONS	08:00						
DATE / ROUTE	12:00						
PRESCRIBER'S SIGNATURE	18:00						
PRESCRIBER'S NAME AND BLEEP	22:00						

NAME OF DRUG	TIME	DATE → / DOSE ↓					
ADDITIONAL INSTRUCTIONS	08:00						
DATE / ROUTE	12:00						
PRESCRIBER'S SIGNATURE	18:00						
PRESCRIBER'S NAME AND BLEEP	22:00						

NAME OF DRUG	TIME	DATE → / DOSE ↓					
ADDITIONAL INSTRUCTIONS	08:00						
DATE / ROUTE	12:00						
PRESCRIBER'S SIGNATURE	18:00						
PRESCRIBER'S NAME AND BLEEP	22:00						

AS REQUIRED PRESCRIPTIONS

NAME OF DRUG		DATE					
INDICATION/ INSTRUCTION	DOSE	TIME					
FREQUENCY	ROUTE	DOSE					
PRESCRIBER'S SIGNATURE		ROUTE					
PRESCRIBER'S NAME AND BLEEP		GIVEN BY					
START DATE	STOP DATE						

PATIENT NAME JAMES ROTHSTEIN   HOSPITAL NO.   178412

NAME OF DRUG		DATE						
INDICATION/ INSTRUCTION	DOSE	TIME						
FREQUENCY	ROUTE	DOSE						
PRESCRIBER'S SIGNATURE		ROUTE						
PRESCRIBER'S NAME AND BLEEP		GIVEN BY						
START DATE	STOP DATE							

INTRAVENOUS FLUIDS

DATE	FLUID	ADDITIVE & DOSE	VOLUME	RATE/ DURATION	PRESCRIBER'S SIGNATURE	GIVEN BY	START TIME	END TIME

Record of signatures. ALL prescribers MUST complete.

DATE	NAME	DESIGNATION	SIGNATURE	BLEEP NUMBER
04/03	KENNETH CHO	SHO	KCho	5765

Step 2: Now check your work overleaf

Answer 32

Stopping anti-Parkinson's disease medication suddenly should be avoided because patients become bradykinetic very quickly. If a patient is nil-by-mouth because of an unsafe swallow, levodopa-containing medications, such as co-beneldopa, should be given nasogastrically in a dispersible form dissolved in a minimal amount of water. However, in this exercise, the patient is vomiting profusely due to bowel obstruction and the enteral route is therefore contraindicated.

Step 3: Compare your answer to the checklist below and the chart opposite ☑

D Details	Checked patient details Used capital letters throughout Used correct abbreviations	☐
R Regular medications	Prescribed alternative to oral anti-Parkinson's medications Prescribed parenteral antibiotic for urinary tract infection Prescribed cyclizine or ondansetron PRN (avoid metoclopramide)	☐
U Unpleasant reactions	None	☐
G Gravid?	No	☐

C Contra-indications	Did not stop Parkinson's disease medications. Did not prescribe metoclopramide	☐
H Hydration	Prescribed maintenance fluid	☐
A Analgesia	Not required	☐
R Renal function	Not required	☐
T Thrombo-prophylaxis	Continued enoxaparin	☐
S Signature box	Signed signature box	☐

Rationale

The two non-oral medications for Parkinson's disease are apomorphine (subcutaneous injection) and rotigotine (transdermal patch). Apomorphine is given by subcutaneous infusion and would only be initiated by a Parkinson's disease specialist. Some hospitals have guidelines for converting from levodopa to rotigotine so it would be prudent to contact a specialist team. The important point is to recognise that a patient cannot go without an element of anti-Parkinson's medication simply because he or she has lost the oral route of administration. There is little evidence showing how to convert doses from levodopa to rotigotine. Start with a low dose patch and review their symptoms: the strength of the patch can be increased as necessary.

This patient will also be unable to take trimethoprim for his urinary tract infection, as trimethoprim is only available orally. Antibiotics such as co-amoxiclav, amoxicillin and gentamicin cover typical urinary pathogens and are available intravenously.

KEY POINTS

- Abrupt withdrawal of anti-Parkinson's medication should be avoided. Look to replace the medication via alternative routes in those who cannot take oral medication
- Not all antibiotics are available in intravenous form

LONGBURY HOSPITAL TRUST			HOSPITAL NUMBER	178412
			SURNAME	ROTHSTEIN
			FIRST NAME	JAMES
			ADDRESS	89 BARRINGTON AVENUE, LONGBURY LB22 9HL
			D.O.B	04/05/YYYY (62 YEARS AGO)

DATE OF ADMISSION	04/03/YYYY	ADMISSION WEIGHT (KG)	71kg	WARD	MEDICAL ASSESSMENT
ALLERGIES			CONSULTANT		ERIN JOHNSON
NKDA			CHART NO		1...OF...1

ONCE ONLY PRESCRIPTIONS

DATE	TIME	NAME OF DRUG	DOSE	ROUTE	PRESCRIBER'S SIGNATURE	GIVEN BY	TIME GIVEN

REGULAR MEDICATIONS

NAME OF DRUG ENOXAPARIN	TIME	DATE → DOSE ↓	04/03	05/03	06/03		
ADDITIONAL INSTRUCTIONS	08:00						
DATE 04/03 ROUTE SC	12:00						
PRESCRIBER'S SIGNATURE KCho	18:00	40mg	RN	RN			
PRESCRIBER'S NAME AND BLEEP KENNETH CHO 5765	22:00						

NAME OF DRUG MADOPAR (CO-BENELDOPA)	TIME	DATE → DOSE ↓	04/03	05/03	06/03		
ADDITIONAL INSTRUCTIONS	08:00	125mg	RN	RN	WITHHELD		
					STOP		
DATE 04/03 ROUTE PO	12:00				ALewis		
PRESCRIBER'S SIGNATURE KCho	14:00	125mg	RN	RN	06/03		
	18:00						
PRESCRIBER'S NAME AND BLEEP KENNETH CHO 5765	22:00	125mg	TJ	WITHHELD			

NAME OF DRUG TRIMETHOPRIM	TIME	DATE → DOSE ↓	04/03	05/03	06/03		
ADDITIONAL INSTRUCTIONS UTI 5 days	08:00	200mg	RN	RN	WITHHELD		
					STOP		
DATE 04/03 ROUTE PO	12:00				ALewis		
PRESCRIBER'S SIGNATURE KCho	18:00				06/03		
PRESCRIBER'S NAME AND BLEEP KENNETH CHO 5765	22:00	200mg	TJ	WITHHELD			

264

PATIENT NAME JAMES ROTHSTEIN   HOSPITAL NO. 178412

NAME OF DRUG ROTIGOTINE 4mg/24 HOURS	TIME	DATE → DOSE ↓			06/03		
ADDITIONAL INSTRUCTIONS NEW APPLICATION EACH DAY	08:00	ONE PATCH	——	——			
DATE 06/03 ROUTE PATCH	12:00						
PRESCRIBER'S SIGNATURE ALewis	18:00						
PRESCRIBER'S NAME AND BLEEP ALEX LEWIS 4567	22:00						

NAME OF DRUG CO-AMOXICLAV	TIME	DATE → DOSE ↓			06/03		
ADDITIONAL INSTRUCTIONS UTI 5 DAYS	08:00	1.2g	——	——			
DATE 06/03 ROUTE IV	12:00						
PRESCRIBER'S SIGNATURE ALewis	14:00	1.2g	——	——			
	18:00						
PRESCRIBER'S NAME AND BLEEP ALEX LEWIS 4567	22:00	1.2g	——	——			

NAME OF DRUG	TIME	DATE → DOSE ↓					
ADDITIONAL INSTRUCTIONS	08:00						
DATE ROUTE	12:00						
PRESCRIBER'S SIGNATURE	18:00						
PRESCRIBER'S NAME AND BLEEP	22:00						

AS REQUIRED PRESCRIPTIONS

NAME OF DRUG CYCLIZINE		DATE					
INDICATION/ INSTRUCTION NAUSEA	DOSE 50mg	TIME					
FREQUENCY TDS	ROUTE IM/SC/IV	DOSE					
PRESCRIBER'S SIGNATURE ALewis		ROUTE					
PRESCRIBER'S NAME AND BLEEP ALEX LEWIS 4567		GIVEN BY					
START DATE 06/03	STOP DATE						

PATIENT NAME JAMES ROTHSTEIN   HOSPITAL NO.   178412

NAME OF DRUG		DATE						
INDICATION/ INSTRUCTION	DOSE	TIME						
FREQUENCY	ROUTE	DOSE						
PRESCRIBER'S SIGNATURE		ROUTE						
PRESCRIBER'S NAME AND BLEEP		GIVEN BY						
START DATE	STOP DATE							

INTRAVENOUS FLUIDS

DATE	FLUID	ADDITIVE & DOSE	VOLUME	RATE/ DURATION	PRESCRIBER'S SIGNATURE	GIVEN BY	START TIME	END TIME
06/03	0.9% NaCl	————	1000ml	100ml/h	ALewis			

Record of signatures. ALL prescribers MUST complete.

DATE	NAME	DESIGNATION	SIGNATURE	BLEEP NUMBER
04/03	KENNETH CHO	SHO	KCho	5765
06/03	ALEX LEWIS	F1	ALewis	4567

Harveer Dev (hospital number: 198623, DOB 14/03/YYYY [78 years old], address: 10 Degalare Road, Longbury LB2 6SE) is suffering from heart failure and was recently treated on the intensive care unit (ITU) with new atrial fibrillation with intravenous amiodarone. He is now on the medical assessment ward. His past medical history includes a metallic mitral valve and mild asthma.

On the ward round today, Mr Dev is comfortable and has no new issues. He is looking forward to going home after his occupational therapist and physiotherapist sign him off.

Routine blood test results, taken this morning:
Sodium 132mmol/L
Potassium 3.3mmol/L
Creatinine 130μmol/L
Haemoglobin 116g/L
Platelets 180 x10⁹/L
International normalised ratio (INR) 6.5

Mr Dev's high INR is noted. On direct questioning he denies any bleeding. He has not started any new drugs since his return from ITU. His normal warfarin dose is 4mg.

Your task is to manage his warfarin therapy.
It is 08:30 on 9th June.

Notes

Step 1: Complete your answers in the drug chart opposite and overleaf

LONGBURY HOSPITAL TRUST			HOSPITAL NUMBER	198623		
			SURNAME	DEV		
			FIRST NAME	HARVEER		
			ADDRESS	10 DEGALARE ROAD, LONGBURY LB2 6SE		
			D.O.B	14/03/YYYY (78 YEARS AGO)		
DATE OF ADMISSION 02/06/YYYY	ADMISSION WEIGHT (KG)	79kg	WARD	MEDICAL ASSESSMENT		
ALLERGIES			CONSULTANT	ERIN JOHNSON		
LATEX – RASH			CHART NO	1…OF…1		

ONCE ONLY PRESCRIPTIONS

DATE	TIME	NAME OF DRUG	DOSE	ROUTE	PRESCRIBER'S SIGNATURE	GIVEN BY	TIME GIVEN

REGULAR MEDICATIONS

NAME OF DRUG RAMIPRIL	TIME	DATE → DOSE ↓	06/06	07/06	08/06	09/06	
ADDITIONAL INSTRUCTIONS	08:00	5 mg	RN	RN	FR	FR	
DATE 06/06 ROUTE PO	12:00						
PRESCRIBER'S SIGNATURE BFord	18:00						
PRESCRIBER'S NAME AND BLEEP BEN FORD 1569	22:00						

NAME OF DRUG DIGOXIN	TIME	DATE → DOSE ↓	06/06	07/06	08/06	09/06	
ADDITIONAL INSTRUCTIONS	08:00	62.5 micrograms	RN	RN	FR	FR	
DATE 06/06 ROUTE PO	12:00						
PRESCRIBER'S SIGNATURE BFord	18:00						
PRESCRIBER'S NAME AND BLEEP BEN FORD 1569	22:00						

NAME OF DRUG FUROSEMIDE	TIME	DATE → DOSE ↓	06/06	07/06	08/06	09/06	
ADDITIONAL INSTRUCTIONS	08:00	80mg	RN	RN	FR	FR	
DATE 06/06 ROUTE PO	12:00	40mg	RN	RN	FR		
PRESCRIBER'S SIGNATURE BFord	18:00						
PRESCRIBER'S NAME AND BLEEP BEN FORD 1569	22:00						

PATIENT NAME HARVEER DEV   HOSPITAL NO.   198623

NAME OF DRUG ISOSORBIDE MONONITRATE MR	TIME	DATE → DOSE ↓	06/06	07/06	08/06	09/06	
ADDITIONAL INSTRUCTIONS	08:00	30mg	RN	RN	FR	FR	
DATE 06/06 ROUTE PO	12:00						
PRESCRIBER'S SIGNATURE BFord	18:00						
PRESCRIBER'S NAME AND BLEEP BEN FORD 1569	22:00						

NAME OF DRUG WARFARIN	TIME	DATE → DOSE ↓	06/06	07/06	08/06	09/06	
ADDITIONAL INSTRUCTIONS	08:00						
DATE 06/06 ROUTE PO	12:00						
PRESCRIBER'S SIGNATURE BFord	18:00	VARIABLE SEE BELOW	RN	RN	FR		
PRESCRIBER'S NAME AND BLEEP BEN FORD 1569	22:00						

NAME OF DRUG ATENOLOL	TIME	DATE → DOSE ↓	06/06	07/06	08/06	09/06	
ADDITIONAL INSTRUCTIONS	08:00	50mg	RN	RN	FR	FR	
DATE 06/06 ROUTE PO	12:00						
PRESCRIBER'S SIGNATURE BFord	18:00						
PRESCRIBER'S NAME AND BLEEP BEN FORD 1569	22:00						

AS REQUIRED PRESCRIPTIONS

NAME OF DRUG SALBUTAMOL		DATE					
INDICATION/ INSTRUCTION S.O.B/ BREATHLESSNESS	DOSE 5mg	TIME					
FREQUENCY PRN	ROUTE NEB	DOSE					
PRESCRIBER'S SIGNATURE BFord		ROUTE					
PRESCRIBER'S NAME AND BLEEP BEN FORD 1569		GIVEN BY					
START DATE 06/06	STOP DATE						

PATIENT NAME HARVEER DEV   HOSPITAL NO.   198623

NAME OF DRUG		DATE					
INDICATION/ INSTRUCTION	DOSE	TIME					
FREQUENCY	ROUTE	DOSE					
PRESCRIBER'S SIGNATURE		ROUTE					
PRESCRIBER'S NAME AND BLEEP		GIVEN BY					
START DATE	STOP DATE						

ANTICOAGULATION CHART

DATE	6/6	7/6	8/6	9/6	10/6	11/6
INR	3.7			6.5		
WARFARIN DOSE	4mg	4mg	4mg	4mg		
PRESCRIBER'S SIGNATURE	BFord	BFord	BFord			
GIVEN BY	RN	RN	FR			
TIME	18:00	18:00	18:00			

INTRAVENOUS FLUIDS

DATE	FLUID	ADDITIVE & DOSE	VOLUME	RATE/ DURATION	PRESCRIBER'S SIGNATURE	GIVEN BY	START TIME	END TIME

Record of signatures. ALL prescribers MUST complete.

DATE	NAME	DESIGNATION	SIGNATURE	BLEEP NUMBER
06/06	BEN FORD	F2	BFord	1569

Step 2: Now check your work overleaf

Answer 33

Managing a deranged INR is a common task for junior doctors and often crops up in OSCEs. This exercise is about applying a strategy for managing deranged INR results and considering what caused them.

Step 3: Compare your answer to the checklist below and the chart opposite ☑

D Details	Checked patient details Used capital letters throughout Used correct abbreviations	☐
R Regular medications	Continued regular medications	☐
U Unpleasant reactions	Noticed that Latex had been documented	☐
G Gravid?	No	☐

C Contra-indications	None	☐
H Hydration	Not required	☐
A Analgesia	Not required	☐
R Renal function	OK	☐
T Thrombo-prophylaxis	Omitted warfarin for 1–2 days	☐
S Signature box	Signed signature box	☐

Rationale

A good starting point for learning how to manage a deranged INR is to consult a national formulary. As this patient's INR is between 5.0 and 8.0 and as there is no evidence of bleeding one or two doses of warfarin are withheld.

It is important to review the INR over the next few days to confirm that it is falling and to monitor the patient for signs of bleeding, which, if present, should be treated with phytomenadione (vitamin K) and/or prothrombin concentrate (Beriplex). The warfarin maintenance dose may need to be reduced to keep the INR within preferred range.

The next step is to consider why this patient's INR has become deranged despite the fact he his on a stable dose of his normal medication. It is worth checking his liver function tests and looking at the medication administered during his intensive care unit (ITU) stay. One potential cause could be use of amiodarone in the ITU, in practice you would check this patient's first chart from the ITU (the exercise shows his second chart). Amiodarone has very long half-life (weeks to months if used chronically) and may continue to increase the effect of warfarin after it has been stopped. This means that the patient will require a lower than usual maintenance dose of warfarin for the next few weeks and requires more frequent monitoring. As this patient has a metallic mitral heart valve it is also worth remembering that his target INR is 3.0–3.5, depending on type of valve used.

KEY POINTS

- Use formularies and local guidance in correcting a deranged INR
- Look for causes of deranged INR, e.g. liver dysfunction, interacting medications, poor compliance/absorption

LONGBURY HOSPITAL TRUST		HOSPITAL NUMBER	198623			
		SURNAME	DEV			
		FIRST NAME	HARVEER			
		ADDRESS	10 DEGALARE ROAD, LONGBURY LB2 6SE			
		D.O.B	14/03/YYYY (78 YEARS AGO)			

DATE OF ADMISSION	02/06/YYYY	ADMISSION WEIGHT (KG)	79kg	WARD	MEDICAL ASSESSMENT
ALLERGIES			CONSULTANT		ERIN JOHNSON
LATEX - RASH			CHART NO		1...OF...1

ONCE ONLY PRESCRIPTIONS

DATE	TIME	NAME OF DRUG	DOSE	ROUTE	PRESCRIBER'S SIGNATURE	GIVEN BY	TIME GIVEN

REGULAR MEDICATIONS

NAME OF DRUG RAMIPRIL	TIME	DATE → DOSE ↓	06/06	07/06	08/06	09/06	
ADDITIONAL INSTRUCTIONS	08:00	5mg	RN	RN	FR	FR	
DATE 06/06 ROUTE PO	12:00						
PRESCRIBER'S SIGNATURE BFord	18:00						
PRESCRIBER'S NAME AND BLEEP BEN FORD 1569	22:00						

NAME OF DRUG DIGOXIN	TIME	DATE → DOSE ↓	06/06	07/06	08/06	09/06	
ADDITIONAL INSTRUCTIONS	08:00	62.5 micrograms	RN	RN	FR	FR	
DATE 06/06 ROUTE PO	12:00						
PRESCRIBER'S SIGNATURE BFord	18:00						
PRESCRIBER'S NAME AND BLEEP BEN FORD 1569	22:00						

NAME OF DRUG FUROSEMIDE	TIME	DATE → DOSE ↓	06/06	07/06	08/06	09/06	
ADDITIONAL INSTRUCTIONS	08:00	80mg	RN	RN	FR	FR	
DATE 06/06 ROUTE PO	12:00	40mg	RN	RN	FR		
PRESCRIBER'S SIGNATURE BFord	18:00						
PRESCRIBER'S NAME AND BLEEP BEN FORD 1569	22:00						

PATIENT NAME HARVEER DEV   HOSPITAL NO. 198623

NAME OF DRUG ISOSORBIDE MONONITRATE MR	TIME	DATE → DOSE ↓	06/06	07/06	08/06	09/06	
ADDITIONAL INSTRUCTIONS	08:00	30mg	RN	RN	FR	FR	
DATE 06/06 ROUTE PO	12:00						
PRESCRIBER'S SIGNATURE BFord	18:00						
PRESCRIBER'S NAME AND BLEEP BEN FORD 1569	22:00						

NAME OF DRUG WARFARIN	TIME	DATE → DOSE ↓	06/06	07/06	08/06	09/06	
ADDITIONAL INSTRUCTIONS	08:00						
DATE 06/06 ROUTE PO	12:00						
PRESCRIBER'S SIGNATURE BFord	18:00	VARIABLE SEE BELOW	RN	RN	FR	OMIT ALewis	OMIT
PRESCRIBER'S NAME AND BLEEP BEN FORD 1569	22:00						

NAME OF DRUG ATENOLOL	TIME	DATE → DOSE ↓	06/06	07/06	08/06	09/06	
ADDITIONAL INSTRUCTIONS	08:00	50mg	RN	RN	FR	FR	
DATE 06/06 ROUTE PO	12:00						
PRESCRIBER'S SIGNATURE BFord	18:00						
PRESCRIBER'S NAME AND BLEEP BEN FORD 1569	22:00						

AS REQUIRED PRESCRIPTIONS

NAME OF DRUG SALBUTAMOL		DATE					
INDICATION/ INSTRUCTION S.O.B/ BREATHLESSNESS	DOSE 5mg	TIME					
FREQUENCY PRN	ROUTE NEB	DOSE					
PRESCRIBER'S SIGNATURE BFord		ROUTE					
PRESCRIBER'S NAME AND BLEEP BEN FORD 1569		GIVEN BY					
START DATE 06/06	STOP DATE						

PATIENT NAME HARVEER DEV   HOSPITAL NO.   198623

NAME OF DRUG		DATE					
INDICATION/ INSTRUCTION	DOSE	TIME					
FREQUENCY	ROUTE	DOSE					
PRESCRIBER'S SIGNATURE		ROUTE					
PRESCRIBER'S NAME AND BLEEP		GIVEN BY					
START DATE	STOP DATE						

ANTICOAGULATION CHART

DATE	6/6	7/6	8/6	9/6	10/6	11/6
INR	3.7			6.5		
WARFARIN DOSE	4mg	4mg	4mg	~~4mg~~		
PRESCRIBER'S SIGNATURE	BFord	BFord	BFord	OMIT	OMIT	REVIEW
GIVEN BY	RN	RN	FR	ALewis		
TIME	18:00	18:00	18:00			

INTRAVENOUS FLUIDS

DATE	FLUID	ADDITIVE & DOSE	VOLUME	RATE/ DURATION	PRESCRIBER'S SIGNATURE	GIVEN BY	START TIME	END TIME

Record of signatures. ALL prescribers MUST complete.

DATE	NAME	DESIGNATION	SIGNATURE	BLEEP NUMBER
06/06	BEN FORD	F2	BFord	1569
09/06	ALEX LEWIS	F1	ALewis	4567

Doreen Finch (hospital number: 709114, DOB 28/02/YYYY [82 years old], address: 31 Lake Close, Longbury LB13 8TW) is being treated for a urinary tract infection with intravenous gentamicin. She had her first dose yesterday at 18:00. Blood was taken to check her gentamicin level this morning at 02:00. It is reported to be gentamicin 6.9microgram/mL Mrs Finch's renal function is stable, with eGFR >60mL /min/1.73m². She weighs 64kg.

Your task is to prescribe a course of gentamicin (dose 5mg/kg) for the next 6 days. Use the dosing nomogram on page 6 to help you. Indicate on the drug chart when the gentamicin level should next be checked.
It is 10:00 on 12th June.

Notes

LONGBURY HOSPITAL TRUST		HOSPITAL NUMBER	709114
		SURNAME	FINCH
		FIRST NAME	DOREEN
		ADDRESS	31 LAKE CLOSE, LONGBURY LB13 8TW
		D.O.B	28/02/YYYY (82 YEARS AGO)

DATE OF ADMISSION	11/06/YYYY	ADMISSION WEIGHT (KG)	64kg	WARD	MEDICAL ASSESSMENT
ALLERGIES			CONSULTANT		ERIN JOHNSON
NKDA			CHART NO		1...OF...1

ONCE ONLY PRESCRIPTIONS

DATE	TIME	NAME OF DRUG	DOSE	ROUTE	PRESCRIBER'S SIGNATURE	GIVEN BY	TIME GIVEN
11/06	18.00	GENTAMICIN	320mg	IV	MHughes	RN	18:05

REGULAR MEDICATIONS

NAME OF DRUG	TIME	DATE → DOSE ↓	11/06			
ENOXAPARIN						
ADDITIONAL INSTRUCTIONS	08:00					
DATE 11/06 ROUTE S/C	12:00					
PRESCRIBER'S SIGNATURE MHughes	18:00	40mg	RN			
PRESCRIBER'S NAME AND BLEEP MICHELLE HUGHES 2357	22:00					

NAME OF DRUG	TIME	DATE → DOSE ↓				
ADDITIONAL INSTRUCTIONS	08:00					
DATE ROUTE	12:00					
PRESCRIBER'S SIGNATURE	18:00					
PRESCRIBER'S NAME AND BLEEP	22:00					

NAME OF DRUG	TIME	DATE → DOSE ↓				
ADDITIONAL INSTRUCTIONS	08:00					
DATE ROUTE	12:00					
PRESCRIBER'S SIGNATURE	18:00					
PRESCRIBER'S NAME AND BLEEP	22:00					

PATIENT NAME DOREEN FINCH   HOSPITAL NO.   709114

NAME OF DRUG		TIME	DATE → DOSE ↓						
ADDITIONAL INSTRUCTIONS		08:00							
DATE	ROUTE	12:00							
PRESCRIBER'S SIGNATURE									
		18:00							
PRESCRIBER'S NAME AND BLEEP		22:00							

NAME OF DRUG		TIME	DATE → DOSE ↓						
ADDITIONAL INSTRUCTIONS		08:00							
DATE	ROUTE	12:00							
PRESCRIBER'S SIGNATURE									
		18:00							
PRESCRIBER'S NAME AND BLEEP		22:00							

NAME OF DRUG		TIME	DATE → DOSE ↓						
ADDITIONAL INSTRUCTIONS		08:00							
DATE	ROUTE	12:00							
PRESCRIBER'S SIGNATURE									
		18:00							
PRESCRIBER'S NAME AND BLEEP		22:00							

AS REQUIRED PRESCRIPTIONS

NAME OF DRUG		DATE					
INDICATION/ INSTRUCTION	DOSE	TIME					
FREQUENCY	ROUTE	DOSE					
PRESCRIBER'S SIGNATURE		ROUTE					
PRESCRIBER'S NAME AND BLEEP		GIVEN BY					
START DATE	STOP DATE						

PATIENT NAME DOREEN FINCH   HOSPITAL NO.   709114

NAME OF DRUG		DATE					
INDICATION/ INSTRUCTION	DOSE	TIME					
FREQUENCY	ROUTE	DOSE					
PRESCRIBER'S SIGNATURE		ROUTE					
PRESCRIBER'S NAME AND BLEEP		GIVEN BY					
START DATE	STOP DATE						

INTRAVENOUS FLUIDS

DATE	FLUID	ADDITIVE & DOSE	VOLUME	RATE/ DURATION	PRESCRIBER'S SIGNATURE	GIVEN BY	START TIME	END TIME

Record of signatures. ALL prescribers MUST complete.

DATE	NAME	DESIGNATION	SIGNATURE	BLEEP NUMBER
11/06	MICHELLE HUGHES	F2	MHughes	2357

Answer 34

Correctly dosing gentamicin is often a daunting task for junior doctors. In this case the patient has already received her first dose of 320mg (at 5mg/kg body weight). Serum gentamicin was assessed 8 hours later to determine when the next dose should be given.

Step 3: Compare your answer to the checklist below and the chart opposite ✔

D Details	Checked patient details Used capital letters throughout Used correct abbreviations	☐
R Regular medications	Correctly interpreted the gentamicin level and prescribed 320mg gentamicin to be given every 36 hours	☐
U Unpleasant reactions	NKDA	☐
G Gravid?	No	☐

C Contra-indications	Risk of overdosing in interpreting the level and the way 36 hourly dosing is written	☐
H Hydration	Not required	☐
A Analgesia	Not required	☐
R Renal function	Her renal function was normal	☐
T Thrombo-prophylaxis	Already prescribed	☐
S Signature box	Signed signature box	☐

Rationale

When plotted on the gentamicin nomogram (page 6) this patient's level is above the line for safe 24-hourly dosing and is in the sector which indicates that gentamicin should be given every 36 hours. The dose given each time does not change (in this case 320mg). Formulae based on creatinine clearance also exist which can predict the dose interval for gentamicin, however information from a timed level always overrules any predicted regimen.

The next doses should be at 08.00 on 13th June (i.e. there should be no gentamicin dose today, 12 June) and at 18:00 the following day (14th June). Practically this may be prescribed with both 6am and 6pm doses on one line or alternatively as two different entries for gentamicin: morning doses on one line and evening on another. In either case, it is essential to clearly cross through boxes when doses are not required. Drawing round boxes for times when a dose is required can also help to make the prescription clear.

Levels need to be checked 6–12 hours after each gentamicin dose is given. Indicating when a level is to be checked can be done by drawing around a box 6–12 hours after a dose. Patients with stable renal function levels should be checked twice each week, while patients with renal impairment should be checked more frequently.

The nomogram method used here is a common basis for hospital guidelines in the UK. Other systems based on trough levels (measured before the next dose) are also used. Check the guidelines used at your hospital.

KEY POINTS

- Calculate initial dose based on GFR and ideal body weight
- An initial level taken 6–12 hours after first dose is required to determine how frequently IV gentamicin can be given safely
- 36 or 48 hourly dosing requires clear prescribing to avoid errors

LONGBURY HOSPITAL TRUST	HOSPITAL NUMBER	709114
	SURNAME	FINCH
	FIRST NAME	DOREEN
	ADDRESS	31 LAKE CLOSE, LONGBURY LB13 8TW
	D.O.B	28/02/YYYY (82 YEARS AGO)

DATE OF ADMISSION	11/06/YYYY	ADMISSION WEIGHT (KG)	64kg	WARD	MEDICAL ASSESSMENT
ALLERGIES NKDA			CONSULTANT		ERIN JOHNSON
			CHART NO		1...OF...1

ONCE ONLY PRESCRIPTIONS

DATE	TIME	NAME OF DRUG	DOSE	ROUTE	PRESCRIBER'S SIGNATURE	GIVEN BY	TIME GIVEN
11/06	18:00	GENTAMICIN	320mg	IV	MHughes	RN	18:05

REGULAR MEDICATIONS

NAME OF DRUG ENOXAPARIN	TIME	DATE → DOSE ↓	11/06				
ADDITIONAL INSTRUCTIONS	08:00						
DATE 11/06 ROUTE S/C	12:00						
PRESCRIBER'S SIGNATURE MHughes	18:00	40mg	RN				
PRESCRIBER'S NAME AND BLEEP MICHELLE HUGHES 2357	22:00						

NAME OF DRUG GENTAMICIN	TIME	DATE → DOSE ↓	11/06	12/06	13/06	14/06	15/06
	06:00	320mg	X	X		X	X
ADDITIONAL INSTRUCTIONS EVERY 36 HOURS	08:00						
DATE 12/06 ROUTE IV	12:00						
PRESCRIBER'S SIGNATURE ALewis					LEVEL		
	18:00	320mg	X	X	X		X
PRESCRIBER'S NAME AND BLEEP ALEX LEWIS 4567	22:00						

NAME OF DRUG	TIME	DATE → DOSE ↓					
ADDITIONAL INSTRUCTIONS	08:00						
DATE ROUTE	12:00						
PRESCRIBER'S SIGNATURE	18:00						
PRESCRIBER'S NAME AND BLEEP	22:00						

PATIENT NAME DOREEN FINCH   HOSPITAL NO.   709114

NAME OF DRUG		TIME	DATE → DOSE ↓					
ADDITIONAL INSTRUCTIONS		08:00						
DATE	ROUTE	12:00						
PRESCRIBER'S SIGNATURE								
		18:00						
PRESCRIBER'S NAME AND BLEEP		22:00						

NAME OF DRUG		TIME	DATE → DOSE ↓					
ADDITIONAL INSTRUCTIONS		08:00						
DATE	ROUTE	12:00						
PRESCRIBER'S SIGNATURE								
		18:00						
PRESCRIBER'S NAME AND BLEEP		22:00						

NAME OF DRUG		TIME	DATE → DOSE ↓					
ADDITIONAL INSTRUCTIONS		08:00						
DATE	ROUTE	12:00						
PRESCRIBER'S SIGNATURE								
		18:00						
PRESCRIBER'S NAME AND BLEEP		22:00						

AS REQUIRED PRESCRIPTIONS

NAME OF DRUG		DATE					
INDICATION/ INSTRUCTION	DOSE	TIME					
FREQUENCY	ROUTE	DOSE					
PRESCRIBER'S SIGNATURE		ROUTE					
PRESCRIBER'S NAME AND BLEEP		GIVEN BY					
START DATE	STOP DATE						

PATIENT NAME DOREEN FINCH   HOSPITAL NO.   709114

NAME OF DRUG		DATE					
INDICATION/ INSTRUCTION	DOSE	TIME					
FREQUENCY	ROUTE	DOSE					
PRESCRIBER'S SIGNATURE		ROUTE					
PRESCRIBER'S NAME AND BLEEP		GIVEN BY					
START DATE	STOP DATE						

INTRAVENOUS FLUIDS

DATE	FLUID	ADDITIVE & DOSE	VOLUME	RATE/ DURATION	PRESCRIBER'S SIGNATURE	GIVEN BY	START TIME	END TIME

Record of signatures. ALL prescribers MUST complete.

DATE	NAME	DESIGNATION	SIGNATURE	BLEEP NUMBER
11/06	MICHELLE HUGHES	F2	MHughes	2357
12/06	ALEX LEWIS	F1	ALewis	4567

Josie Fox (hospital number: 455443, DOB 12/04/YYYY [24 years old], address: 14 Princes' Way, Longbury LB11 3TL) has been brought to the hospital by one of her flatmates. She has a 2-day history of fever, headache and photophobia. Her friend also reports that she seems a little confused. She thinks it may have started with a sore throat around a week ago. She has not noticed a rash. She is not known to be allergic to any medications. Her weight is 71kg.

On examination Miss Fox is pyrexial with marked neck stiffness and photophobia. The rest of her examination is unremarkable. She is known not to be pregnant. Her Glasgow Coma Score is 15. Miss Fox's consultant on the medical assessment ward is Dr Erin Johnson.

A lumbar puncture is carried out, the results show:

Opening pressure 26cmH$_2$O
White cells 1200/mm^3
Polymorphs >95%
Red cells 5/mm^3

CSF protein 1100mg/L (normal 140–450mg/L)
CSF glucose 2.3mmol/L (normal 2.3–4.0mmol/L)
Serum glucose 5.4mmol/L

Gram stain: no organisms seen

Your task is to prescribe appropriate therapy, based on the likely diagnosis.
It is 11:00 on 30th June.

Notes

Step 1: Complete your answers in the drug chart opposite and overleaf

LONGBURY HOSPITAL TRUST				HOSPITAL NUMBER SURNAME FIRST NAME ADDRESS		
				D.O.B		
DATE OF ADMISSION			ADMISSION WEIGHT (KG)		WARD	
ALLERGIES				CONSULTANT		
				CHART NO		...OF...

ONCE ONLY PRESCRIPTIONS

DATE	TIME	NAME OF DRUG	DOSE	ROUTE	PRESCRIBER'S SIGNATURE	GIVEN BY	TIME GIVEN

REGULAR MEDICATIONS

NAME OF DRUG		TIME	DATE → DOSE ↓				
ADDITIONAL INSTRUCTIONS		08:00					
DATE	ROUTE	12:00					
PRESCRIBER'S SIGNATURE		18:00					
PRESCRIBER'S NAME AND BLEEP		22:00					

NAME OF DRUG		TIME	DATE → DOSE ↓				
ADDITIONAL INSTRUCTIONS		08:00					
DATE	ROUTE	12:00					
PRESCRIBER'S SIGNATURE		18:00					
PRESCRIBER'S NAME AND BLEEP		22:00					

NAME OF DRUG		TIME	DATE → DOSE ↓				
ADDITIONAL INSTRUCTIONS		08:00					
DATE	ROUTE	12:00					
PRESCRIBER'S SIGNATURE		18:00					
PRESCRIBER'S NAME AND BLEEP		22:00					

PATIENT NAME HOSPITAL NO.

NAME OF DRUG		TIME	DATE → DOSE ↓						
ADDITIONAL INSTRUCTIONS		08:00							
DATE	ROUTE	12:00							
PRESCRIBER'S SIGNATURE									
		18:00							
PRESCRIBER'S NAME AND BLEEP									
		22:00							

NAME OF DRUG		TIME	DATE → DOSE ↓						
ADDITIONAL INSTRUCTIONS		08:00							
DATE	ROUTE	12:00							
PRESCRIBER'S SIGNATURE									
		18:00							
PRESCRIBER'S NAME AND BLEEP									
		22:00							

NAME OF DRUG		TIME	DATE → DOSE ↓						
ADDITIONAL INSTRUCTIONS		08:00							
DATE	ROUTE	12:00							
PRESCRIBER'S SIGNATURE									
		18:00							
PRESCRIBER'S NAME AND BLEEP									
		22:00							

AS REQUIRED PRESCRIPTIONS

NAME OF DRUG		DATE						
INDICATION/ INSTRUCTION	DOSE	TIME						
FREQUENCY	ROUTE	DOSE						
PRESCRIBER'S SIGNATURE		ROUTE						
PRESCRIBER'S NAME AND BLEEP		GIVEN BY						
START DATE	STOP DATE							

PATIENT NAME   HOSPITAL NO.

NAME OF DRUG		DATE					
INDICATION/ INSTRUCTION	DOSE	TIME					
FREQUENCY	ROUTE	DOSE					
PRESCRIBER'S SIGNATURE		ROUTE					
PRESCRIBER'S NAME AND BLEEP		GIVEN BY					
START DATE	STOP DATE						

INTRAVENOUS FLUIDS

DATE	FLUID	ADDITIVE & DOSE	VOLUME	RATE/ DURATION	PRESCRIBER'S SIGNATURE	GIVEN BY	START TIME	END TIME

Record of signatures. ALL prescribers MUST complete.

DATE	NAME	DESIGNATION	SIGNATURE	BLEEP NUMBER

Answer 35

This young woman has history and examination findings typical of meningitis. Excluding the rarer causes, meningitis falls into two main groups; viral and bacterial. History alone is often not enough to tell them apart. A lumbar puncture is the key investigation to confirm the diagnosis and cause.

Step 3: Compare your answer to the checklist below and the chart opposite ☑

D	Details	Checked patient details Used capital letters throughout Used correct abbreviations	☐
R	Regular medications	Prescribed a stat dose of cefotaxime	☐
U	Unpleasant reactions	Wrote NKDA	☐
G	Gravid?	No	☐

C	Contra-indications	None	☐
H	Hydration	Not required	☐
A	Analgesia	Prescribed analgesia according to pain ladder	☐
R	Renal function	Cephalosporins are safe outside of severe renal impairment	☐
T	Thrombo-prophylaxis	Recognised that a severe debilitating infection is a risk factor for thrombosis	☐
S	Signature box	Signed signature box	☐

Rationale

The characteristic CSF pattern associated with bacterial meningitis is raised protein, raised white cell count (mostly neutrophils) and glucose <60% of serum. The gram stain may be diagnostic, however it can be misleadingly negative in the presence of infection.

Bacterial meningitis in adults is most commonly caused by *Streptococcus pneumoniae* or *Neisseria meningitidis*, both of which are sensitive to third generation cephalosporins. High-dose cefotaxime or ceftriaxone is recommended for the treatment of meningitis. Individual hospitals may vary as to which cephalosporin is used as first line. Cefotaxime or ceftriaxone are used in preference to Tazocin or co-amoxiclav as they have better CSF penetration. In patients over 50 years old, *Listeria monocytogenes* is a major cause of bacterial meningitis and requires a prolonged course of high-dose amoxicillin (14–21 days).

In viral meningitis the lumbar puncture findings are a raised white cell count of mostly lymphocytes with mildly raised CSF protein. CSF glucose is not reduced. The most common causes are enterovirus and herpes simplex virus. Treatment is supportive: intravenous aciclovir is commonly given for herpes meningitis but evidence for its effectiveness is limited.

KEY POINTS

- A lack of observable bacteria on gram stain does not rule out bacterial meningitis
- Once a diagnosis of bacterial meningitis has been made antimicrobial therapy must begin immediately: treatment should not be delayed to perform a lumbar puncture
- Acute meningitis is a notifiable disease and must be reported to the regional public health laboratory

LONGBURY HOSPITAL TRUST				HOSPITAL NUMBER	455443	
				SURNAME	FOX	
				FIRST NAME	JOSIE	
				ADDRESS	14 PRINCES' WAY, LONGBURY LB11 3TL	
				D.O.B	12/04/YYYY (24 YEARS AGO)	
DATE OF ADMISSION	30/06/YYYY	ADMISSION WEIGHT (KG)	71kg	WARD	MEDICAL ASSESSMENT	
ALLERGIES			CONSULTANT	ERIN JOHNSON		
NKDA			CHART NO	1...OF...1		

ONCE ONLY PRESCRIPTIONS

DATE	TIME	NAME OF DRUG	DOSE	ROUTE	PRESCRIBER'S SIGNATURE	GIVEN BY	TIME GIVEN
30/06	11:00	CEFOTAXIME	2g	IV	ALewis		

REGULAR MEDICATIONS

		DATE →	30/06				
NAME OF DRUG CEFOTAXIME	**TIME**	DOSE ↓					
	06:00	2g	X				
ADDITIONAL INSTRUCTIONS MENINGITIS	**08:00**						
DATE 30/06 ROUTE IV	**12:00**	2g	X				
PRESCRIBER'S SIGNATURE ALewis	**18:00**	2g					
PRESCRIBER'S NAME AND BLEEP ALEX LEWIS 4567	**22:00**	2g					

		DATE →	30/06				
NAME OF DRUG ENOXAPARIN	**TIME**	DOSE ↓					
ADDITIONAL INSTRUCTIONS	**08:00**						
DATE 30/06 ROUTE SC	**12:00**						
PRESCRIBER'S SIGNATURE ALewis	**18:00**	40mg					
PRESCRIBER'S NAME AND BLEEP ALEX LEWIS 4567	**22:00**						

		DATE →	30/06				
NAME OF DRUG PARACETAMOL	**TIME**	DOSE ↓					
ADDITIONAL INSTRUCTIONS	**08:00**	1g	X				
DATE 30/6 ROUTE IV/ PO/PR	**12:00**	1g					
PRESCRIBER'S SIGNATURE ALewis	**18:00**	1g					
PRESCRIBER'S NAME AND BLEEP ALEX LEWIS 4567	**22:00**	1g					

PATIENT NAME *JOSIE FOX*　　　　　　HOSPITAL NO.　455443

NAME OF DRUG CODEINE		TIME	DATE → DOSE ↓	30/06				
ADDITIONAL INSTRUCTIONS		**08:00**	30 - 60mg	X				
DATE 30/06	ROUTE PO	**12:00**	30 - 60mg					
PRESCRIBER'S SIGNATURE ALewis		**18:00**	30 - 60mg					
PRESCRIBER'S NAME AND BLEEP ALEX LEWIS 4567		**22:00**	30 - 60mg					

NAME OF DRUG		TIME	DATE → DOSE ↓					
ADDITIONAL INSTRUCTIONS		**08:00**						
DATE	ROUTE	**12:00**						
PRESCRIBER'S SIGNATURE		**18:00**						
PRESCRIBER'S NAME AND BLEEP		**22:00**						

NAME OF DRUG		TIME	DATE → DOSE ↓					
ADDITIONAL INSTRUCTIONS		**08:00**						
DATE	ROUTE	**12:00**						
PRESCRIBER'S SIGNATURE		**18:00**						
PRESCRIBER'S NAME AND BLEEP		**22:00**						

AS REQUIRED PRESCRIPTIONS

NAME OF DRUG CYCLIZINE		DATE					
INDICATION/ INSTRUCTION NAUSEA	DOSE 50mg	TIME					
FREQUENCY TDS	ROUTE IM/PO/IV	DOSE					
PRESCRIBER'S SIGNATURE ALewis		ROUTE					
PRESCRIBER'S NAME AND BLEEP ALEX LEWIS 4567		GIVEN BY					
START DATE 30/06	STOP DATE						

PATIENT NAME *JOSIE FOX*   HOSPITAL NO.   *455443*

NAME OF DRUG		DATE					
INDICATION/ INSTRUCTION	DOSE	TIME					
FREQUENCY	ROUTE	DOSE					
PRESCRIBER'S SIGNATURE		ROUTE					
PRESCRIBER'S NAME AND BLEEP		GIVEN BY					
START DATE	STOP DATE						

INTRAVENOUS FLUIDS

DATE	FLUID	ADDITIVE & DOSE	VOLUME	RATE/ DURATION	PRESCRIBER'S SIGNATURE	GIVEN BY	START TIME	END TIME

Record of signatures. ALL prescribers MUST complete.

DATE	NAME	DESIGNATION	SIGNATURE	BLEEP NUMBER
30/06	ALEX LEWIS	F1	ALewis	4567

Dylan Stephens (hospital number: 101034, 29/03/YYYY [13 weeks old]; address: 21 Abbey Lane, Longbury LB1 6CY) has been admitted to the paediatric ward for repair of a large inguinal hernia. The operation is scheduled for this afternoon and Dylan has been nil by mouth since midnight. Apart from his inguinal hernia, he has no other known medical problems or allergies. He has a prescription for E45 cream for dry skin on his ears. Dylan's consultant is Dr Carol Wyke.

On examination Dylan is settled and sleeping comfortably; he weighs 6kg.

Observations:
Heart rate 110bpm
Respiratory rate 33 breaths/minute
SpO_2 100% on air
Temperature 37.1°C

Dylan has a capillary refill time of 2 seconds and moist mucous membranes. He has produced two wet nappies with approximately 40mL in each since midnight.

Fluid prescription is required and some ranitidine perioperatively.

Your task is to prescribe perioperative management.
It is 07:30 on 15th June.

Notes

Step 1: Complete your answers in the drug chart opposite and overleaf

LONGBURY HOSPITAL TRUST			HOSPITAL NUMBER SURNAME FIRST NAME ADDRESS D.O.B		
DATE OF ADMISSION		ADMISSION WEIGHT (KG)		WARD	
ALLERGIES			CONSULTANT		
			CHART NO		...OF...

ONCE ONLY PRESCRIPTIONS

DATE	TIME	NAME OF DRUG	DOSE	ROUTE	PRESCRIBER'S SIGNATURE	GIVEN BY	TIME GIVEN

REGULAR MEDICATIONS

NAME OF DRUG	TIME	DATE → DOSE ↓				
ADDITIONAL INSTRUCTIONS	08:00					
DATE ROUTE	12:00					
PRESCRIBER'S SIGNATURE						
	18:00					
PRESCRIBER'S NAME AND BLEEP						
	22:00					

NAME OF DRUG	TIME	DATE → DOSE ↓				
ADDITIONAL INSTRUCTIONS	08:00					
DATE ROUTE	12:00					
PRESCRIBER'S SIGNATURE						
	18:00					
PRESCRIBER'S NAME AND BLEEP						
	22:00					

NAME OF DRUG	TIME	DATE → DOSE ↓				
ADDITIONAL INSTRUCTIONS	08:00					
DATE ROUTE	12:00					
PRESCRIBER'S SIGNATURE						
	18:00					
PRESCRIBER'S NAME AND BLEEP						
	22:00					

PATIENT NAME   HOSPITAL NO.

NAME OF DRUG		TIME	DATE → DOSE ↓					
ADDITIONAL INSTRUCTIONS		08:00						
DATE	ROUTE	12:00						
PRESCRIBER'S SIGNATURE		18:00						
PRESCRIBER'S NAME AND BLEEP		22:00						

NAME OF DRUG		TIME	DATE → DOSE ↓					
ADDITIONAL INSTRUCTIONS		08:00						
DATE	ROUTE	12:00						
PRESCRIBER'S SIGNATURE		18:00						
PRESCRIBER'S NAME AND BLEEP		22:00						

NAME OF DRUG		TIME	DATE → DOSE ↓					
ADDITIONAL INSTRUCTIONS		08:00						
DATE	ROUTE	12:00						
PRESCRIBER'S SIGNATURE		18:00						
PRESCRIBER'S NAME AND BLEEP		22:00						

AS REQUIRED PRESCRIPTIONS

NAME OF DRUG		DATE					
INDICATION/ INSTRUCTION	DOSE	TIME					
FREQUENCY	ROUTE	DOSE					
PRESCRIBER'S SIGNATURE		ROUTE					
PRESCRIBER'S NAME AND BLEEP		GIVEN BY					
START DATE	STOP DATE						

PATIENT NAME   HOSPITAL NO.

NAME OF DRUG		DATE					
INDICATION/ INSTRUCTION	DOSE	TIME					
FREQUENCY	ROUTE	DOSE					
PRESCRIBER'S SIGNATURE		ROUTE					
PRESCRIBER'S NAME AND BLEEP		GIVENS BY					
START DATE	STOP DATE						

INTRAVENOUS FLUIDS

DATE	FLUID	ADDITIVE & DOSE	VOLUME	RATE/ DURATION	PRESCRIBER'S SIGNATURE	GIVEN BY	START TIME	END TIME

Record of signatures. ALL prescribers MUST complete.

DATE	NAME	DESIGNATION	SIGNATURE	BLEEP NUMBER

Step 2: Now check your work overleaf

Answer 36

This exercise requires interpretation of the patient's clinical information to find that they are euvolaemic and to prescribe fluid appropriately. Normal ranges for vital signs vary in different age groups for patients, e.g. normal urine output is closer to 1–2mL/kg/h in infants than the 0.5mL/kg/h expected in adults.

Step 3: Compare your answer to the checklist below and the chart opposite ☑

D Details	Checked patient details Used capital letters throughout Used correct abbreviations	☐
R Regular medications	Prescribed E45 cream b.d.	☐
U Unpleasant reactions	None	☐
G Gravid?	No	☐

C Contra-indications	Checked drug dosing in paediatric formulary	☐
H Hydration	Prescribed maintenance regime for euvolaemic baby based on 100mL/kg	☐
A Analgesia	Prescribed postoperative paracetamol	☐
R Renal function	Not required	☐
T Thrombo-prophylaxis	Not required	☐
S Signature box	Signed signature box	☐

Rationale

The fluid calculation for this patient was based on the following:
- Normal 24 hour requirements are 100mL for each 10kg of a child's weight
- Given that this baby weighs 6kg we calculate a fluid requirement of:
  100mL x 6kg = 600mL over 24 hours
  　　　　　 = 25mL/h

Potassium has not been added to this bag of fluid but it would be acceptable to do so in line with daily requirements. Ranitidine has been prescribed intravenously while this patient is nil-by-mouth. Paracetamol has been prescribed per rectum for the same reason. It would be acceptable to prescribe intravenously but remember that intravenous access is often difficult to obtain and cannulas often do not work very long before failing in children of this age. The priority is to use this child's cannula for maintenance fluid. Postoperatively it would be acceptable to prescribe oral paracetamol when the patient is tolerating feeds but the administration of rectal analgesia will not be dependent on the timing of this. Check the strengths of suppository available: they influence the dose prescribed. When prescribing for children, especially when prescribing an oral liquid formulation, ensure that the dose will be measurable by the parents.

KEY POINTS

- Assess a paediatric patient's fluid status before prescribing
- Perform a fluid calculation for all paediatric patients who need fluid
- Check every medication in a paediatric formulary and ensure the calculated dose can be administered
- Intravenous access is often difficult in children, where practical seek other routes for giving drugs

LONGBURY HOSPITAL TRUST					
		HOSPITAL NUMBER	101034		
		SURNAME	STEPHENS		
		FIRST NAME	DYLAN		
		ADDRESS	21 ABBEY LANE, LONGBURY LB1 6CY		
		D.O.B	29/03/YYYY (13 WEEKS AGO)		

DATE OF ADMISSION	15/06/YYYY	ADMISSION WEIGHT (KG)	6kg	WARD	PAEDIATRIC
ALLERGIES			CONSULTANT		CAROL WYKE
NKDA			CHART NO		1...OF...1

ONCE ONLY PRESCRIPTIONS

DATE	TIME	NAME OF DRUG	DOSE	ROUTE	PRESCRIBER'S SIGNATURE	GIVEN BY	TIME GIVEN

REGULAR MEDICATIONS

NAME OF DRUG	TIME	DATE → / DOSE ↓	15/06				
RANITIDINE							
ADDITIONAL INSTRUCTIONS	08:00	6mg					
DATE 15/06 ROUTE IV	12:00						
PRESCRIBER'S SIGNATURE ALewis	14:00	6mg					
	18:00						
PRESCRIBER'S NAME AND BLEEP ALEX LEWIS 4567	22:00	6mg					

NAME OF DRUG	TIME	DATE → / DOSE ↓	15/06				
PARACETAMOL							
ADDITIONAL INSTRUCTIONS	08:00	60mg					
DATE 15/06 ROUTE PR	12:00	60mg					
PRESCRIBER'S SIGNATURE ALewis	18:00	60mg					
PRESCRIBER'S NAME AND BLEEP ALEX LEWIS 4567	22:00	60mg					

NAME OF DRUG	TIME	DATE → / DOSE ↓	15/06				
E45 CREAM							
ADDITIONAL INSTRUCTIONS EARS	08:00	ṫ					
DATE 15/06 ROUTE TOP	12:00						
PRESCRIBER'S SIGNATURE ALewis	18:00						
PRESCRIBER'S NAME AND BLEEP ALEX LEWIS 4567	22:00	ṫ					

PATIENT NAME *DYLAN STEPHENS* **HOSPITAL NO.** *101034*

NAME OF DRUG		TIME	DATE → DOSE ↓					
ADDITIONAL INSTRUCTIONS		08:00						
DATE	ROUTE	12:00						
PRESCRIBER'S SIGNATURE		18:00						
PRESCRIBER'S NAME AND BLEEP		22:00						

NAME OF DRUG		TIME	DATE → DOSE ↓					
ADDITIONAL INSTRUCTIONS		08:00						
DATE	ROUTE	12:00						
PRESCRIBER'S SIGNATURE		18:00						
PRESCRIBER'S NAME AND BLEEP		22:00						

NAME OF DRUG		TIME	DATE → DOSE ↓					
ADDITIONAL INSTRUCTIONS		08:00						
DATE	ROUTE	12:00						
PRESCRIBER'S SIGNATURE		18:00						
PRESCRIBER'S NAME AND BLEEP		22:00						

AS REQUIRED PRESCRIPTIONS

NAME OF DRUG		DATE					
INDICATION/ INSTRUCTION	DOSE	TIME					
FREQUENCY	ROUTE	DOSE					
PRESCRIBER'S SIGNATURE		ROUTE					
PRESCRIBER'S NAME AND BLEEP		GIVEN BY					
START DATE	STOP DATE						

PATIENT NAME *DYLAN STEPHENS*   HOSPITAL NO.   *101034*

NAME OF DRUG		DATE						
INDICATION/ INSTRUCTION	DOSE	TIME						
FREQUENCY	ROUTE	DOSE						
PRESCRIBER'S SIGNATURE		ROUTE						
PRESCRIBER'S NAME AND BLEEP		GIVEN BY						
START DATE	STOP DATE							

INTRAVENOUS FLUIDS

DATE	FLUID	ADDITIVE & DOSE	VOLUME	RATE/ DURATION	PRESCRIBER'S SIGNATURE	GIVEN BY	START TIME	END TIME
15/06	0.45% NaCl AND 5% DEXTROSE	——————	500ml	25ml/hr	ALewis			

Record of signatures. ALL prescribers MUST complete.

DATE	NAME	DESIGNATION	SIGNATURE	BLEEP NUMBER
15/06	ALEX LEWIS	F1	ALewis	4567

Robin Green (hospital number: 005729, DOB 12/03/YYYY [75 years old], address: 5 Marina Drive, Longbury LB17 1NO) has been admitted to hospital with worsening confusion, breathlessness and a decreased level of consciousness. Initial investigations including a CT scan showed lung cancer with cerebral metastases. His condition has continued to decline and after discussions with the family the consultant has decided to start a palliative care pathway.

The consultant has asked for a syringe driver to be set up, containing diamorphine and midazolam. Mr Green has been receiving subcutaneous doses of both and currently appears settled.

The most recent blood tests demonstrated normal renal function.

Your task is to prescribe the syringe driver.
It is 10:15 on 10th July.

Notes

LONGBURY HOSPITAL TRUST			HOSPITAL NUMBER	005729		
			SURNAME	GREEN		
			FIRST NAME	ROBIN		
			ADDRESS	5 MARINA DRIVE, LONGBURY LB17 1NO		
			D.O.B	12/03/YYYY (75 YEARS AGO)		

DATE OF ADMISSION	08/07/YYYY	ADMISSION WEIGHT (KG)	70kg	WARD	MEDICAL ASSESSMENT
ALLERGIES			CONSULTANT		ERIN JOHNSON
NKDA			CHART NO		1...OF...1

ONCE ONLY PRESCRIPTIONS

DATE	TIME	NAME OF DRUG	DOSE	ROUTE	PRESCRIBER'S SIGNATURE	GIVEN BY	TIME GIVEN

REGULAR MEDICATIONS

NAME OF DRUG		TIME	DATE → DOSE ↓				
ADDITIONAL INSTRUCTIONS		08:00					
DATE	ROUTE	12:00					
PRESCRIBER'S SIGNATURE		18:00					
PRESCRIBER'S NAME AND BLEEP		22:00					

NAME OF DRUG		TIME	DATE → DOSE ↓				
ADDITIONAL INSTRUCTIONS		08:00					
DATE	ROUTE	12:00					
PRESCRIBER'S SIGNATURE		18:00					
PRESCRIBER'S NAME AND BLEEP		22:00					

NAME OF DRUG		TIME	DATE → DOSE ↓				
ADDITIONAL INSTRUCTIONS		08:00					
DATE	ROUTE	12:00					
PRESCRIBER'S SIGNATURE		18:00					
PRESCRIBER'S NAME AND BLEEP		22:00					

PATIENT NAME ROBIN GREEN   HOSPITAL NO.   005729

NAME OF DRUG	TIME	DATE → / DOSE ↓					
ADDITIONAL INSTRUCTIONS	08:00						
DATE ROUTE	12:00						
PRESCRIBER'S SIGNATURE							
	18:00						
PRESCRIBER'S NAME AND BLEEP							
	22:00						

NAME OF DRUG	TIME	DATE → / DOSE ↓					
ADDITIONAL INSTRUCTIONS	08:00						
DATE ROUTE	12:00						
PRESCRIBER'S SIGNATURE							
	18:00						
PRESCRIBER'S NAME AND BLEEP							
	22:00						

NAME OF DRUG	TIME	DATE → / DOSE ↓					
ADDITIONAL INSTRUCTIONS	08:00						
DATE ROUTE	12:00						
PRESCRIBER'S SIGNATURE							
	18:00						
PRESCRIBER'S NAME AND BLEEP							
	22:00						

AS REQUIRED PRESCRIPTIONS

NAME OF DRUG DIAMORPHINE		DATE	08/07	08/07	09/07	09/07	09/07	09/07	10/07
INDICATION/ INSTRUCTION PAIN	DOSE 2.5mg	TIME	14:15	20:15	06:30	10:15	15:30	21:00	08:00
FREQUENCY 2HRLY	ROUTE S/C	DOSE	2.5mg	2.5mg	2.5mg	2.5mg	2.5mg	2.5mg	2.5mg
PRESCRIBER'S SIGNATURE NShah		ROUTE	S/C	S/C	S/C	S/C	S/C	S/C	S/C
PRESCRIBER'S NAME AND BLEEP NAZIA SHAH 9761		GIVEN BY	CF	TO	TO	CF	CF	TO	JC
START DATE 08/07	STOP DATE								

PATIENT NAME ROBIN GREEN   HOSPITAL NO.   005729

NAME OF DRUG MIDAZOLAM		DATE	08/07	09/07	09/07		
INDICATION/ INSTRUCTION AGITATION	DOSE 2.5-5mg	TIME	14:15	10:30	20:15		
FREQUENCY 4HRLY	ROUTE' S/C	DOSE	2.5mg	2.5mg	2.5mg		
PRESCRIBER'S SIGNATURE NShah		ROUTE	S/C	S/C	S/C		
PRESCRIBER'S NAME AND BLEEP NAZIA SHAH 9761		GIVEN BY	CF	CF	TO		
START DATE 08/07	STOP DATE						

INFUSIONS

DATE	DRUG	DILUTION FLUID	TOTAL VOLUME	RATE/ DURATION	PRESCRIBER'S SIGNATURE	GIVEN BY	START TIME	END TIME

Record of signatures. ALL prescribers MUST complete.

DATE	NAME	DESIGNATION	SIGNATURE	BLEEP NUMBER
08/07	NAZIA SHAH	F2	NShah	9761

Answer 37

The main objectives of palliative prescribing are to make sure the patient is as symptom-free, comfortable and retains as much dignity as possible. Good palliative prescribing is anticipatory and should have provision for worsening of symptoms. It is important to know how to prescribe syringe drivers for this reason.

Step 3: Compare your answer to the checklist below and the chart opposite ✔

D	Details	Checked patient details Used capital letters throughout Used correct abbreviations	☐
R	Regular medications	Prescribed a SC syringe driver containing 10mg diamorphine and 5mg midazolam	☐
U	Unpleasant reactions	NKDA already entered	☐
G	Gravid?	Not required	☐

C	Contra-indications	Noticed that diamorphine and midazolam can both cause respiratory depression	☐
H	Hydration	Not required	☐
A	Analgesia	Continue as-required diamorphine	☐
R	Renal function	OK	☐
T	Thrombo-prophylaxis	Not appropriate for patients being palliated	☐
S	Signature box	Signed signature box	☐

Rationale

A syringe driver allows continuous subcutaneous administration of symptom-control medications in palliative care. Advantages of the syringe driver are that it avoids variable levels that would occur when giving divided doses spaced through the day and that it anticipates the symptoms, meaning that the patient does not need to alert a member of staff to obtain more pain relief. In this exercise, calculating doses for the syringe driver is straightforward. This patient required a total of 10mg of diamorphine and 5mg of midazolam every 24 hours to remain comfortable. This indicates the doses that should be prescribed for the 24 hour syringe driver. As these doses are being given subcutaneously they can be added up and put in the syringe driver. Prescribe water for injections as the diluent, as some medicines precipitate if sodium chloride 0.9% is used (the situation is more complicated when converting transdermal patches or oral preparations).

When patients are having analgesia delivered by continuous subcutaneous infusion they should still have as-required doses prescribed. These can be used for breakthrough pain not controlled by the infusion. If a patient regularly requires extra breakthrough doses each day it is a sign the dose needs to be increased. As-required doses should be approximately one sixth of the total daily infusion dose.

Be careful when prescribing opiates in patients with poor renal function: opiates are renally excreted and thus accumulate in renal failure. Be aware of the signs of opiate toxicity: pinpoint pupils, reduced respiratory rate and reduced consciousness level. Naloxone is used to reverse the effects of opiate toxicity but bear in mind that it also reverses the analgesic effect.

KEY POINTS

- Calculate doses for syringe drivers based on previous requirements or hospital guidance
- Use water for injections as the diluent
- Retain breakthrough PRN prescriptions and monitor their usage. Review the clinical effect of the syringe driver and exercise caution in renal failure
- Do not increase opiate dose by more than 50% at a time

LONGBURY HOSPITAL TRUST

HOSPITAL NUMBER	005729
SURNAME	GREEN
FIRST NAME	ROBIN
ADDRESS	5 MARINA DRIVE, LONGBURY LB17 1NO
D.O.B	12/03/YYYY (75 YEARS AGO)

DATE OF ADMISSION	08/07/YYYY	ADMISSION WEIGHT (KG)	70kg	WARD	MEDICAL ASSESSMENT

ALLERGIES		CONSULTANT	ERIN JOHNSON
NKDA		CHART NO	1...OF...1

ONCE ONLY PRESCRIPTIONS

DATE	TIME	NAME OF DRUG	DOSE	ROUTE	PRESCRIBER'S SIGNATURE	GIVEN BY	TIME GIVEN

REGULAR MEDICATIONS

NAME OF DRUG		TIME	DATE → DOSE ↓					
ADDITIONAL INSTRUCTIONS		08:00						
DATE	ROUTE	12:00						
PRESCRIBER'S SIGNATURE		18:00						
PRESCRIBER'S NAME AND BLEEP		22:00						

NAME OF DRUG		TIME	DATE → DOSE ↓					
ADDITIONAL INSTRUCTIONS		08:00						
DATE	ROUTE	12:00						
PRESCRIBER'S SIGNATURE		18:00						
PRESCRIBER'S NAME AND BLEEP		22:00						

NAME OF DRUG		TIME	DATE → DOSE ↓					
ADDITIONAL INSTRUCTIONS		08:00						
DATE	ROUTE	12:00						
PRESCRIBER'S SIGNATURE		18:00						
PRESCRIBER'S NAME AND BLEEP		22:00						

PATIENT NAME ROBIN GREEN   HOSPITAL NO.   005729

NAME OF DRUG		TIME	DATE → DOSE ↓						
ADDITIONAL INSTRUCTIONS		08:00							
DATE	ROUTE	12:00							
PRESCRIBER'S SIGNATURE		18:00							
PRESCRIBER'S NAME AND BLEEP		22:00							

NAME OF DRUG		TIME	DATE → DOSE ↓						
ADDITIONAL INSTRUCTIONS		08:00							
DATE	ROUTE	12:00							
PRESCRIBER'S SIGNATURE		18:00							
PRESCRIBER'S NAME AND BLEEP		22:00							

NAME OF DRUG		TIME	DATE → DOSE ↓						
ADDITIONAL INSTRUCTIONS		08:00							
DATE	ROUTE	12:00							
PRESCRIBER'S SIGNATURE		18:00							
PRESCRIBER'S NAME AND BLEEP		22:00							

AS REQUIRED PRESCRIPTIONS

NAME OF DRUG DIAMORPHINE		DATE	08/07	08/07	09/07	09/07	09/07	09/07	10/07
INDICATION/ INSTRUCTION PAIN	DOSE 2.5mg	TIME	14:15	20:15	06:30	10:15	15:30	21:00	08:00
FREQUENCY 2HRLY	ROUTE S/C	DOSE	2.5mg	2.5mg	2.5mg	2.5mg	2.5mg	2.5mg	2.5mg
PRESCRIBER'S SIGNATURE NShah		ROUTE	S/C	S/C	S/C	S/C	S/C	S/C	S/C
PRESCRIBER'S NAME AND BLEEP NAZIA SHAH 9761		GIVEN BY	CF	TO	TO	CF	CF	TO	JC
START DATE 08/07	STOP DATE								

PATIENT NAME ROBIN GREEN   HOSPITAL NO.   005729

NAME OF DRUG MIDAZOLAM		DATE	08/07	09/07	09/07		
INDICATION/ INSTRUCTION AGITATION	DOSE 2.5-5mg	TIME	14:15	10:30	20:15		
FREQUENCY 4HRLY	ROUTE' S/C	DOSE	2.5mg	2.5mg	2.5mg		
PRESCRIBER'S SIGNATURE NShah		ROUTE	S/C	S/C	S/C		
PRESCRIBER'S NAME AND BLEEP NAZIA SHAH 9761		GIVEN BY	CF	CF	TO		
START DATE 08/07	STOP DATE						

INFUSIONS

DATE	DRUG	DILUTION FLUID	TOTAL VOLUME	RATE/ DURATION	PRESCRIBER'S SIGNATURE	GIVEN BY	START TIME	END TIME
10/07	MIDAZOLAM	H_2O	20ml	5mg OVER 24 hours	ALewis			
10/07	DIAMORPHINE	H_2O	20ml	10mg OVER 24 hours	ALewis			

Record of signatures. ALL prescribers MUST complete.

DATE	NAME	DESIGNATION	SIGNATURE	BLEEP NUMBER
08/07	NAZIA SHAH	F2	NShah	9761
10/07	ALEX LEWIS	F1	ALewis	4567

Oliver Stewart (hospital number: 654211, DOB 13/12/YYYY [19 years old], address: 36 Amber Road, Longbury LB8 7AM) has arrived on the surgical ward. He is being admitted for an elective anterior cruciate ligament repair. As the clerking is being completed he remarks that he has a terrible sore throat which has been bothering him for a few days. He does not take any medication on a regular basis.

On examination Mr Stewart's tonsils are enlarged, erythematous and covered in a white exudate. He has a few small palpable cervical lymph nodes. He has a low-grade fever: his temperature is 37.6°C.

He says that he is intolerant of doxycycline and that it brings him out in a rash. He weighs 64kg. The consultant, Mr Joshua Gibb, has asked you to prescribe medication for Mr Stewart's sore throat.

His admission blood test results show:
Haemoglobin 145g/L
White cell count 7.6 x10^9/L
Neutrophils 6.1 x10^9/L
Lymphocytes 1.2 x10^9/L
Monocytes 0.2 x10^9/L
Platelets 485 x10^9/L
Bilirubin 40mmol/L
Alkaline phosphatase 98iU/L
Alanine transaminase 109iU/L

Your task is to prescribe the appropriate medication.
It is 10:00 on 9th June.

Notes

Step 1: Complete your answers in the drug chart opposite and overleaf

LONGBURY HOSPITAL TRUST			HOSPITAL NUMBER SURNAME FIRST NAME ADDRESS D.O.B			
DATE OF ADMISSION		ADMISSION WEIGHT (KG)		WARD		
ALLERGIES			CONSULTANT			
			CHART NO		...OF...	

ONCE ONLY PRESCRIPTIONS

DATE	TIME	NAME OF DRUG	DOSE	ROUTE	PRESCRIBER'S SIGNATURE	GIVEN BY	TIME GIVEN

REGULAR MEDICATIONS

NAME OF DRUG		**TIME**	DATE → DOSE ↓				
ADDITIONAL INSTRUCTIONS		**08:00**					
DATE	ROUTE	**12:00**					
PRESCRIBER'S SIGNATURE		**18:00**					
PRESCRIBER'S NAME AND BLEEP		**22:00**					

NAME OF DRUG		**TIME**	DATE → DOSE ↓				
ADDITIONAL INSTRUCTIONS		**08:00**					
DATE	ROUTE	**12:00**					
PRESCRIBER'S SIGNATURE		**18:00**					
PRESCRIBER'S NAME AND BLEEP		**22:00**					

NAME OF DRUG		**TIME**	DATE → DOSE ↓				
ADDITIONAL INSTRUCTIONS		**08:00**					
DATE	ROUTE	**12:00**					
PRESCRIBER'S SIGNATURE		**18:00**					
PRESCRIBER'S NAME AND BLEEP		**22:00**					

PATIENT NAME   HOSPITAL NO.

NAME OF DRUG		TIME	DATE →					
			DOSE ↓					
ADDITIONAL INSTRUCTIONS		08:00						
DATE	ROUTE	12:00						
PRESCRIBER'S SIGNATURE								
		18:00						
PRESCRIBER'S NAME AND BLEEP								
		22:00						

NAME OF DRUG		TIME	DATE →					
			DOSE ↓					
ADDITIONAL INSTRUCTIONS		08:00						
DATE	ROUTE	12:00						
PRESCRIBER'S SIGNATURE								
		18:00						
PRESCRIBER'S NAME AND BLEEP								
		22:00						

NAME OF DRUG		TIME	DATE →					
			DOSE ↓					
ADDITIONAL INSTRUCTIONS		08:00						
DATE	ROUTE	12:00						
PRESCRIBER'S SIGNATURE								
		18:00						
PRESCRIBER'S NAME AND BLEEP								
		22:00						

AS REQUIRED PRESCRIPTIONS

NAME OF DRUG		DATE					
INDICATION/ INSTRUCTION	DOSE	TIME					
FREQUENCY	ROUTE	DOSE					
PRESCRIBER'S SIGNATURE		ROUTE					
PRESCRIBER'S NAME AND BLEEP		GIVEN BY					
START DATE	STOP DATE						

PATIENT NAME   HOSPITAL NO.

NAME OF DRUG		DATE					
INDICATION/ INSTRUCTION	DOSE	TIME					
FREQUENCY	ROUTE	DOSE					
PRESCRIBER'S SIGNATURE		ROUTE					
PRESCRIBER'S NAME AND BLEEP		GIVEN BY					
START DATE	STOP DATE						

INTRAVENOUS FLUIDS

DATE	FLUID	ADDITIVE & DOSE	VOLUME	RATE/ DURATION	PRESCRIBER'S SIGNATURE	GIVEN BY	START TIME	END TIME

Record of signatures. ALL prescribers MUST complete.

DATE	NAME	DESIGNATION	SIGNATURE	BLEEP NUMBER

Answer 38

Not all infections require antibiotics. At best prescribing inappropriate antibiotics will do nothing for the patient, at worst they can cause serious adverse effects.

Step 3: Compare your answer to the checklist below and the chart opposite ☑

D Details	Checked patient details Used capital letters throughout Used correct abbreviations	☐
R Regular medications	Prescribed simple analgesia, e.g. paracetamol and/or ibuprofen	☐
U Unpleasant reactions	Correctly entered doxycycline in allergies box	☐
G Gravid?	No	☐

C Contra-indications	Noted that amoxicillin can cross react with Epstein–Barr virus to produce a rash	☐
H Hydration	Not required	☐
A Analgesia	Prescribed an analgesic throat spray or mouth rinse	☐
R Renal function	Not required	☐
T Thrombo-prophylaxis	Prescribed enoxaparin because the patient is going to have knee surgery	☐
S Signature box	Signed signature box	☐

Rationale

Exudates covering the tonsils are not a reliable sign of bacterial tonsillitis: they are a general sign of inflammation and may be present in viral illnesses. The majority of sore throats do not require antibiotics. Scoring systems such as the Centor score can be used to guide decision-making.

In this patient, the mildly raised bilirubin and ALT suggest an Epstein–Barr virus infection. This would cause all of his symptoms, including the tonsillar exudate, and he is in the most likely age group to be infected. Patients with Epstein–Barr virus are often mistakenly given amoxicillin to treat a presumed bacterial sore throat. Unfortunately, amoxicillin reacts with the virus and can cause a florid rash. This reaction often results in patients being labelled with a penicillin allergy. Epstein–Barr virus infection is diagnosed by positive serology. Treatment is supportive.

Another thing to consider in this exercise is the need for analgesia. Regular paracetamol would be an appropriate starting point and ibuprofen can be used in conjunction. Here, an anti-inflammatory throat spray has been prescribed to provide local analgesia. Intravenous fluids would only be necessary if the patient could not eat or drink, or was nil-by-mouth preoperatively. It would also be prudent to inform the anaesthetist and the surgeon of the working diagnosis, as they may want to consider delaying the operation.

KEY POINTS

- Sore throats rarely require treatment with antibiotics
- Consider topical therapy in addition to other analgesics
- Epstein–Barr virus cross-reacts with amoxicillin, producing a rash

LONGBURY HOSPITAL TRUST				HOSPITAL NUMBER	654211		
				SURNAME	STEWART		
				FIRST NAME	OLIVER		
				ADDRESS	36 AMBER ROAD, LONGBURY LB8 7AM		
				D.O.B	13/12/YYYY (19 YEARS AGO)		
DATE OF ADMISSION	09/06/YYYY	ADMISSION WEIGHT (KG)		64kg	WARD	SURGICAL	
ALLERGIES				CONSULTANT		JOSHUA GIBB	
DOXYCYCLINE - RASH				CHART NO		1...OF...1	

ONCE ONLY PRESCRIPTIONS

DATE	TIME	NAME OF DRUG	DOSE	ROUTE	PRESCRIBER'S SIGNATURE	GIVEN BY	TIME GIVEN

REGULAR MEDICATIONS

NAME OF DRUG	TIME	DATE → DOSE ↓	09/06				
ENOXAPARIN							
ADDITIONAL INSTRUCTIONS	08:00						
DATE 09/06 ROUTE SC	12:00						
PRESCRIBER'S SIGNATURE ALewis	18:00	40mg					
PRESCRIBER'S NAME AND BLEEP ALEX LEWIS 4567	22:00						

NAME OF DRUG	TIME	DATE → DOSE ↓	09/06				
PARACETAMOL							
ADDITIONAL INSTRUCTIONS	08:00	1g	X				
DATE 09/06 ROUTE PO	12:00	1g					
PRESCRIBER'S SIGNATURE ALewis	18:00	1g					
PRESCRIBER'S NAME AND BLEEP ALEX LEWIS 4567	22:00	1g					

NAME OF DRUG	TIME	DATE → DOSE ↓	09/06				
IBUPROFEN							
ADDITIONAL INSTRUCTIONS	08:00	400mg	X				
DATE 09/06 ROUTE PO	12:00						
PRESCRIBER'S SIGNATURE ALewis	14:00	400mg					
	18:00						
PRESCRIBER'S NAME AND BLEEP ALEX LEWIS 4567	22:00	400mg					

PATIENT NAME *OLIVER STEWART* HOSPITAL NO. *654211*

NAME OF DRUG DIFFLAM SPRAY (BENZYDAMINE HYDROCHLORIDE)	TIME	DATE → / DOSE ↓	09/06				
ADDITIONAL INSTRUCTIONS	08:00	4 SPRAYS	X				
DATE 09/06 ROUTE MOUTH SPRAY	12:00						
PRESCRIBER'S SIGNATURE ALewis	14:00	4 SPRAYS					
	18:00						
PRESCRIBER'S NAME AND BLEEP ALEX LEWIS 4567	22:00	4 SPRAYS					

NAME OF DRUG	TIME	DATE → / DOSE ↓					
ADDITIONAL INSTRUCTIONS	08:00						
DATE ROUTE	12:00						
PRESCRIBER'S SIGNATURE	18:00						
PRESCRIBER'S NAME AND BLEEP	22:00						

NAME OF DRUG	TIME	DATE → / DOSE ↓					
ADDITIONAL INSTRUCTIONS	08:00						
DATE ROUTE	12:00						
PRESCRIBER'S SIGNATURE	18:00						
PRESCRIBER'S NAME AND BLEEP	22:00						

AS REQUIRED PRESCRIPTIONS

NAME OF DRUG BENZYDAMINE HYDROCHLORIDE SPRAY		DATE					
INDICATION/ INSTRUCTION SORE THROAT	DOSE 4 – 8 SPRAYS	TIME					
FREQUENCY 1.5 – 3 HOURS	ROUTE MOUTH SPRAY	DOSE					
PRESCRIBER'S SIGNATURE ALewis		ROUTE					
PRESCRIBER'S NAME AND BLEEP ALEX LEWIS 4567		GIVEN BY					
START DATE 09/06	STOP DATE						

PATIENT NAME *OLIVER STEWART*   HOSPITAL NO.   *654211*

NAME OF DRUG		DATE						
INDICATION/ INSTRUCTION	DOSE	TIME						
FREQUENCY	ROUTE	DOSE						
PRESCRIBER'S SIGNATURE		ROUTE						
PRESCRIBER'S NAME AND BLEEP		GIVEN BY						
START DATE	STOP DATE							

INTRAVENOUS FLUIDS

DATE	FLUID	ADDITIVE & DOSE	VOLUME	RATE/ DURATION	PRESCRIBER'S SIGNATURE	GIVEN BY	START TIME	END TIME

Record of signatures. ALL prescribers MUST complete.

DATE	NAME	DESIGNATION	SIGNATURE	BLEEP NUMBER
09/06	ALEX LEWIS	F1	ALewis	4567

Glenda Roberts (hospital number: 784634, DOB 13/04/YYYY [78 years old], address: 2 Pensum Avenue, Longbury LB20 3WL) was admitted over 2 weeks ago in an acute confusional state. She was treated with trimethoprim for an urinary tract infection and has been medically fit for discharge for 10 days. She is due to go home tomorrow or the day after when her care package is put in place.

Mrs Roberts is reviewed during the ward round. She is well orientated, and feeling well. Her examination is normal and her observations stable. She takes warfarin for atrial fibrillation, normally has a stable international normalised ratio and has been taking her usual dose of 5mg since admission. She was also started on ramipril for hypertension by her general practitioner a while ago.

Blood test results from this morning:
Sodium: 133mmol/L
Potassium 3.6mmol/L
Creatinine 89µmol/L
International normalised ratio 3.8

Blood pressure readings over the last 24 hours:
160/90mmHg yesterday morning
158/87mmHg yesterday lunchtime
169/56mmHg yesterday evening
162/88mmHg this morning

Your task is to prescribe appropriately for Mrs Roberts during the ward round.
It is 09:15 on the 21st July.

Notes

Step 1: Complete your answers in the drug chart opposite and overleaf

LONGBURY HOSPITAL TRUST			HOSPITAL NUMBER	784634		
			SURNAME	ROBERTS		
			FIRST NAME	GLENDA		
			ADDRESS	2 PENSUM AVENUE, LONGBURY LB20 3WL		
			D.O.B	13/04/YYYY (78 YEARS AGO)		
DATE OF ADMISSION	03/07/YYYY	ADMISSION WEIGHT (KG)	61kg	WARD	MEDICAL ASSESSMENT	
ALLERGIES			CONSULTANT		ERIN JOHNSON	
PENICILLIN - RASH, STATINS - MYALGIA			CHART NO		1...OF...1	

ONCE ONLY PRESCRIPTIONS

DATE	TIME	NAME OF DRUG	DOSE	ROUTE	PRESCRIBER'S SIGNATURE	GIVEN BY	TIME GIVEN
18/07	2330	ZOPICLONE	3.75mg	PO	EJones	WP	2350

REGULAR MEDICATIONS

NAME OF DRUG RAMIPRIL	TIME	DATE → DOSE ↓	18/07	19/07	20/07	21/07	
ADDITIONAL INSTRUCTIONS	08:00	1.25mg	RN	RN	BE	BE	
DATE 03/07 ROUTE PO	12:00						
PRESCRIBER'S SIGNATURE EJones	18:00						
PRESCRIBER'S NAME AND BLEEP EMMA JONES 4876	22:00						

NAME OF DRUG OMEPRAZOLE	TIME	DATE → DOSE ↓	18/07	19/07	20/07	21/07	
ADDITIONAL INSTRUCTIONS	08:00	20mg	RN	RN	BE	BE	
DATE 03/07 ROUTE PO	12:00						
PRESCRIBER'S SIGNATURE EJones	18:00						
PRESCRIBER'S NAME AND BLEEP EMMA JONES 4876	22:00						

NAME OF DRUG CITALOPRAM	TIME	DATE → DOSE ↓	18/07	19/07	20/07	21/07	
ADDITIONAL INSTRUCTIONS	08:00	20mg	RN	RN	BE	BE	
DATE 03/07 ROUTE PO	12:00						
PRESCRIBER'S SIGNATURE EJones	18:00						
PRESCRIBER'S NAME AND BLEEP EMMA JONES 4876	22:00						

PATIENT NAME GLENDA ROBERTS   HOSPITAL NO.   784634

NAME OF DRUG	TIME	DATE → DOSE ↓					
ADDITIONAL INSTRUCTIONS	08:00						
DATE	ROUTE	12:00						
PRESCRIBER'S SIGNATURE							
	18:00						
PRESCRIBER'S NAME AND BLEEP							
	22:00						

NAME OF DRUG	TIME	DATE → DOSE ↓					
ADDITIONAL INSTRUCTIONS	08:00						
DATE	ROUTE	12:00						
PRESCRIBER'S SIGNATURE							
	18:00						
PRESCRIBER'S NAME AND BLEEP							
	22:00						

NAME OF DRUG	TIME	DATE → DOSE ↓					
ADDITIONAL INSTRUCTIONS	08:00						
DATE	ROUTE	12:00						
PRESCRIBER'S SIGNATURE							
	18:00						
PRESCRIBER'S NAME AND BLEEP							
	22:00						

AS REQUIRED PRESCRIPTIONS

NAME OF DRUG		DATE					
INDICATION/ INSTRUCTION	DOSE	TIME					
FREQUENCY	ROUTE	DOSE					
PRESCRIBER'S SIGNATURE		ROUTE					
PRESCRIBER'S NAME AND BLEEP		GIVEN BY					
START DATE	STOP DATE						

PATIENT NAME GLENDA ROBERTS   HOSPITAL NO.   784634

NAME OF DRUG		DATE						
INDICATION/ INSTRUCTION	DOSE	TIME						
FREQUENCY	ROUTE	DOSE						
PRESCRIBER'S SIGNATURE		ROUTE						
PRESCRIBER'S NAME AND BLEEP		GIVEN BY						
START DATE	STOP DATE							

ANTICOAGULATION CHART

DATE	18/07	19/07	20/07	21/07	22/07	23/07
INR		2.9		3.8		
WARFARIN DOSE	5mg	5mg	5mg			
PRESCRIBER'S SIGNATURE	EJones	EJones	EJones			
GIVEN BY	RN	RN	BE			
TIME	18:00	18:00	18:00			

INTRAVENOUS FLUIDS

DATE	FLUID	ADDITIVE & DOSE	VOLUME	RATE/ DURATION	PRESCRIBER'S SIGNATURE	GIVEN BY	START TIME	END TIME

Record of signatures. ALL prescribers MUST complete.

DATE	NAME	DESIGNATION	SIGNATURE	BLEEP NUMBER
03/07	EMMA JONES	F2	EJones	4876

Answer 39

These types of 'housekeeping' prescribing tasks are common for the junior doctor. Using the DRUGCHARTS mnemonic in this case is a good 0way of ensuring a holistic approach to this patient's medication review.

Step 3: Compare your answer to the checklist below and the chart opposite ☑

D	Details	Checked patient details Used capital letters throughout Used correct abbreviations	☐
R	Regular medications	Increased ramipril to 2.5mg	☐
U	Unpleasant reactions	Did not start a statin	☐
G	Gravid?	No	☐

C	Contra-indications	Avoided over-anticoagulating the patient	☐
H	Hydration	Not required	☐
A	Analgesia	Not required. Prescribing PRN paracetamol would be acceptable	☐
R	Renal function	OK	☐
T	Thrombo-prophylaxis	On warfarin	☐
S	Signature box	Signed signature box	☐

Rationale

When managing this patient's INR, remember that she has relatively stable warfarin control. Although her INR today is raised beyond her likely target of 2–3, it is not high enough to warrant concern and she is asymptomatic. There are no new interacting medications on her drug chart therefore no big changes should be made to her prescription. The prescriber has reduced the warfarin dose slightly to 4mg instead of making a large dose reduction or omitting the drug. If the dose was omitted then the risk would be that her next INR would be too low and then the following day she would be over-anticoagulated in response, creating a see-saw like effect and unstable INR control. The new dose of 4mg has been prescribed for at least 2 days, giving time to properly assess the effect this will have on the INR. An alternative option would be to prescribe the usual 5mg and check the INR again the following morning and see if it is still increasing. Some hospitals will have a specialist anticoagulation service and their own guidelines, which can be invaluable.

The other task in this exercise is the adjustment of rampiril. This is a medication newly started by the patient's general practitioner for hypertension diagnosed prior to admission. The patient's blood pressure is still high and it falls to the prescriber to recognise this and increase the dose of ramipril accordingly. Check the patient has good renal function and stable urea and electrolytes before doing this.

KEY POINTS

- Correct slight derangeements of INR with minor adjustments: avoid destabilising control by overcorrecting the warfarin dose
- Check if doses need adjusting as part of the regular medication review, in this case the ramipiril

LONGBURY HOSPITAL TRUST

HOSPITAL NUMBER	784634
SURNAME	ROBERTS
FIRST NAME	GLENDA
ADDRESS	2 PENSUM AVENUE, LONGBURY LB20 3WL
D.O.B	13/04/YYYY (78 YEARS AGO)

DATE OF ADMISSION	03/07/YYYY	ADMISSION WEIGHT (KG)	61kg	WARD	MEDICAL ASSESSMENT

ALLERGIES	CONSULTANT	ERIN JOHNSON
PENICILLIN - RASH; STATINS - MYALGIA	CHART NO	1...OF...1

ONCE ONLY PRESCRIPTIONS

DATE	TIME	NAME OF DRUG	DOSE	ROUTE	PRESCRIBER'S SIGNATURE	GIVEN BY	TIME GIVEN
18/07	2330	ZOPICLONE	3.75mg	PO	EJones	WP	2350

REGULAR MEDICATIONS

NAME OF DRUG RAMIPRIL	TIME	DATE → DOSE ↓	18/07	19/07	20/07	21/07	
ADDITIONAL INSTRUCTIONS	08:00	1.25mg	RN	RN	BE	BE	STOP ALewis 21/07
DATE 03/07 ROUTE PO	12:00						
PRESCRIBER'S SIGNATURE EJones	18:00						
PRESCRIBER'S NAME AND BLEEP EMMA JONES 4876	22:00						

NAME OF DRUG OMEPRAZOLE	TIME	DATE → DOSE ↓	18/07	19/07	20/07	21/07	
ADDITIONAL INSTRUCTIONS	08:00	20mg	RN	RN	BE	BE	
DATE 03/07 ROUTE PO	12:00						
PRESCRIBER'S SIGNATURE EJones	18:00						
PRESCRIBER'S NAME AND BLEEP EMMA JONES 4876	22:00						

NAME OF DRUG CITALOPRAM	TIME	DATE → DOSE ↓	18/07	19/07	20/07	21/07	
ADDITIONAL INSTRUCTIONS	08:00	20mg	RN	RN	BE	BE	
DATE 03/07 ROUTE PO	12:00						
PRESCRIBER'S SIGNATURE EJones	18:00						
PRESCRIBER'S NAME AND BLEEP EMMA JONES 4876	22:00						

PATIENT NAME GLENDA ROBERTS   HOSPITAL NO.   784634

NAME OF DRUG		TIME	DATE → DOSE ↓					22/07
RAMIPRIL								
ADDITIONAL INSTRUCTIONS		08:00	2.5mg	X	X	X	X	
DATE 21/07	ROUTE PO	12:00						
PRESCRIBER'S SIGNATURE ALewis		18:00						
PRESCRIBER'S NAME AND BLEEP ALEX LEWIS 4567		22:00						

NAME OF DRUG		TIME	DATE → DOSE ↓					
ADDITIONAL INSTRUCTIONS		08:00						
DATE	ROUTE	12:00						
PRESCRIBER'S SIGNATURE		18:00						
PRESCRIBER'S NAME AND BLEEP		22:00						

NAME OF DRUG		TIME	DATE → DOSE ↓					
ADDITIONAL INSTRUCTIONS		08:00						
DATE	ROUTE	12:00						
PRESCRIBER'S SIGNATURE		18:00						
PRESCRIBER'S NAME AND BLEEP		22:00						

AS REQUIRED PRESCRIPTIONS

NAME OF DRUG		DATE					
INDICATION/ INSTRUCTION	DOSE	TIME					
FREQUENCY	ROUTE	DOSE					
PRESCRIBER'S SIGNATURE		ROUTE					
PRESCRIBER'S NAME AND BLEEP		GIVEN BY					
START DATE	STOP DATE						

PATIENT NAME GLENDA ROBERTS   HOSPITAL NO.   784634

NAME OF DRUG		DATE					
INDICATION/ INSTRUCTION	DOSE	TIME					
FREQUENCY	ROUTE	DOSE					
PRESCRIBER'S SIGNATURE		ROUTE					
PRESCRIBER'S NAME AND BLEEP		GIVEN BY					
START DATE	STOP DATE						

ANTICOAGULATION CHART

DATE	18/07	19/07	20/07	21/07	22/07	23/07
INR		2.9		3.8		
WARFARIN DOSE	5mg	5mg	5mg	4mg	4mg	
PRESCRIBER'S SIGNATURE	EJones	EJones	EJones	ALewis	ALewis	
GIVEN BY	RN	RN	BE			
TIME	18:00	18:00	18:00			

INTRAVENOUS FLUIDS

DATE	FLUID	ADDITIVE & DOSE	VOLUME	RATE/ DURATION	PRESCRIBER'S SIGNATURE	GIVEN BY	START TIME	END TIME

Record of signatures. ALL prescribers MUST complete.

DATE	NAME	DESIGNATION	SIGNATURE	BLEEP NUMBER
03/07	EMMA JONES	F2	E Jones	4876
09/06	ALEX LEWIS	F1	ALewis	4567

Exercise 40　Pain management

Gerald Bell (hospital number: 153647, DOB 11/02/YYYY [64 years old], address: 307 Potters Street, Longbury LB6 5LK) is diabetic. He is on the surgical ward recovering from a left above knee amputation carried out 3 days ago. A postoperative sciatic nerve catheter has been left in his wound to provide local anaesthesia. He has been making good progress and during the ward round the consultant asks for the catheter to be removed. Mr Bell's renal function is OK.

　(A sciatic catheter is a small clear plastic tube which is left in the surgical site. Local anaesthetic is then injected by syringe into the tube, delivering analgesia directly to the stump.)

Your task is to stop the bupivacaine and add any new prescriptions as necessary.
It is 08:45 on 16th June.

Notes

Step 1: Complete your answers in the drug chart opposite and overleaf

LONGBURY HOSPITAL TRUST		HOSPITAL NUMBER	153647		
		SURNAME	BELL		
		FIRST NAME	GERALD		
		ADDRESS	307 POTTERS STREET, LONGBURY LB6 5LK		
		D.O.B	11/02/YYYY (64 YEARS AGO)		
DATE OF ADMISSION	13/06/YYYY	ADMISSION WEIGHT (KG)	87kg	WARD	SURGICAL
ALLERGIES		CONSULTANT		JOSHUA GIBB	
CODEINE - 'FEELS DIZZY'		CHART NO		1...OF...1	

ONCE ONLY PRESCRIPTIONS

DATE	TIME	NAME OF DRUG	DOSE	ROUTE	PRESCRIBER'S SIGNATURE	GIVEN BY	TIME GIVEN

REGULAR MEDICATIONS

NAME OF DRUG BUPIVACAINE 1.25mg/ml	TIME	DATE → DOSE ↓	13/06	14/06	15/06	16/06	
ADDITIONAL INSTRUCTIONS TO STUMP	08:00	10ml	——	PU	WP	WP	
DATE 13/06 ROUTE CATHETER	12:00	10ml	——	PU	WP		
PRESCRIBER'S SIGNATURE KCho	18:00	10ml	PU	PU	WP		
PRESCRIBER'S NAME AND BLEEP KENNETH CHO 5765	22:00	10ml	SS	PM	PM		

NAME OF DRUG SIMVASTATIN	TIME	DATE → DOSE ↓	13/06	14/06	15/06	16/06	
ADDITIONAL INSTRUCTIONS	08:00						
DATE 13/06 ROUTE PO	12:00						
PRESCRIBER'S SIGNATURE KCho	18:00						
PRESCRIBER'S NAME AND BLEEP KENNETH CHO 5765	22:00	40mg	SS	PM	PM		

NAME OF DRUG RAMIPRIL	TIME	DATE → DOSE ↓	13/06	14/06	15/06	16/06	
ADDITIONAL INSTRUCTIONS	08:00	5mg	——	PU	WP	WP	
DATE 13/06 ROUTE PO	12:00		PRE-OP				
PRESCRIBER'S SIGNATURE KCho	18:00						
PRESCRIBER'S NAME AND BLEEP KENNETH CHO 5765	22:00						

PATIENT NAME GERALD BELL   HOSPITAL NO.   153647

NAME OF DRUG METFORMIN	TIME	DATE → DOSE ↓	13/06	14/06	15/06	16/06	
ADDITIONAL INSTRUCTIONS	08:00	1g	————	————	————	WP	
DATE 13/06 ROUTE PO	12:00						
PRESCRIBER'S SIGNATURE KCho	18:00	1g	————	————	WP		
PRESCRIBER'S NAME AND BLEEP KENNETH CHO 5765	22:00		POST-OP				

NAME OF DRUG ENOXAPARIN	TIME	DATE → DOSE ↓	13/06	14/06	15/06	16/06	
ADDITIONAL INSTRUCTIONS	08:00						
DATE 13/06 ROUTE S/C	12:00						
PRESCRIBER'S SIGNATURE KCho	18:00	40mg	————	PU	WP		
PRESCRIBER'S NAME AND BLEEP KENNETH CHO 5765	22:00		POST OP				

NAME OF DRUG	TIME	DATE → DOSE ↓					
ADDITIONAL INSTRUCTIONS	08:00						
DATE ROUTE	12:00						
PRESCRIBER'S SIGNATURE	18:00						
PRESCRIBER'S NAME AND BLEEP	22:00						

NAME OF DRUG	TIME	DATE → DOSE ↓					
ADDITIONAL INSTRUCTIONS	08:00						
DATE ROUTE	12:00						
PRESCRIBER'S SIGNATURE	18:00						
PRESCRIBER'S NAME AND BLEEP	22:00						

PATIENT NAME GERALD BELL   HOSPITAL NO.   153647

AS REQUIRED PRESCRIPTIONS

NAME OF DRUG		DATE						
INDICATION/ INSTRUCTION	DOSE	TIME						
FREQUENCY	ROUTE	DOSE						
PRESCRIBER'S SIGNATURE		ROUTE						
PRESCRIBER'S NAME AND BLEEP		GIVEN BY						
START DATE	STOP DATE							

NAME OF DRUG		DATE						
INDICATION/ INSTRUCTION	DOSE	TIME						
FREQUENCY	ROUTE	DOSE						
PRESCRIBER'S SIGNATURE		ROUTE						
PRESCRIBER'S NAME AND BLEEP		GIVEN BY						
START DATE	STOP DATE							

INTRAVENOUS FLUIDS

DATE	FLUID	ADDITIVE & DOSE	VOLUME	RATE/ DURATION	PRESCRIBER'S SIGNATURE	GIVEN BY	START TIME	END TIME
13/06	HARTMANN'S	——————	1 litre	10 hrs	KCho	PU	1600	0200
14/06	N SALINE 0.9%	20mmol KCl	1 litre	10 hrs	KCho	SS	0500	1500

Record of signatures. ALL prescribers MUST complete.

DATE	NAME	DESIGNATION	SIGNATURE	BLEEP NUMBER
13/06	KENNETH CHO	CT2	KCho	5765

Step 2: Now check your work overleaf

Answer 40

This exercise demonstrates the importance of applying the principles of the WHO pain ladder in both directions. Just as the pain ladder is used as a guide to increasing analgesia, it is also used to decrease analgesia.

Step 3: Compare your answer to the checklist below and the chart opposite ☑

D Details	Checked patient details Used capital letters throughout Used correct abbreviations	☐
R Regular medications	Stopped bupivacaine	☐
U Unpleasant reactions	Noticed that codeine has been documented	☐
G Gravid?	No	☐

C Contra-indications	None	☐
H Hydration	Not required	☐
A Analgesia	Prescribed step-down analgesia: regular paracetamol and considered a mild to moderate opiate	☐
R Renal function	OK	☐
T Thrombo-prophylaxis	Continued enoxaparin	☐
S Signature box	Signed signature box	☐

Rationale

This patient was receiving no analgesia apart from the local supply of bupivacaine into his catheter. It is important to allow the new analgesic prescription to take effect before depriving him of the cover he is receiving from the bupivacaine, so do not stop the bupivacaine until he has received his paracetamol at least once.

This patient has said that he gets a reaction with codeine. The dizziness listed on his drug chart is unlikely to represent a true allergy: therefore you can assume that opiates are safe. However, if an alternative can be found, it is worth trying a drug that isn't known to cause problems for the patient. In this case tramadol has been used. Meptazinol or another weak opiate would be suitable. This patient has diabetes, which has likely led to him requiring an amputation. NSAIDs should be avoided in this patient because of the added risk of renal injury in diabetes and because they contribute to cardiovascular risk.

Don't forget to prescribe as-required analgesia with antiemetic cover and consider laxatives. Many of this patient's medications have been stopped in the perioperative period. Metformin has been stopped pre- and postoperatively because of the potential to exacerbate lactic acidosis brought about by surgery. The angiotensin-converting enzyme inhibitor (ramipril) has also been stopped as it can cause hypotension during surgery.

KEY POINTS

- Remember to use the pain ladder in both directions
- Allow your step-down analgesia to take effect before withdrawing the initial analgesia

LONGBURY HOSPITAL TRUST		HOSPITAL NUMBER	153647
		SURNAME	BELL
		FIRST NAME	GERALD
		ADDRESS	307 POTTERS STREET, LONGBURY LB6 5LK
		D.O.B	11/02/YYYY (64 YEARS AGO)

DATE OF ADMISSION	13/06/YYYY	ADMISSION WEIGHT (KG)	87kg	WARD	SURGICAL
ALLERGIES			CONSULTANT		JOSHUA GIBB
CODEINE - 'FEELS DIZZY'			CHART NO		1...OF...1

ONCE ONLY PRESCRIPTIONS

DATE	TIME	NAME OF DRUG	DOSE	ROUTE	PRESCRIBER'S SIGNATURE	GIVEN BY	TIME GIVEN

REGULAR MEDICATIONS

NAME OF DRUG BUPIVACAINE 1.25mg/ml	TIME	DATE → DOSE ↓	13/06	14/06	15/06	16/06	
ADDITIONAL INSTRUCTIONS TO STUMP	08:00	10ml	——	PU	WP	WP	——
DATE 13/06 ROUTE CATHETER	12:00	10ml	——	PU	WP		——
PRESCRIBER'S SIGNATURE KCho	18:00	10ml	PU	PU	WP	ALewis ‾‾‾‾ STOP	16/06 ——
PRESCRIBER'S NAME AND BLEEP KENNETH CHO 5765	22:00	10ml	SS	PM	PM	——	——

NAME OF DRUG SIMVASTATIN	TIME	DATE → DOSE ↓	13/06	14/06	15/06	16/06	
ADDITIONAL INSTRUCTIONS	08:00						
DATE 13/06 ROUTE PO	12:00						
PRESCRIBER'S SIGNATURE KCho	18:00						
PRESCRIBER'S NAME AND BLEEP KENNETH CHO 5765	22:00	40mg	SS	PM	PM		

NAME OF DRUG RAMIPRIL	TIME	DATE → DOSE ↓	13/06	14/06	15/06	16/06	
ADDITIONAL INSTRUCTIONS	08:00	5mg	—— PRE-OP	PU	WP	WP	
DATE 13/06 ROUTE PO	12:00						
PRESCRIBER'S SIGNATURE KCho	18:00						
PRESCRIBER'S NAME AND BLEEP KENNETH CHO 5765	22:00						

PATIENT NAME GERALD BELL   HOSPITAL NO.   153647

NAME OF DRUG METFORMIN	TIME	DATE → DOSE ↓	13/06	14/06	15/06	16/06	
ADDITIONAL INSTRUCTIONS	08:00	1g	——	——	——	WP	
DATE 13/06 ROUTE PO	12:00						
PRESCRIBER'S SIGNATURE KCho	18:00	1g	——	——	WP		
PRESCRIBER'S NAME AND BLEEP KENNETH CHO 5765	22:00		POST-OP				

NAME OF DRUG ENOXAPARIN	TIME	DATE → DOSE ↓	13/06	14/06	15/06	16/06	
ADDITIONAL INSTRUCTIONS	08:00						
DATE 13/06 ROUTE S/C	12:00						
PRESCRIBER'S SIGNATURE KCho	18:00	40mg	——	PU	WP		
PRESCRIBER'S NAME AND BLEEP KENNETH CHO 5765	22:00		POST OP				

NAME OF DRUG PARACETAMOL	TIME	DATE → DOSE ↓				16/06	
ADDITIONAL INSTRUCTIONS	08:00	1g					
DATE 16/06 ROUTE O/IV	12:00	1g					
PRESCRIBER'S SIGNATURE ALewis	18:00	1g					
PRESCRIBER'S NAME AND BLEEP ALEX LEWIS 4567	22:00	1g					

NAME OF DRUG TRAMADOL	TIME	DATE → DOSE ↓				16/06	
ADDITIONAL INSTRUCTIONS	08:00	50–100mg					
DATE 16/06 ROUTE PO	12:00	50–100mg					
PRESCRIBER'S SIGNATURE ALewis	18:00	50–100mg					
PRESCRIBER'S NAME AND BLEEP ALEX LEWIS 4567	22:00	50–100mg					

PATIENT NAME GERALD BELL   HOSPITAL NO.   153647

AS REQUIRED PRESCRIPTIONS

NAME OF DRUG ORAMORPH		DATE					
INDICATION/ INSTRUCTION PAIN	DOSE 5–10mg	TIME					
FREQUENCY 2 HRLY	ROUTE PO	DOSE					
PRESCRIBER'S SIGNATURE ALewis		ROUTE					
PRESCRIBER'S NAME AND BLEEP ALEX LEWIS 4567		GIVEN BY					
START DATE 16/06	STOP DATE						

NAME OF DRUG CYCLIZINE		DATE					
INDICATION/ INSTRUCTION NAUSEA	DOSE 50mg	TIME					
FREQUENCY TDS	ROUTE PO/IM/IV	DOSE					
PRESCRIBER'S SIGNATURE ALewis		ROUTE					
PRESCRIBER'S NAME AND BLEEP ALEX LEWIS 4567		GIVEN BY					
START DATE 16/06	STOP DATE						

INTRAVENOUS FLUIDS

DATE	FLUID	ADDITIVE & DOSE	VOLUME	RATE/ DURATION	PRESCRIBER'S SIGNATURE	GIVEN BY	START TIME	END TIME
13/06	HARTMANN'S	————	1 litre	10 hrs	KCho	PU	1600	0200
14/06	N SALINE 0.9%	20mmol KCl	1 litre	10 hrs	KCho	SS	0500	1500

Record of signatures. ALL prescribers MUST complete.

DATE	NAME	DESIGNATION	SIGNATURE	BLEEP NUMBER
13/06	KENNETH CHO	CT2	KCho	5765
16/06	ALEX LEWIS	F1	ALewis	4567

Gladys Adams (hospital number: 649375, DOB 02/05/YYYY [74 years old], address: 89C Bocca Street, Longbury LB9 0FP) was admitted 2 days ago having had a fall that resulted in a femoral neck fracture. She had a dynamic hip screw performed yesterday. She has previously had a heart attack but has no other medical problems. The nurses on the ward have asked for review because urine output has dropped to 5mL/h.

On examination Mrs Adams's jugular venous pressure is not visible, her chest is clear and there is no peripheral oedema.

Recent blood test results:
Sodium 141mmol/L
Potassium 3.9mmol/L
Urea 9.8mmol/L
Creatinine 135μmol/L

Your task is to review the chart and prescribe appropriate treatment for low urine output.
It is 16:30 on 19th June.

Notes

Step 1: Complete your answers in the drug chart opposite and overleaf

LONGBURY HOSPITAL TRUST

HOSPITAL NUMBER	649375
SURNAME	ADAMS
FIRST NAME	GLADYS
ADDRESS	89C BOCCA STREET, LONGBURY LB9 0FP
D.O.B	02/05/YYYY (74 YEARS AGO)

DATE OF ADMISSION	17/06/YYYY	ADMISSION WEIGHT (KG)	82kg	WARD	SURGICAL

ALLERGIES	CONSULTANT	JOSHUA GIBB
PENICILLIN - RASH	CHART NO	1...OF...1

ONCE ONLY PRESCRIPTIONS

DATE	TIME	NAME OF DRUG	DOSE	ROUTE	PRESCRIBER'S SIGNATURE	GIVEN BY	TIME GIVEN

REGULAR MEDICATIONS

NAME OF DRUG ENOXAPARIN	TIME	DATE → DOSE ↓	17/06	18/06	19/06		
ADDITIONAL INSTRUCTIONS	08:00						
DATE 17/06 ROUTE SC	12:00						
PRESCRIBER'S SIGNATURE BFord	18:00	40mg	CG	CG			
PRESCRIBER'S NAME AND BLEEP BEN FORD 1569	22:00						

NAME OF DRUG FUROSEMIDE	TIME	DATE → DOSE ↓	17/06	18/06	19/06		
ADDITIONAL INSTRUCTIONS	08:00	20mg	CG	X	TO		
DATE 17/06 ROUTE PO	12:00						
PRESCRIBER'S SIGNATURE BFord	14:00	20mg	CG	CG			
	18:00						
PRESCRIBER'S NAME AND BLEEP BEN FORD 1569	22:00						

NAME OF DRUG ASPIRIN DISPERSIBLE	TIME	DATE → DOSE ↓	17/06	18/06	19/06		
ADDITIONAL INSTRUCTIONS	08:00	75mg	X	X	TO		
DATE 17/06 ROUTE PO	12:00						
PRESCRIBER'S SIGNATURE BFord	18:00						
PRESCRIBER'S NAME AND BLEEP BEN FORD 1569	22:00						

PATIENT NAME GLADYS ADAMS   HOSPITAL NO.   649375

NAME OF DRUG PARACETAMOL	TIME	DATE → DOSE ↓	17/06	18/06	19/06		
ADDITIONAL INSTRUCTIONS	08:00	1g	CG	CG	TO		
DATE 17/06 ROUTE PO	12:00	1g	CG	CG	TO		
PRESCRIBER'S SIGNATURE BFord	18:00	1g	CG	CG			
PRESCRIBER'S NAME AND BLEEP BEN FORD 1569	22:00	1g	TJ	RC			

NAME OF DRUG RAMIPRIL	TIME	DATE → DOSE ↓	17/06	18/06	19/06		
ADDITIONAL INSTRUCTIONS	08:00	2.5mg		CG	TO		
DATE 17/06 ROUTE PO	12:00						
PRESCRIBER'S SIGNATURE BFord	18:00						
PRESCRIBER'S NAME AND BLEEP BEN FORD 1569	22:00						

NAME OF DRUG SIMVASTATIN	TIME	DATE → DOSE ↓	17/06	18/06	19/06		
ADDITIONAL INSTRUCTIONS	08:00						
DATE 17/06 ROUTE PO	12:00						
PRESCRIBER'S SIGNATURE BFord	18:00						
PRESCRIBER'S NAME AND BLEEP BEN FORD 1569	22:00	20mg	TJ	RC			

AS REQUIRED PRESCRIPTIONS

NAME OF DRUG CODEINE		DATE					
INDICATION/ INSTRUCTION PAIN	DOSE 30–60mg	TIME					
FREQUENCY QDS	ROUTE PO	DOSE					
PRESCRIBER'S SIGNATURE BFord		ROUTE					
PRESCRIBER'S NAME AND BLEEP BEN FORD		GIVEN BY					
START DATE 19/06	STOP DATE						

PATIENT NAME GLADYS ADAMS   HOSPITAL NO.   649375

NAME OF DRUG		DATE					
INDICATION/ INSTRUCTION	DOSE	TIME					
FREQUENCY	ROUTE	DOSE					
PRESCRIBER'S SIGNATURE		ROUTE					
PRESCRIBER'S NAME AND BLEEP		GIVEN BY					
START DATE	STOP DATE						

INTRAVENOUS FLUIDS

DATE	FLUID	ADDITIVE & DOSE	VOLUME	RATE/ DURATION	PRESCRIBER'S SIGNATURE	GIVEN BY	START TIME	END TIME
17/06	0.9% NaCl	————————	1000ml	125ml/hr	BFord	CG	16:30	00:30

Record of signatures. ALL prescribers MUST complete.

DATE	NAME	DESIGNATION	SIGNATURE	BLEEP NUMBER
17/06	BEN FORD	SpR	BFord	1569

Answer 41

This is a common scenario in postoperative patients. In this case the patient has become dehydrated.

Step 3: Compare your answer to the checklist below and the chart opposite ☑

D Details	Checked patient details Used capital letters throughout Used correct abbreviations	☐
R Regular medications	Crossed off or suspended furosemide and prescribed IV fluids	☐
U Unpleasant reactions	None	☐
G Gravid?	No	☐

C Contra-indications	This patient's previous cardiovascular history means fluids should be given cautiously	☐
H Hydration	Prescribed 2L of fluid no faster than 125mL/h	☐
A Analgesia	Not required	☐
R Renal function	Continued ramipril	☐
T Thrombo-prophylaxis	Continued enoxaparin	☐
S Signature box	Signed signature box	☐

Rationale

This patient has become dehydrated. She has had 1L of intravenous fluid since admission, however she will have been nil-by-mouth before the operation on her hip. Her diuretics have been continued and will be contributing to the dehydration. Urinary retention is common in the postoperative period but can be quickly ruled out with a bladder scan, which should be done immediately.

While the patient is being rehydrated her diuretics should be withheld because fluids and diuretics together will cancel each other out. It is tempting to use diuretics to increase a patient's urine output, however this is only beneficial if there is fluid overload. Diuretics can be restarted once the patient is eating and drinking normally, and is euvolaemic.

This patient's previous cardiovascular history and the fact that she was admitted on diuretics should prompt caution when prescribing intravenous fluids. She is likely to have a degree of ventricular impairment and could easily become fluid overloaded.

KEY POINTS

- Stop diuretics in dehydrated patients
- Patients should not receive diuretics and intravenous fluid at the same time
- Consider other causes for low urine output, e.g. a blocked catheter or urinary retention

LONGBURY HOSPITAL TRUST

HOSPITAL NUMBER	649375
SURNAME	ADAMS
FIRST NAME	GLADYS
ADDRESS	89C BOCCA STREET, LONGBURY LB9 0FP
D.O.B	02/05/YYYY (74 YEARS AGO)

DATE OF ADMISSION	17/06/YYYY	ADMISSION WEIGHT (KG)	82kg	WARD	SURGICAL
ALLERGIES			CONSULTANT		JOSHUA GIBB
PENICILLIN - RASH			CHART NO		1…OF…1

ONCE ONLY PRESCRIPTIONS

DATE	TIME	NAME OF DRUG	DOSE	ROUTE	PRESCRIBER'S SIGNATURE	GIVEN BY	TIME GIVEN

REGULAR MEDICATIONS

NAME OF DRUG ENOXAPARIN	TIME	DATE → DOSE ↓	17/06	18/06			
ADDITIONAL INSTRUCTIONS	08:00						
DATE 17/06 ROUTE SC	12:00						
PRESCRIBER'S SIGNATURE BFord	18:00	40mg	CG	CG			
PRESCRIBER'S NAME AND BLEEP BEN FORD 1569	22:00						

NAME OF DRUG FUROSEMIDE	TIME	DATE → DOSE ↓	17/06	18/06	19/06		
ADDITIONAL INSTRUCTIONS	08:00	20mg	CG	X	TO	———	———
DATE 17/06 ROUTE PO	12:00						
PRESCRIBER'S SIGNATURE BFord	18:00	20mg	CG	CG	———	———	———
PRESCRIBER'S NAME AND BLEEP BEN FORD 1569	22:00					STOP 19/06	ALewis 19/06

NAME OF DRUG ASPIRIN DISPERSIBLE	TIME	DATE → DOSE ↓	17/06	18/06	19/06		
ADDITIONAL INSTRUCTIONS	08:00	75mg	X	X	TO		
DATE 17/06 ROUTE PO	12:00						
PRESCRIBER'S SIGNATURE BFord	18:00						
PRESCRIBER'S NAME AND BLEEP BEN FORD 1569	22:00						

PATIENT NAME GLADYS ADAMS   HOSPITAL NO. 649375

NAME OF DRUG PARACETAMOL	TIME	DATE → DOSE ↓	17/06	18/06	19/06		
ADDITIONAL INSTRUCTIONS	08:00	1g	CG	CG	TO		
DATE 17/06 ROUTE PO	12:00	1g	CG	CG	TO		
PRESCRIBER'S SIGNATURE BFord	18:00	1g	CG	CG			
PRESCRIBER'S NAME AND BLEEP BEN FORD 1569	22:00	1g	TJ	RC			

NAME OF DRUG RAMIPRIL	TIME	DATE → DOSE ↓	17/06	18/06	19/06		
ADDITIONAL INSTRUCTIONS	08:00	2.5mg		CG	TO		
DATE 17/06 ROUTE PO	12:00						
PRESCRIBER'S SIGNATURE BFord	18:00						
PRESCRIBER'S NAME AND BLEEP BEN FORD 1569	22:00						

NAME OF DRUG SIMVASTATIN	TIME	DATE → DOSE ↓	17/06	18/06	19/06		
ADDITIONAL INSTRUCTIONS	08:00						
DATE 17/06 ROUTE PO	12:00						
PRESCRIBER'S SIGNATURE BFord	18:00						
PRESCRIBER'S NAME AND BLEEP BEN FORD 1569	22:00	20mg	TJ	RC			

AS REQUIRED PRESCRIPTIONS

NAME OF DRUG CODEINE		DATE					
INDICATION/ INSTRUCTION PAIN	DOSE 30–60mg	TIME					
FREQUENCY QDS	ROUTE PO	DOSE					
PRESCRIBER'S SIGNATURE BFord		ROUTE					
PRESCRIBER'S NAME AND BLEEP BEN FORD		GIVEN BY					
START DATE 19/06	STOP DATE						

PATIENT NAME GERALD SMITH   HOSPITAL NO.   649375

NAME OF DRUG		DATE						
INDICATION/ INSTRUCTION	DOSE	TIME						
FREQUENCY	ROUTE	DOSE						
PRESCRIBER'S SIGNATURE		ROUTE						
PRESCRIBER'S NAME AND BLEEP		GIVEN BY						
START DATE	STOP DATE							

INTRAVENOUS FLUIDS

DATE	FLUID	ADDITIVE & DOSE	VOLUME	RATE/ DURATION	PRESCRIBER'S SIGNATURE	GIVEN BY	START TIME	END TIME
17/06	0.9% NaCl	——————	1000ml	125ml/hr	BFord	CG	16:30	00:30
19/06	0.9% NaCl	——————	1000ml	83ml/h	ALewis			
19/06	5% DEXTROSE	——————	1000ml	83ml/h	ALewis			

Record of signatures. ALL prescribers MUST complete.

DATE	NAME	DESIGNATION	SIGNATURE	BLEEP NUMBER
17/06	BEN FORD	SPR	BFord	1569
19/06	ALEX LEWIS	F1	ALewis	4567

Paramjit Ahlawat (hospital number: 669250, DOB 03/04/YYYY [92 years old], address: 6 Libra Park, Longbury LB5 8WC) was admitted 3 days ago with chest pain which was found to be musculoskeletal. The nursing staff have asked for a review as she has become confused and is calling out for her son. The nurses are concerned that she is disturbing the other patients in the bay and are asking whether she could be given anything to calm her down.

At review Mrs Ahlawat is disorientated and distressed. Unfortunately the nurses have been unable to do any observations as she is too agitated.

Examination of her cardiovascular and respiratory systems is unremarkable. Her abdomen is soft and non tender with her bladder palpable suprapubically.

Your task is to review the chart and prescribe any medication you feel is necessary.
It is 19:15 on 15th May.

Notes

LONGBURY HOSPITAL TRUST			HOSPITAL NUMBER	669250	
			SURNAME	AHLAWAT	
			FIRST NAME	PARAMJIT	
			ADDRESS	6 LIBRA PARK, LONGBURY LB5 8WC	
			D.O.B	03/04/YYYY (92 YEARS AGO)	
DATE OF ADMISSION 12/05/YYYY	ADMISSION WEIGHT (KG)	54kg	WARD	MEDICAL ASSESSMENT	
ALLERGIES		CONSULTANT	ERIN JOHNSON		
PENICILLIN - ANAPHYLAXIS		CHART NO	1...OF...1		

ONCE ONLY PRESCRIPTIONS

DATE	TIME	NAME OF DRUG	DOSE	ROUTE	PRESCRIBER'S SIGNATURE	GIVEN BY	TIME GIVEN

REGULAR MEDICATIONS

NAME OF DRUG ENOXAPARIN	TIME	DATE → DOSE ↓	12/05	13/05	14/05	15/05	
ADDITIONAL INSTRUCTIONS	08:00						
DATE 12/05 ROUTE SC	12:00						
PRESCRIBER'S SIGNATURE MHughes	18:00	40mg	RN	NC	NC	RN	
PRESCRIBER'S NAME AND BLEEP MICHELLE HUGHES 2357	22:00						

NAME OF DRUG PARACETAMOL	TIME	DATE → DOSE ↓	12/05	13/05	14/05	15/05	
ADDITIONAL INSTRUCTIONS	08:00	1g	RN	NC	NC	RN	
DATE 12/05 ROUTE PO	12:00	1g	RN	NC	NC	RN	
PRESCRIBER'S SIGNATURE MHughes	18:00	1g	RN	NC	NC	RN	
PRESCRIBER'S NAME AND BLEEP MICHELLE HUGHES 2357	22:00	1g	CB	TO	CB		

NAME OF DRUG CODEINE	TIME	DATE → DOSE ↓	12/05	13/05	14/05	15/05	
ADDITIONAL INSTRUCTIONS	08:00	60mg	RN	NC	NC	RN	
DATE 12/05 ROUTE PO	12:00	60mg	RN	NC	NC	RN	
PRESCRIBER'S SIGNATURE MHughes	18:00	60mg	RN	NC	NC	RN	
PRESCRIBER'S NAME AND BLEEP MICHELLE HUGHES 2357	22:00	60mg	CB	TO	CB		

PATIENT NAME PARAMJIT AHLAWAT   HOSPITAL NO.   669250

NAME OF DRUG SOLIFENACIN	TIME	DATE → DOSE ↓	12/05	13/05	14/05	15/05	
ADDITIONAL INSTRUCTIONS	08:00	10mg	RN	NC	NC	RN	
DATE 12/05 ROUTE PO	12:00						
PRESCRIBER'S SIGNATURE MHughes	18:00						
PRESCRIBER'S NAME AND BLEEP MICHELLE HUGHES 2357	22:00						

NAME OF DRUG LEVOTHYROXINE	TIME	DATE → DOSE ↓	12/05	13/05	14/05	15/05	
ADDITIONAL INSTRUCTIONS	08:00	250 micrograms	RN	NC	NC	RN	
DATE 12/05 ROUTE PO	12:00						
PRESCRIBER'S SIGNATURE MHughes	18:00						
PRESCRIBER'S NAME AND BLEEP MICHELLE HUGHES 2357	22:00						

NAME OF DRUG	TIME	DATE → DOSE ↓					
ADDITIONAL INSTRUCTIONS	08:00						
DATE ROUTE	12:00						
PRESCRIBER'S SIGNATURE	18:00						
PRESCRIBER'S NAME AND BLEEP	22:00						

AS REQUIRED PRESCRIPTIONS

NAME OF DRUG TRAMADOL		DATE	14/05	14/05	14/05	15/05	15/05	15/05
INDICATION/ INSTRUCTION PAIN	DOSE 50–100mg	TIME	08:00	12:00	18:00	04:00	11:00	15:30
FREQUENCY QDS	ROUTE PO	DOSE	100mg	100mg	100mg	100mg	100mg	100mg
PRESCRIBER'S SIGNATURE NShah		ROUTE	PO	PO	PO	PO	PO	PO
PRESCRIBER'S NAME AND BLEEP NAZIA SHAH 9761		GIVEN BY	NC	NC	NC	CB	RN	RN
START DATE 14/05	STOP DATE							

PATIENT NAME PARAMJIT AHLAWAT   HOSPITAL NO.   669250

NAME OF DRUG		DATE						
INDICATION/ INSTRUCTION	DOSE	TIME						
FREQUENCY	ROUTE	DOSE						
PRESCRIBER'S SIGNATURE		ROUTE						
PRESCRIBER'S NAME AND BLEEP		GIVEN BY						
START DATE	STOP DATE							

INTRAVENOUS FLUIDS

DATE	FLUID	ADDITIVE & DOSE	VOLUME	RATE/ DURATION	PRESCRIBER'S SIGNATURE	GIVEN BY	START TIME	END TIME

Record of signatures. ALL prescribers MUST complete.

DATE	NAME	DESIGNATION	SIGNATURE	BLEEP NUMBER
12/05	MICHELLE HUGHES	SpR	MHughes	2357
14/05	NAZIA SHAH	F2	NShah	9761

Step 2: Now check your work overleaf

Answer 42

This elderly woman has delirium. Delirium is common in older patients and can have many triggers. It is often not possible to be absolutely sure what the cause of delirium is. Remember delirium can be multifactorial and requires a comprehensive review of the patient.

Step 3: Compare your answer to the checklist below and the chart opposite ✔

D	Details	Checked patient details Used capital letters throughout Used correct abbreviations	☐
R	Regular medications	Stopped tramadol Did not prescribe more than 0.5mg haloperidol Wrote that solifenacin is to be reviewed	☐
U	Unpleasant reactions	NKDA	☐
G	Gravid?	No	☐

C	Contra-indications	None	☐
H	Hydration	Not required	☐
A	Analgesia	Continued paracetamol	☐
R	Renal function	Not required	☐
T	Thrombo-prophylaxis	Continued enoxaparin	☐
S	Signature box	Signed signature box	☐

Rationale

A key part of assessing a patient with delirium is a review of current medication. In this exercise the patient has been prescribed codeine and tramadol. These are weak opiates and there is no benefit to using both concurrently. Tramadol also causes confusion in older patients and is a potential cause of this woman's delirium. Urinary retention is another common cause of delirium: this woman has a palpable bladder which implies she may be in retention. She is also taking solifenacin, an antimuscarinic drug used for urinary incontinence and which can also cause urinary retention; it is appropriate to consider stopping it.

If it becomes necessary sedative medications like haloperidol should be used at the lowest possible dose. They should also used only when a patient is at risk of self-harm or is in considerable distress. In this case it could be argued that the patient is distressed and therefore this is an indication for haloperidol. Conversely, it could be argued that the factors driving the delirium should be treated first before resorting to sedation. The administration of sedative medication such as haloperidol increases the risk of falls, particularly in confused patients.

KEY POINTS

- Delirium is common among elderly patients in hospital
- Review medications that may contribute to confusion
- Rule out any all medical causes of delirium before considering prescribing sedatives

LONGBURY HOSPITAL TRUST

HOSPITAL NUMBER	669250
SURNAME	AHLAWAT
FIRST NAME	PARAMJIT
ADDRESS	6 LIBRA PARK, LONGBURY LB5 8WC
D.O.B	03/04/YYYY (92 YEARS AGO)

DATE OF ADMISSION	12/05/YYYY	ADMISSION WEIGHT (KG)	54kg	WARD	MEDICAL ASSESSMENT

ALLERGIES	CONSULTANT	ERIN JOHNSON
PENICILLIN - ANAPHYLAXIS	CHART NO	1...OF...1

ONCE ONLY PRESCRIPTIONS

DATE	TIME	NAME OF DRUG	DOSE	ROUTE	PRESCRIBER'S SIGNATURE	GIVEN BY	TIME GIVEN

REGULAR MEDICATIONS

NAME OF DRUG ENOXAPARIN	TIME	DATE → DOSE ↓	12/05	13/05	14/05	15/05	
ADDITIONAL INSTRUCTIONS	08:00						
DATE 12/05 ROUTE SC	12:00						
PRESCRIBER'S SIGNATURE MHughes	18:00	40mg	RN	NC	NC	RN	
PRESCRIBER'S NAME AND BLEEP MICHELLE HUGHES 2357	22:00						

NAME OF DRUG PARACETAMOL	TIME	DATE → DOSE ↓	12/05	13/05	14/05	15/05	
ADDITIONAL INSTRUCTIONS	08:00	1g	RN	NC	NC	RN	
DATE 12/05 ROUTE PO	12:00	1g	RN	NC	NC	RN	
PRESCRIBER'S SIGNATURE MHughes	18:00	1g	RN	NC	NC	RN	
PRESCRIBER'S NAME AND BLEEP MICHELLE HUGHES 2357	22:00	1g	CB	TO	CB		

NAME OF DRUG CODEINE	TIME	DATE → DOSE ↓	12/05	13/05	14/05	15/05	
ADDITIONAL INSTRUCTIONS	08:00	60mg	RN	NC	NC	RN	
DATE 12/05 ROUTE PO	12:00	60mg	RN	NC	NC	RN	
PRESCRIBER'S SIGNATURE MHughes	18:00	60mg	RN	NC	NC	RN	
PRESCRIBER'S NAME AND BLEEP MICHELLE HUGHES 2357	22:00	60mg	CB	TO	CB		

PATIENT NAME PARAMJIT AHLAWAT   HOSPITAL NO.   669250

NAME OF DRUG SOLIFENACIN	TIME	DATE → DOSE ↓	12/05	13/05	14/05	15/05	
ADDITIONAL INSTRUCTIONS	08:00	10mg	RN	NC	NC	RN	
							REVIEW ALewis 15/05
DATE 12/05 ROUTE PO	12:00						
PRESCRIBER'S SIGNATURE MHughes	18:00						
PRESCRIBER'S NAME AND BLEEP MICHELLE HUGHES 2357	22:00						

NAME OF DRUG LEVOTHYROXINE	TIME	DATE → DOSE ↓	12/05	13/05	14/05	15/05	
ADDITIONAL INSTRUCTIONS	08:00	250 micrograms	RN	NC	NC	RN	
DATE 12/05 ROUTE PO	12:00						
PRESCRIBER'S SIGNATURE MHughes	18:00						
PRESCRIBER'S NAME AND BLEEP MICHELLE HUGHES 2357	22:00						

NAME OF DRUG	TIME	DATE → DOSE ↓					
ADDITIONAL INSTRUCTIONS	08:00						
DATE ROUTE	12:00						
PRESCRIBER'S SIGNATURE	18:00						
PRESCRIBER'S NAME AND BLEEP	22:00						

AS REQUIRED PRESCRIPTIONS

NAME OF DRUG TRAMADOL		DATE	14/05	14/05	14/05	15/05	15/05	15/05
INDICATION/ INSTRUCTION PAIN	DOSE 50–100mg	TIME	08:00	12:00	18:00	04:00	11:00	15:30
FREQUENCY QDS	ROUTE PO	DOSE	100mg	100mg	100mg	100mg	100mg	100mg
PRESCRIBER'S SIGNATURE NShah		ROUTE	PO	PO	PO	PO	PO	PO
PRESCRIBER'S NAME AND BLEEP NAZIA SHAH 9761		GIVEN BY	NC	NC	NC	CB STOP	RN ALewis	RN 15/05
START DATE 14/05	STOP DATE							

PATIENT NAME PARAMJIT AHLAWAT   HOSPITAL NO.   669250

NAME OF DRUG		DATE					
INDICATION/ INSTRUCTION	DOSE	TIME					
FREQUENCY	ROUTE	DOSE					
PRESCRIBER'S SIGNATURE		ROUTE					
PRESCRIBER'S NAME AND BLEEP		GIVEN BY					
START DATE	STOP DATE						

INTRAVENOUS FLUIDS

DATE	FLUID	ADDITIVE & DOSE	VOLUME	RATE/ DURATION	PRESCRIBER'S SIGNATURE	GIVEN BY	START TIME	END TIME

Record of signatures. ALL prescribers MUST complete.

DATE	NAME	DESIGNATION	SIGNATURE	BLEEP NUMBER
12/05	MICHELLE HUGHES	SpR	MHughes	2357
14/05	NAZIA SHAH	F2	NShah	9761
15/05	ALEX LEWIS	F1	ALewis	4567

Kayleigh Mason-Dunn (hospital number: 458112, DOB 14/12/YYYY [23 years old], address: 42 Law Close, Longbury LB19 2ZQ) has been admitted to the medical assessment ward with a severe sore throat which prevents her from eating but not from taking her medication. She has a history of fibromyalgia, chronic low back pain and non-epileptic attack disorder. She says that the regular painkillers she takes are not controlling the pain and asks if she can have some morphine. She is also feeling sick and asks if she can have some cyclizine. She is not pregnant. Her weight is 124kg and her consultant is Dr Erin Johnson.

Mrs Mason-Dunn's list of medications is as follows:
Morphine sulphate modified release tablets 40mg twice daily
Gabapentin 300mg three times daily
She comments that she is 'allergic' to ibuprofen, tramadol and codeine as they all make her feel sick.

Your task is to prescribe the appropriate medication.
It is 08:00 on 23rd June.

Notes

Step 1: Complete your answers in the drug chart opposite and overleaf

LONGBURY HOSPITAL TRUST			HOSPITAL NUMBER SURNAME FIRST NAME ADDRESS D.O.B		
DATE OF ADMISSION		ADMISSION WEIGHT (KG)		WARD	
ALLERGIES			CONSULTANT		
			CHART NO		...OF...

ONCE ONLY PRESCRIPTIONS

DATE	TIME	NAME OF DRUG	DOSE	ROUTE	PRESCRIBER'S SIGNATURE	GIVEN BY	TIME GIVEN

REGULAR MEDICATIONS

NAME OF DRUG		TIME	DATE → DOSE ↓				
ADDITIONAL INSTRUCTIONS		08:00					
DATE	ROUTE	12:00					
PRESCRIBER'S SIGNATURE		18:00					
PRESCRIBER'S NAME AND BLEEP		22:00					

NAME OF DRUG		TIME	DATE → DOSE ↓				
ADDITIONAL INSTRUCTIONS		08:00					
DATE	ROUTE	12:00					
PRESCRIBER'S SIGNATURE		18:00					
PRESCRIBER'S NAME AND BLEEP		22:00					

NAME OF DRUG		TIME	DATE → DOSE ↓				
ADDITIONAL INSTRUCTIONS		08:00					
DATE	ROUTE	12:00					
PRESCRIBER'S SIGNATURE		18:00					
PRESCRIBER'S NAME AND BLEEP		22:00					

PATIENT NAME   HOSPITAL NO.

NAME OF DRUG		TIME	DATE → DOSE ↓					
ADDITIONAL INSTRUCTIONS		08:00						
DATE	ROUTE	12:00						
PRESCRIBER'S SIGNATURE		18:00						
PRESCRIBER'S NAME AND BLEEP		22:00						

NAME OF DRUG		TIME	DATE → DOSE ↓					
ADDITIONAL INSTRUCTIONS		08:00						
DATE	ROUTE	12:00						
PRESCRIBER'S SIGNATURE		18:00						
PRESCRIBER'S NAME AND BLEEP		22:00						

NAME OF DRUG		TIME	DATE → DOSE ↓					
ADDITIONAL INSTRUCTIONS		08:00						
DATE	ROUTE	12:00						
PRESCRIBER'S SIGNATURE		18:00						
PRESCRIBER'S NAME AND BLEEP		22:00						

AS REQUIRED PRESCRIPTIONS

NAME OF DRUG		DATE					
INDICATION/ INSTRUCTION	DOSE	TIME					
FREQUENCY	ROUTE	DOSE					
PRESCRIBER'S SIGNATURE		ROUTE					
PRESCRIBER'S NAME AND BLEEP		GIVEN BY					
START DATE	STOP DATE						

PATIENT NAME   HOSPITAL NO.

NAME OF DRUG		DATE					
INDICATION/ INSTRUCTION	DOSE	TIME					
FREQUENCY	ROUTE	DOSE					
PRESCRIBER'S SIGNATURE		ROUTE					
PRESCRIBER'S NAME AND BLEEP		GIVEN BY					
START DATE	STOP DATE						

INTRAVENOUS FLUIDS

DATE	FLUID	ADDITIVE & DOSE	VOLUME	RATE/ DURATION	PRESCRIBER'S SIGNATURE	GIVEN BY	START TIME	END TIME

Record of signatures. ALL prescribers MUST complete.

DATE	NAME	DESIGNATION	SIGNATURE	BLEEP NUMBER

Patients with chronic pain or medically unexplained symptoms are challenging. In this exercise the patient is already taking substantial doses of morphine; adding more is unlikely to improve her pain relief. Instead it is better to explore alternative modes of analgesia. Sore throats are ideal for topical treatment as the affected area is small. Benzydamine has anti-inflammatory properties which makes it perfect for a scenario like this.

Step 3: Compare your answer to the checklist below and the chart opposite ✔

D Details	Checked patient details Used capital letters throughout Used correct abbreviations	☐
R Regular medications	Prescribed the patient's usual doses of morphine and gabapentin	☐
U Unpleasant reactions	Recorded the patient's sensitivities to ibuprofen, codeine and tramadol	☐
G Gravid?	No	☐

C Contra-indications	None	☐
H Hydration	Not required	☐
A Analgesia	Prescribed alternative analgesia, e.g. paracetamol or a throat spray	☐
R Renal function	Not required	☐
T Thrombo-prophylaxis	Not required: this patient has no risk factors	☐
S Signature box	Signed signature box	☐

Rationale

Cyclizine can cause a mild euphoria, particularly when given intravenously. It can also potentiate the central effects of strong opioids like morphine. This can cause dependence problems, particularly in those who have frequent admissions.

If simple analgesia is not helping, the next step would be to take advice from the chronic pain team. These teams of specialist nurses and anaesthetists are experts in managing difficult pain syndromes and can often help to rationalise a patient's analgesia. The patient has reported the nausea she suffers when taking ibuprofen, codeine and tramadol as an allergy. Patients often think of allergies in different terms to medical staff. Taking a clear history of what happens when the patient takes the drug will help determine if they truly do have an allergy or are experiencing side effects that they find intolerable.

KEY POINTS

- Think of alternative modes of analgesia before increasing doses of morphine
- Cyclizine can interact with opiates and some patients may seek it out for this reason
- Don't forget there are expert pain teams to help with difficult pain problems

LONGBURY HOSPITAL TRUST						
			HOSPITAL NUMBER	458112		
			SURNAME	MASON-DUNN		
			FIRST NAME	KAYLEIGH		
			ADDRESS	42 LAW CLOSE, LONGBURY LB19 2ZQ		
			D.O.B	14/12/YYYY (23 YEARS AGO)		
DATE OF ADMISSION	23/06/YYYY	ADMISSION WEIGHT (KG)	124kg	WARD	MEDICAL ASSESSMENT	
ALLERGIES IBUPROFEN – NAUSEA CODEINE – NAUSEA TRAMADOL – NAUSEA			CONSULTANT	ERIN JOHNSON		
			CHART NO		1...OF...1	

ONCE ONLY PRESCRIPTIONS

DATE	TIME	NAME OF DRUG	DOSE	ROUTE	PRESCRIBER'S SIGNATURE	GIVEN BY	TIME GIVEN

REGULAR MEDICATIONS

NAME OF DRUG MORPHINE SULPHATE MODIFIED RELEASE TABLETS	TIME	DATE → DOSE ↓	23/06				
ADDITIONAL INSTRUCTIONS	08:00	40mg					
DATE 23/06 ROUTE PO	12:00						
PRESCRIBER'S SIGNATURE ALewis	18:00	40mg					
PRESCRIBER'S NAME AND BLEEP ALEX LEWIS 4567	22:00						

NAME OF DRUG GABAPENTIN	TIME	DATE → DOSE ↓	23/06				
ADDITIONAL INSTRUCTIONS	08:00	300mg					
DATE 23/06 ROUTE PO	12:00						
PRESCRIBER'S SIGNATURE ALewis	14:00	300mg					
	18:00						
PRESCRIBER'S NAME AND BLEEP ALEX LEWIS 4567	22:00	300mg					

NAME OF DRUG PARACETAMOL	TIME	DATE → DOSE ↓	23/06				
ADDITIONAL INSTRUCTIONS	08:00	1g					
DATE 23/06 ROUTE PO	12:00	1g					
PRESCRIBER'S SIGNATURE ALewis	18:00	1g					
PRESCRIBER'S NAME AND BLEEP ALEX LEWIS 4567	22:00	1g					

PATIENT NAME *KAYLEIGH MASON-DUNN*   HOSPITAL NO.   *458112*

NAME OF DRUG *BENZYDAMINE 0.15% ORAL SPRAY*		TIME	DATE → DOSE ↓	*23/06*					
ADDITIONAL INSTRUCTIONS		**08:00**	*4-8 SPRAYS*						
DATE *23/06*	ROUTE *MOUTH SPRAY*	**12:00**							
PRESCRIBER'S SIGNATURE *ALewis*		*14:00*	*4-8 SPRAYS*						
		18:00							
PRESCRIBER'S NAME AND BLEEP *ALEX LEWIS 4567*		**22:00**	*4-8 SPRAYS*						

NAME OF DRUG		TIME	DATE → DOSE ↓						
ADDITIONAL INSTRUCTIONS		**08:00**							
DATE	ROUTE	**12:00**							
PRESCRIBER'S SIGNATURE									
		18:00							
PRESCRIBER'S NAME AND BLEEP		**22:00**							

NAME OF DRUG		TIME	DATE → DOSE ↓						
ADDITIONAL INSTRUCTIONS		**08:00**							
DATE	ROUTE	**12:00**							
PRESCRIBER'S SIGNATURE									
		18:00							
PRESCRIBER'S NAME AND BLEEP		**22:00**							

AS REQUIRED PRESCRIPTIONS

NAME OF DRUG *ONDANSETRON*		DATE						
INDICATION/ INSTRUCTION *NAUSEA*	DOSE *4mg*	TIME						
FREQUENCY *TDS*	ROUTE *PO*	DOSE						
PRESCRIBER'S SIGNATURE *ALewis*		ROUTE						
PRESCRIBER'S NAME AND BLEEP *ALEX LEWIS 4567*		GIVEN BY						
START DATE *23/06*	STOP DATE							

PATIENT NAME   *KAYLEIGH MASON-DUNN*   HOSPITAL NO.   *458112*

NAME OF DRUG *BENZYDAMINE 0.15% ORAL SPRAY*		DATE					
INDICATION/ INSTRUCTION *PAIN*	DOSE *4-8 SPRAYS*	TIME					
FREQUENCY *1.5 – 3 HOURLY*	ROUTE *MOUTH SPRAY*	DOSE					
PRESCRIBER'S SIGNATURE *ALewis*		ROUTE					
PRESCRIBER'S NAME AND BLEEP *ALEX LEWIS 4567*		GIVEN BY					
START DATE *23/06*	STOP DATE						

INTRAVENOUS FLUIDS

DATE	FLUID	ADDITIVE & DOSE	VOLUME	RATE/ DURATION	PRESCRIBER'S SIGNATURE	GIVEN BY	START TIME	END TIME

Record of signatures. ALL prescribers MUST complete.

DATE	NAME	DESIGNATION	SIGNATURE	BLEEP NUMBER
23/06	*ALEX LEWIS*	*F1*	*ALewis*	*4567*

Leonard Nash (hospital number: 411973, DOB 31/12/YYYY [68 years old], address: 18 Upper Lane, Longbury LB5 4BH) is being treated on the respiratory ward for type two respiratory failure and is receiving BiPAP non-invasive ventilation overnight. He says he finds he cannot sleep with the BiPAP machine on and is at his wits end, having struggled to sleep for the last two nights. He admits he normally takes one of his wife's sleeping tablets without any problems and is desperate for some sleep. He is a smoker with advanced chronic obstructive pulmonary disease (COPD). His usual COPD therapy has been replaced with oral steroid, and inhaled salbutamol and ipratropium.

During the night the nursing staff ask for sleeping tablets to be prescribed.

Mr Nash's most recent (2 hours ago) arterial blood gases are:

pH 7.34
PaO_2 8.1kPa
$PaCO_2$ 9.30kPa
HCO_3 34mmol/L
On 1L O_2
BiPAP set at 14/8

Your task is to review the chart and prescribe appropriately.
It is 23:30 on 13th April.

Notes

Step 1: Complete your answers in the drug chart opposite and overleaf

LONGBURY HOSPITAL TRUST				
	HOSPITAL NUMBER	411973		
	SURNAME	NASH		
	FIRST NAME	LEONARD		
	ADDRESS	18 UPPER LANE, LONGBURY LB5 4BH		
	D.O.B	31/12/YYYY (68 YEARS AGO)		

DATE OF ADMISSION	11/04/YYYY	ADMISSION WEIGHT (KG)	81kg	WARD	MEDICAL ASSESSMENT
ALLERGIES			CONSULTANT		ERIN JOHNSON
LATEX - RASH			CHART NO		1...OF...1

ONCE ONLY PRESCRIPTIONS

DATE	TIME	NAME OF DRUG	DOSE	ROUTE	PRESCRIBER'S SIGNATURE	GIVEN BY	TIME GIVEN
11/04	2200	ZOPICLONE	3.75mg	PO	KCho	WP	2300
12/04	2350	ZOPICLONE	7.5mg	PO	KCho	WP	0100

REGULAR MEDICATIONS

NAME OF DRUG PREDNISOLONE	TIME	DATE → DOSE ↓	11/04	12/04	13/04		15/04
ADDITIONAL INSTRUCTIONS	08:00						
DATE 11/04 ROUTE PO	12:00						
PRESCRIBER'S SIGNATURE EJones	18:00	40mg	FR	FR	TJ		
PRESCRIBER'S NAME AND BLEEP EMMA JONES 4876	22:00						REVIEW

NAME OF DRUG SALBUTAMOL	TIME	DATE → DOSE ↓	11/04	12/04	13/04		
ADDITIONAL INSTRUCTIONS	08:00	2.5mg	FR	FR	TJ		
DATE 11/04 ROUTE NEB	12:00	2.5mg	FR	FR	TJ		
PRESCRIBER'S SIGNATURE EJones	18:00	2.5mg	FR	FR	TJ		
PRESCRIBER'S NAME AND BLEEP EMMA JONES 4876	22:00	2.5mg	WP	WP	TO		

NAME OF DRUG IPRATROPIUM	TIME	DATE → DOSE ↓	11/04	12/04	13/04		
ADDITIONAL INSTRUCTIONS	08:00	500 micrograms	FR	FR	TJ		
DATE 11/04 ROUTE NEB	12:00	500 micrograms	FR	FR	TJ		
PRESCRIBER'S SIGNATURE EJones	18:00	500 micrograms	FR	FR	TJ		
PRESCRIBER'S NAME AND BLEEP EMMA JONES 4876	22:00	500 micrograms	WP	WP	TO		

PATIENT NAME LEONARD NASH   HOSPITAL NO.   411973

NAME OF DRUG SIMVASTATIN	TIME	DATE → DOSE ↓	11/04	12/04	13/04		
ADDITIONAL INSTRUCTIONS	08:00						
DATE 11/04 ROUTE PO	12:00						
PRESCRIBER'S SIGNATURE EJones	18:00						
PRESCRIBER'S NAME AND BLEEP EMMA JONES 4876	22:00	40mg	WP	WP	TO		

NAME OF DRUG ENOXAPARIN	TIME	DATE → DOSE ↓	11/04	12/04	13/04		
ADDITIONAL INSTRUCTIONS	08:00						
DATE 11/04 ROUTE S/C	12:00						
PRESCRIBER'S SIGNATURE EJones	18:00	40mg	FR	FR	TJ		
PRESCRIBER'S NAME AND BLEEP EMMA JONES 4876	22:00						

NAME OF DRUG	TIME	DATE → DOSE ↓					
ADDITIONAL INSTRUCTIONS	08:00						
DATE ROUTE	12:00						
PRESCRIBER'S SIGNATURE	18:00						
PRESCRIBER'S NAME AND BLEEP	22:00						

AS REQUIRED PRESCRIPTIONS

NAME OF DRUG SALBUTAMOL		DATE					
INDICATION/ INSTRUCTION SOB	DOSE 2.5mg	TIME					
FREQUENCY PRN	ROUTE NEB	DOSE					
PRESCRIBER'S SIGNATURE EJones		ROUTE					
PRESCRIBER'S NAME AND BLEEP EMMA JONES 4876		GIVEN BY					
START DATE 11/04	STOP DATE						

PATIENT NAME LEONARD NASH   HOSPITAL NO.   411973

NAME OF DRUG		DATE						
INDICATION/ INSTRUCTION	DOSE	TIME						
FREQUENCY	ROUTE	DOSE						
PRESCRIBER'S SIGNATURE		ROUTE						
PRESCRIBER'S NAME AND BLEEP		GIVEN BY						
START DATE	STOP DATE							

INTRAVENOUS FLUIDS

DATE	FLUID	ADDITIVE & DOSE	VOLUME	RATE/ DURATION	PRESCRIBER'S SIGNATURE	GIVEN BY	START TIME	END TIME

Record of signatures. ALL prescribers MUST complete.

DATE	NAME	DESIGNATION	SIGNATURE	BLEEP NUMBER
11/04	EMMA JONES	F2	EJones	4876
11/04	KENNETH CHO	F1	KCho	5765

Answer 44

Being asked to prescribe sleeping tablets is a common task for a junior doctor on a night shift and there is often pressure from patients and nursing staff to prescribe them. Like any medication, consider the indication, side effects and physiology of each patient for who you prescribe them.

Step 3: Compare your answer to the checklist below and the chart opposite ✔

D Details	Checked patient details Used capital letters throughout Used correct abbreviations	☐
R Regular medications	Changed prednisolone prescription from the evening to the morning	☐
U Unpleasant reactions	Noticed the latex allergy	☐
G Gravid?	No	☐

C Contra-indications	Danger: avoid respiratory depressants in respiratory failure	☐
H Hydration	Not required	☐
A Analgesia	Not required. Prescribing PRN paracetamol would be acceptable	☐
R Renal function	Not required	☐
T Thrombo-prophylaxis	Continued enoxaparin 40mg	☐
S Signature box	Signed signature box	☐

Rationale

In this exercise, the patient has type 2 respiratory failure which has decompensated to the point where he requires noninvasive ventilation overnight. Prescribing a respiratory depressant such as zopiclone could exacerbate his respiratory failure and worsen his condition. A precedent has been set by previous doctors who have prescribed zopiclone, and the patient himself is directly asking you to prescribe it. It would be better help him by explaining why zopiclone is an unsafe prescription in his case and by thinking of other ways you could help him sleep.

The drug chart shows prednisolone is being prescribed in the evening. This is unusual as steroids disrupt the circadian cycle and an evening spike in the cortisol will disturb sleep. For this reason, it would be prudent to amend the prednisolone prescription, specifying morning administration. There is little that can be done about the uncomfortable and sleep-depriving effects of wearing the BiPAP mask but it is important to emphasise to patients the importance of wearing it to speed recovery. It is worth considering alternative approaches, e.g. eye shades and/or ear plugs.

KEY POINTS

- Continuing to prescribe night sedation is not always the correct answer
- Don't give in to staff or patient pressure; objectively review what is best for the patient
- Think of other ways to help patient if the prescribing is not appropriate

LONGBURY HOSPITAL TRUST

HOSPITAL NUMBER	411973
SURNAME	NASH
FIRST NAME	LEONARD
ADDRESS	18 UPPER LANE, LONGBURY LB5 4BH
D.O.B	31/12/YYYY (68 YEARS AGO)

DATE OF ADMISSION	11/04/YYYY	ADMISSION WEIGHT (KG)	81kg	WARD	MEDICAL ASSESSMENT

ALLERGIES	CONSULTANT	ERIN JOHNSON
LATEX - RASH	CHART NO	1...OF...1

ONCE ONLY PRESCRIPTIONS

DATE	TIME	NAME OF DRUG	DOSE	ROUTE	PRESCRIBER'S SIGNATURE	GIVEN BY	TIME GIVEN
11/04	2200	ZOPICLONE	3.75mg	PO	KCho	WP	2300
12/04	2350	ZOPICLONE	7.5mg	PO	KCho	WP	0100

REGULAR MEDICATIONS

NAME OF DRUG PREDNISOLONE	TIME	DATE → DOSE ↓	11/04	12/04	13/04		15/04
ADDITIONAL INSTRUCTIONS	08:00				STOP ALewis 13/04		
DATE 11/04 ROUTE PO	12:00						
PRESCRIBER'S SIGNATURE EJones	18:00	40mg	FR	FR	TJ		REVIEW
PRESCRIBER'S NAME AND BLEEP EMMA JONES 4876	22:00						REVIEW

NAME OF DRUG SALBUTAMOL	TIME	DATE → DOSE ↓	11/04	12/04	13/04		
ADDITIONAL INSTRUCTIONS	08:00	2.5mg	FR	FR	TJ		
DATE 11/04 ROUTE NEB	12:00	2.5mg	FR	FR	TJ		
PRESCRIBER'S SIGNATURE EJones	18:00	2.5mg	FR	FR	TJ		
PRESCRIBER'S NAME AND BLEEP EMMA JONES 4876	22:00	2.5mg	WP	WP	TO		

NAME OF DRUG IPRATROPIUM	TIME	DATE → DOSE ↓	11/04	12/04	13/04		
ADDITIONAL INSTRUCTIONS	08:00	500 micrograms	FR	FR	TJ		
DATE 11/04 ROUTE NEB	12:00	500 micrograms	FR	FR	TJ		
PRESCRIBER'S SIGNATURE EJones	18:00	500 micrograms	FR	FR	TJ		
PRESCRIBER'S NAME AND BLEEP EMMA JONES 4876	22:00	500 micrograms	WP	WP	TO		

PATIENT NAME LEONARD NASH   HOSPITAL NO. 411973

NAME OF DRUG SIMVASTATIN	TIME	DATE → DOSE ↓	11/04	12/04	13/04		
ADDITIONAL INSTRUCTIONS	08:00						
DATE 11/04 ROUTE PO	12:00						
PRESCRIBER'S SIGNATURE EJones	18:00						
PRESCRIBER'S NAME AND BLEEP EMMA JONES 4876	22:00	40mg	WP	WP	TO		

NAME OF DRUG ENOXAPARIN	TIME	DATE → DOSE ↓	11/04	12/04	13/04		
ADDITIONAL INSTRUCTIONS	08:00						
DATE 11/04 ROUTE S/C	12:00						
PRESCRIBER'S SIGNATURE EJones	18:00	40mg	FR	FR	TJ		
PRESCRIBER'S NAME AND BLEEP EMMA JONES 4876	22:00						

NAME OF DRUG PREDNISOLONE	TIME	DATE → DOSE ↓	11/04	12/04	13/04		
ADDITIONAL INSTRUCTIONS	08:00	40mg	X	X	X		
DATE 14/04 ROUTE PO	12:00						REVIEW
PRESCRIBER'S SIGNATURE ALewis	18:00						
PRESCRIBER'S NAME AND BLEEP ALEX LEWIS 4567	22:00						

AS REQUIRED PRESCRIPTIONS

NAME OF DRUG SALBUTAMOL		DATE					
INDICATION/ INSTRUCTION SOB	DOSE 2.5mg	TIME					
FREQUENCY PRN	ROUTE NEB	DOSE					
PRESCRIBER'S SIGNATURE EJones		ROUTE					
PRESCRIBER'S NAME AND BLEEP EMMA JONES 4876		GIVEN BY					
START DATE 11/04	STOP DATE						

PATIENT NAME LEONARD NASH   HOSPITAL NO.   411973

NAME OF DRUG		DATE						
INDICATION/ INSTRUCTION	DOSE	TIME						
FREQUENCY	ROUTE	DOSE						
PRESCRIBER'S SIGNATURE		ROUTE						
PRESCRIBER'S NAME AND BLEEP		GIVEN BY						
START DATE	STOP DATE							

INTRAVENOUS FLUIDS

DATE	FLUID	ADDITIVE & DOSE	VOLUME	RATE/ DURATION	PRESCRIBER'S SIGNATURE	GIVEN BY	START TIME	END TIME

Record of signatures. ALL prescribers MUST complete.

DATE	NAME	DESIGNATION	SIGNATURE	BLEEP NUMBER
11/04	EMMA JONES	F2	EJones	4876
11/04	KENNETH CHO	F1	KCho	5765
13/04	ALEX LEWIS	F1	ALewis	4567

Francis Freestone (hospital number: 312132, DOB 28/07/YYYY [78 years old], address: 20 Cyril Road, Longbury LB3 1PW) has yet to wake up after returning to the surgery ward from theatre. One hour ago he underwent evacuation of a left sided chronic subdural haematoma after being transferred from a local hospital last night. The ward staff have asked for a review.

The primary survey reveals:
Airway – intact
Breathing – chest clear, SaO_2 93% on air, respiratory rate 9 breaths/minute
Circulation – blood pressure 98/62mmHg, pulse 73bpm, Capillary refill 2 seconds, urine output 40mL last hour
Disability – pupils equal and reactive, size 1 bilaterally
Glasgow coma score: E2V1M5
E – drain in place, no leak from wound, fentanyl patch noted on back

Arterial blood gas results:
pH 7.28
HCO_3 24
PaO_2 12kPa
$PaCO_2$ 7.4kPa

Blood test results:
Sodium 131mmol/L
Potassium 3.4mmol/L
Urea 2.4mmol/L

A CT of the head is done, which excludes any post surgery complications.
The nursing staff have already bleeped the registrar, who will attend when he finishes with a trauma call in the emergency department.

Your task is to prescribe treatment for the unresponsiveness.
It is 19:00 on 4th August.

Notes

Step 1: Complete your answers in the drug chart opposite and overleaf

LONGBURY HOSPITAL TRUST

HOSPITAL NUMBER	312132
SURNAME	FREESTONE
FIRST NAME	FRANCIS
ADDRESS	20 CYRIL ROAD, LONGBURY LB3 1PW
D.O.B	28/07/YYYY (78 YEARS AGO)

DATE OF ADMISSION	04/08/YYYY	ADMISSION WEIGHT (KG)	49kg	WARD	SURGICAL

ALLERGIES	CONSULTANT	JOSHUA GIBB
NIL	CHART NO	1...OF...1

ONCE ONLY PRESCRIPTIONS

DATE	TIME	NAME OF DRUG	DOSE	ROUTE	PRESCRIBER'S SIGNATURE	GIVEN BY	TIME GIVEN
04/08	1200	ORAMORPH	10mg	PO	BFord	BN	12:00
04/08	1500	ORAMORPH	10mg	PO	BFord	BN	15:10

REGULAR MEDICATIONS

NAME OF DRUG PARACETAMOL	TIME	DATE → DOSE ↓	04/08			
ADDITIONAL INSTRUCTIONS	08:00	1g	BN			
DATE 04/08 ROUTE PO/IV	12:00	1g	BN			
PRESCRIBER'S SIGNATURE BFord	18:00	1g				
PRESCRIBER'S NAME AND BLEEP BEN FORD 1569	22:00	1g				

NAME OF DRUG CODEINE	TIME	DATE → DOSE ↓	04/08			
ADDITIONAL INSTRUCTIONS	08:00	60mg	BN			
DATE 04/08 ROUTE PO	12:00	60mg	BN			
PRESCRIBER'S SIGNATURE BFord	18:00	60mg				
PRESCRIBER'S NAME AND BLEEP BEN FORD 1569	22:00	60mg				

NAME OF DRUG FUROSEMIDE	TIME	DATE → DOSE ↓	04/08			
ADDITIONAL INSTRUCTIONS	08:00	20mg	BN			
DATE 04/08 ROUTE PO	12:00					
PRESCRIBER'S SIGNATURE BFord	18:00					
PRESCRIBER'S NAME AND BLEEP BEN FORD 1569	22:00					

PATIENT NAME FRANCIS FREESTONE   HOSPITAL NO.   312132

NAME OF DRUG		TIME	DATE → DOSE ↓					
ADDITIONAL INSTRUCTIONS		08:00						
DATE	ROUTE	12:00						
PRESCRIBER'S SIGNATURE								
		18:00						
PRESCRIBER'S NAME AND BLEEP		22:00						

NAME OF DRUG		TIME	DATE → DOSE ↓					
ADDITIONAL INSTRUCTIONS		08:00						
DATE	ROUTE	12:00						
PRESCRIBER'S SIGNATURE								
		18:00						
PRESCRIBER'S NAME AND BLEEP		22:00						

NAME OF DRUG		TIME	DATE → DOSE ↓					
ADDITIONAL INSTRUCTIONS		08:00						
DATE	ROUTE	12:00						
PRESCRIBER'S SIGNATURE								
		18:00						
PRESCRIBER'S NAME AND BLEEP		22:00						

AS REQUIRED PRESCRIPTIONS

NAME OF DRUG ORAMORPH		DATE	04/08				
INDICATION/ INSTRUCTION PAIN	DOSE 10mg	TIME	1400				
FREQUENCY 2HRLY	ROUTE PO	DOSE	10mg				
PRESCRIBER'S SIGNATURE BFord		ROUTE	PO				
PRESCRIBER'S NAME AND BLEEP BEN FORD 1569		GIVEN BY	BN				
START DATE 04/08	STOP DATE						

PATIENT NAME FRANCIS FREESTONE   HOSPITAL NO.   312132

NAME OF DRUG		DATE					
INDICATION/ INSTRUCTION	DOSE	TIME					
FREQUENCY	ROUTE	DOSE					
PRESCRIBER'S SIGNATURE		ROUTE					
PRESCRIBER'S NAME AND BLEEP		GIVEN BY					
START DATE	STOP DATE						

INTRAVENOUS FLUIDS

DATE	FLUID	ADDITIVE & DOSE	VOLUME	RATE/ DURATION	PRESCRIBER'S SIGNATURE	GIVEN BY	START TIME	END TIME
04/08	HARTMANN'S	——————	1l	12 hrs	BFord	BN	0800	

Record of signatures. ALL prescribers MUST complete.

DATE	NAME	DESIGNATION	SIGNATURE	BLEEP NUMBER
04/08	BEN FORD	F2	BFord	1569

In this scenario the patient is showing signs of postoperative respiratory depression caused by opiate toxicity. Note that he weighs only 49kg and appears to have received significant amounts of opiates in the form of codeine, Oramorph and a fentanyl patch that may have previously gone unnoticed. It is likely that opiates will also have been administered intraoperatively.

Step 3: Compare your answer to the checklist below and the chart opposite ✔

D Details	Checked patient details Used capital letters throughout Used correct abbreviations	☐
R Regular medications	Continued furosemide Reduced paracetamol to weight-appropriate dose	☐
U Unpleasant reactions	NKDA	☐
G Gravid?	No	☐

C Contra-indications	Withheld opiates	☐
H Hydration	Continued fluids at same rate	☐
A Analgesia	Amended paracetamol (as regular medications) Withheld opiates	☐
R Renal function	Unknown but urea and electrolytes normal	☐
T Thrombo-prophylaxis	Not required, in practice this would start the following day	☐
S Signature box	Signed signature box	☐

Rationale

The diagnosis of opiate-related postoperative respiratory depression is complicated by the nature of surgery the patient has experienced. A thorough primary survey and read of the patient's drug chart will help piece together what has happened. Surgical causes are excluded by the CT of the head but getting senior support early is still essential in this scenario. The ABG results show signs of respiratory acidaemia: the low respiratory rate caused by opiates has led to a CO_2 narcosis, which will deepen the patient's drowsiness. His HCO_3 is normal, indicating that this problem has come on quickly and is not chronic.

Treatment includes a prescription of oxygen and if there are any airway concerns an airway adjunct, such as a nasopharyngeal or oropharyngeal airway, should be fitted while help is summoned. Naloxone hydrochloride, a competitive antagonist of opioid receptors, should be prescribed to reverse the opioid toxicity. When looking up naloxone in the poisoning section of the formulary it is easy to mistakenly prescribe too high a dose. As this exercise is postoperative, a lower dose of 100–200 micrograms is recommended. Low dosage is important not only because this patient's body weight is low but also because you need to ensure that when he wakes he is not in pain as a result of a complete removal of the opioid effect. The fentanyl patch is removed, as it is contributing to the patient's opiate toxicity (highlighting the importance of a thorough secondary survey).

Naloxone has a short half-life, so reassess the patient to ensure he has not slipped back into opioid-driven respiratory depression. A repeat ABG test will be needed to demonstrate the CO_2 narcosis is improving.

KEY POINTS

- Exclude surgical and medical causes of low Glasgow Coma Score
- Check naloxone dosing for the correct indication using a formulary
- Reassess patients who have been prescribed naloxone. It is essential to reassess their GCS and evaluate if further naloxone is required. Ensure nursing staff perform regular neurological observations

			HOSPITAL NUMBER	312132		
			SURNAME	FREESTONE		
LONGBURY HOSPITAL TRUST			FIRST NAME	FRANCIS		
			ADDRESS	20 CYRIL ROAD, LONGBURY LB3 1PW		
			D.O.B	28/07/YYYY (78 YEARS AGO)		
DATE OF ADMISSION	04/08/YYYY	ADMISSION WEIGHT (KG)	49kg	WARD	SURGICAL	
ALLERGIES			CONSULTANT		JOSHUA GIBB	
NIL			CHART NO		1...OF...1	

ONCE ONLY PRESCRIPTIONS

DATE	TIME	NAME OF DRUG	DOSE	ROUTE	PRESCRIBER'S SIGNATURE	GIVEN BY	TIME GIVEN
04/08	1200	ORAMORPH	10mg	PO	BFord	BN	12:00
04/08	1500	ORAMORPH	10mg	PO	BFord	BN	15:10
04/08	STAT	NALOXONE	100 micrograms	IV	ALewis		

REGULAR MEDICATIONS

NAME OF DRUG	TIME	DATE → DOSE ↓	04/08				
PARACETAMOL							
ADDITIONAL INSTRUCTIONS	08:00	1g	BN				
					04/08	STOP	ALewis
DATE 04/08 ROUTE PO/IV	12:00	1g	BN		———	———	———
PRESCRIBER'S SIGNATURE BFord	18:00	1g	———	———	———	———	———
PRESCRIBER'S NAME AND BLEEP BEN FORD 1569	22:00	1g	———	———	———	———	———

NAME OF DRUG	TIME	DATE → DOSE ↓	04/08				
CODEINE							
ADDITIONAL INSTRUCTIONS	08:00	60mg	BN ———				
DATE 04/08 ROUTE PO	12:00	60mg	BN				
PRESCRIBER'S SIGNATURE BFord	18:00	60mg	REVIEW ALewis				
PRESCRIBER'S NAME AND BLEEP BEN FORD 1569	22:00	60mg	———				

NAME OF DRUG	TIME	DATE → DOSE ↓	04/08				
FUROSEMIDE							
ADDITIONAL INSTRUCTIONS	08:00	20mg	BN				
DATE 04/08 ROUTE PO	12:00						
PRESCRIBER'S SIGNATURE BFord	18:00						
PRESCRIBER'S NAME AND BLEEP BEN FORD 1569	22:00						

PATIENT NAME FRANCIS FREESTONE   HOSPITAL NO.   312132

NAME OF DRUG PARACETAMOL	TIME	DATE → DOSE ↓	04/08				
ADDITIONAL INSTRUCTIONS	08:00	500mg	——				
DATE 04/08 ROUTE PO/IV	12:00	500mg	——				
PRESCRIBER'S SIGNATURE ALewis	18:00	500mg	——				
PRESCRIBER'S NAME AND BLEEP ALEX LEWIS 4567	22:00	500mg					

NAME OF DRUG	TIME	DATE → DOSE ↓					
ADDITIONAL INSTRUCTIONS	08:00						
DATE ROUTE	12:00						
PRESCRIBER'S SIGNATURE	18:00						
PRESCRIBER'S NAME AND BLEEP	22:00						

NAME OF DRUG	TIME	DATE → DOSE ↓					
ADDITIONAL INSTRUCTIONS	08:00						
DATE ROUTE	12:00						
PRESCRIBER'S SIGNATURE	18:00						
PRESCRIBER'S NAME AND BLEEP	22:00						

AS REQUIRED PRESCRIPTIONS

NAME OF DRUG ORAMORPH		DATE	04/08	——	——		
INDICATION/ INSTRUCTION PAIN	DOSE 10mg	TIME	1400	STOP ALewis 04/08	——		
FREQUENCY 2HRLY	ROUTE PO	DOSE	10mg	——	——		
PRESCRIBER'S SIGNATURE BFord		ROUTE	PO	——	——		
PRESCRIBER'S NAME AND BLEEP BEN FORD 1569		GIVEN BY	BN	——	——		
START DATE 04/08	STOP DATE						

PATIENT NAME FRANCIS FREESTONE   HOSPITAL NO.   312132

NAME OF DRUG		DATE						
INDICATION/ INSTRUCTION	DOSE	TIME						
FREQUENCY	ROUTE	DOSE						
PRESCRIBER'S SIGNATURE		ROUTE						
PRESCRIBER'S NAME AND BLEEP		GIVEN BY						
START DATE	STOP DATE							

INTRAVENOUS FLUIDS

DATE	FLUID	ADDITIVE & DOSE	VOLUME	RATE/ DURATION	PRESCRIBER'S SIGNATURE	GIVEN BY	START TIME	END TIME
04/08	HARTMANNS	————————	1l	12 hrs	BFord	BN	0800	

Record of signatures. ALL prescribers MUST complete.

DATE	NAME	DESIGNATION	SIGNATURE	BLEEP NUMBER
04/08	BEN FORD	F2	BFord	1569
04/08	ALEX LEWIS	F1	ALewis	4567